P9-EEM-093

COMMUNITY PSYCHOLOGY

COMMUNITY PSYCHOLOGY

Concepts and Applications

Philip A. Mann

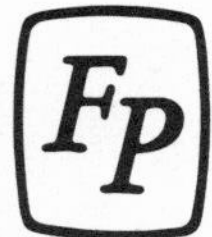

THE FREE PRESS
A Division of Macmillan Publishing Co., Inc.
NEW YORK

Collier Macmillan Publishers
LONDON

The Free Press
A Division of Macmillan Publishing Co., Inc.
866 Third Avenue, New York, N. Y. 10022

Collier Macmillan Canada, Ltd.

Library of Congress Catalog Card Number: 77-83164

Printed in the United States of America

printing number

1 2 3 4 5 6 7 8 9 10

Library of Congress Cataloging in Publication Data

Mann, Philip A
Community psychology.

Includes bibliographies and index.
1. Community psychology. I. Title.
RA790.M328 362.2'04'25 77-83164
ISBN 0-02-920000-8

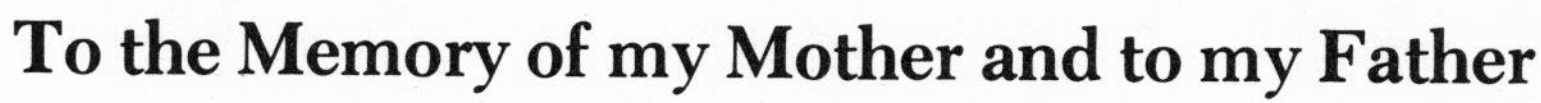
To the Memory of my Mother and to my Father

Contents

Preface

During the tumult and change of the 1960s, social innovations such as community mental health centers, the war on poverty, and civil rights activism mushroomed. One development in the midst of this change was the birth of community psychology, an attempt to adapt psychological knowledge and practices to the challenges of these new programs. Efforts to define and develop this new field have occupied the dedicated efforts of a relatively small group of psychologists for a little more than a decade. Both the newness and the diversity of their activities have made defining the field a difficult task. Development of the field depends in turn upon its definition and the goals that give direction to its activities. The purpose of this book is to further the process of definition.

The task is both challenging and frustrating, constantly demanding a degree of completeness that is not entirely possible in such a new field. The writing of this book has fulfilled a personal need to bring some conceptual integration to the work of community psychologists so as to guide research and practice, to attempt to communicate to students a developing conception of a new form of psychology, and to contribute to a dialogue among colleagues that can enhance the effectiveness of those who identify with community psychology. My personal experience is that this need is widely shared, and how well this effort succeeds in meeting that need must be judged by others.

The history of community psychology shows a change from an initial concern with the application of psychology *in* the community to a broadened conception of a psychology *about* the community in a relatively brief period of time. The first tentative gropings of community psychologists were an effort to extend psychology's traditional concern with the relationship of human beings to themselves and others as individual organisms into new settings in community programs, outside of the traditional clinic and laboratory. Since then, a definite sense has emerged that the problems require a concern with the relationships of individuals to each other as a community; as a differentiated social grouping with elaborate systems of formal and informal relationships.

These developments reflect a shift from the relatively isolated efforts of a set of diverse individuals to an increasing concern with more general conceptual problems. It has been a largely inductive, theory-building effort. Progress in such a field requires periodic reflection and attempts at integration, to be followed by hypothesis testing and further development.

Many other fields, including psychiatry, social work, and urban planning, have undergone similar changes during this same period. Others, such as sociology, can claim a prior and more long-standing interest in the topics with which community psychologists are concerned. Readers from those fields may examine what is to be found here and justifiably reflect, "Oh, yes, my field was concerned with that problem some years ago." No claim to exclusive or superior knowledge is made here for the psychological conceptions of the problems to be discussed. If the important contributions of other fields to these problems appear to have been overlooked in this work, it is because the concern has been with a delineation of the mainly psychological approaches employed by community psychologists. To the extent that these psychological approaches do omit contributions from other fields, it is a reflection of the limited amount of intellectual cross-fertilization that occurs in an age of increasing specialization.

Even within psychology, specialization tends to be quite narrow, and the idea of the community psychologist as a kind of generalist with special interests is difficult to grasp. Such a role cannot be defined with reference to the usual niches of specialization within psychology, but requires a definition of the particular problems and approaches that are the community psychologist's concern. Such roles presently are defined better by example than by prior conception. It is toward this approach, and whatever integration can be derived from it, that this work is committed.

The book consists of three parts. The first part reviews the history of the field and constructs a framework of community and social concepts that form the context for community psychology activities. In the second part, the work of community psychologists is grouped into four models. These models are identified by the assumptions that each makes about human behavior and community processes. The typical research, interventions, and settings associated with each model are described. The third part compares the models on the basis of requirements for integrated approaches to community problems, deriving concepts and principles for research, interventions, and training.

Many of the social programs initiated during the 1960s have become subjects of controversy, and the activities of some of those programs have been reduced or eliminated. Many of the expectations concerning the effects of those programs have not been matched by the results of the relatively few reliable evaluation studies that have been conducted. But while changes in popular emphasis and program strategies have taken place, the social problems that stimulated those programs remain, accompanied now by new and complex challenges. The need for soundly conceived solutions remains great, and grows with each day that action is postponed.

However, the sense of urgency must be accompanied by an adequate conception of the nature of the problems and an awareness of the context in which the problems exist. Most community programs can be questioned as to their definition of community, and their conception of social history. These qualities have particular salience for community psychology, yet both of these features have only gradually evolved in the thoughts and works of community psychologists. As a deliberate effort to underscore this requirement, emphasis has been placed here on the historical origins of each of the models described in this book, as well as on their conceptions of the community.

Both the writing of this book and my own development as a community psychologist are indebted to a diversity of experiences and people. The wish to acknowledge all of them, strong though it is, cannot be fulfilled here. Those sources of inspiration, edification, and support that stand out include the residents of several communities, a number of talented and curious students, the gifted and dedicated teachers in the clinical, social, and community areas of the Department of Psychology at the University of Michigan, and a wonderful variety of professional colleagues.

Special acknowledgments are due James G. Kelly, William C. Rhodes, and Ira Iscoe for their support and guidance as teachers, role models, and colleagues. While they are not responsible for what is written here, they have contributed immeasurably to my desire and ability to write this book. It is my hope that this work may in some small way justify their patience and effort.

The stimulating and insightful comments of Murray Levine, who read the initial manuscript, and the help of Robert Wallace, of The Free Press, in encouraging this book are gratefully acknowledged.

Philip A. Mann

Cedar Falls, Iowa

Part I
Introduction

1. Community Psychology: Origins of a New Approach

Community psychology is a very new term as the history of psychology goes, and one that is difficult to define. In order to approach a definition of community psychology, it is helpful to examine the historical developments that preceded it. Part of these historical developments have to do with the mental health movement, but both that movement and community psychology are also the result of other social forces.

There are some excellent histories that have detailed the origins of the community mental health movement (Schwartz, 1972; Rossi, 1969) more extensively than is necessary here, but the main points of these developments are important to understanding how community psychology came into being.

Federal legislation providing funds for comprehensive community mental health centers was first enacted in 1963 (P. L. 88-164). This legislation was the result of an accumulation of scientific findings, public awareness, and political leadership. At least as early as 1854, mental health workers had documented their concern with the relationship between social conditions and mental illness (Plog, 1969), but one of the most influential studies was Faris and Dunham's (1939) finding of a relationship between hospitalized mental illness and the area of the city in which people lived. This relationship was subsequently traced down to relationships with poverty and social alienation that happened to be concentrated in those areas. Numerous subsequent studies have supported the relationship of mental illness to these latter two factors, although the question of causation, or etiology, has not been resolved.

During and after World War II, there was considerable alarm over the high number of people who were rejected for military service, or were casualties of military service, because of psychiatric impairment. The Joint Commission on Mental Illness and Health was established in 1955 to study mental illness as a national problem. The commission sponsored a number of studies which were published in a seven-volume series, and which culminated in the commission's final report, *Action for Mental Health* (1961). The commission found that mental illness was enormously expensive in both human and economic terms, that the provision of mental health services in the country was woefully inadequate, and, along with other studies done during this same period (Hollingshead and Redlich, 1958), found that mental health services were distributed differently in both frequency and form to some parts of the population than to others.

Poorer persons were found to receive services for more severe problems than those who were not so poor, their services consisted more often of hospitalization and custodial care, as distinguished from outpatient psychotherapy, and there was reason to believe that poorer persons more often put off seeking mental health services until their problems had reached more extreme proportions. The specific interpretations of these findings is a subtle and complex issue that will be considered in a later chapter; here it is sufficient to note that these findings were taken as an indication of a need to increase and redistribute mental health services.

At the same time, there was a recognition that certain social conditions contributed, at the very least, to mental health problems; and some people feel that they play a partly causal role in mental illness. Social conditions of poverty, alienation, isolation, marital disruptions, and, in general, a lack of social resources are clearly implicated in mental health problems in a number of ways. These conditions, along with increased stress, increasingly became the concern of people in the mental health field (Fried, 1964).

These findings suggested the desirability of trying preventive strategies in addition to treating existing cases. However, prevention was a new idea in the mental health field, and it was not clear how such measures might be taken, or how effective they would be. The preventive terminology of public health can be applied to mental health problems to illustrate the alternatives. Primary prevention is an effort to reduce the number of new cases of a disease or, by extrapolation, a problem. It involves effecting the population, or the environment, before problems have occurred. Secondary prevention refers to early identification and treatment of cases in order to reduce severity. Such an approach would involve bringing more of the existing cases into treatment earlier than had been the case before. Tertiary prevention is an attempt to prevent relapses of persons who have recovered from mental illness through rehabilitation and reintegration into the community, so that chronic disability does not develop.

There had been, relative to the first two types of prevention, considerably more research pointing to a tertiary preventive program. Some of the risk of chronicity is associated with the patient's problem itself, some arises from negative social attitudes toward ex-patients, and some is the result of the form of treatment provided. It was recognized that the existing pattern of psychiatric hospital treatment tended to socialize patients into the role of inmates (Goffman, 1961; Stanton and Schwartz, 1954), that prolonged absence from family and community, often aggravated by the remote location of mental hospitals, made reentry into these social systems a risky prospect (Freeman and Simmons, 1958; Yarrow, Clausen, and Robbins, 1955), and that follow-up and after-care services that might improve the chances for reestablishing the former patient in the community were usually nonexistent.

Secondary prevention in mental health was more a hope than a demonstrated fact, but it is a fact that this was the form of activity and the kind of thinking with which most mental health professionals were familiar. The idea of early identification and treatment was consonant with both professional and public expectations and beliefs, *as treatment*, but the preventive prospects of such an approach had not been established.

If this was the case with secondary prevention, there was less clarity about what a program of primary prevention would look like, and what its effects might be. Gerald Caplan (1961, 1964) was a strong advocate of primary prevention, and he outlined courses of social action and interpersonal action that would be required for such programs. However, there was, and is, considerable skepticism over the feasibility of primary prevention. To some extent, primary prevention involves changing social conditions, and it was not clear how such changes might effect rates of mental illness. It should be noted, however, that such changes would be desirable in their own right, whether or not this action has a preventive effect on mental illness.

The Joint Commission placed major emphasis in its recommendations on expanded treatment facilities that could increase the coverage and impact of mental health services with the aim of secondary and tertiary prevention.

The Joint Commission's recommendations were followed by President John F. Kennedy's message to Congress calling for the establishment of comprehensive community mental health and mental retardation centers. President Kennedy was the first president ever to address the Congress on the subject of mental health and mental retardation. The subsequent legislation was a major force for change in the conduct of mental health programs in the United States. It called for a comprehensive mental health facility, located *in* the community, to serve a maximum population of two hundred thousand, and for a design of service delivery that would maximize availability to every member of that population group. In order to qualify for support under this act, a mental health center was required to provide five basic services: inpatient, outpatient, partial hospitalization, twenty-four-hour emergency service, and consultation and education to the community. The latter provision was intended to make mandatory preventive efforts by the community mental health centers (Yolles, 1969) and reflected the intent of one part of President Kennedy's message:

> Prevention will require both selected specific programs directed especially at known causes, and the general strengthening of our fundamental community, social welfare, and education programs which can do much to eliminate or correct the harsh environmental conditions which often are associated with mental retardation and mental illness. (Kennedy, 1963, p. 2)

This historic development caught the professional mental health fields unprepared in many respects. While the critical shortage of professionals in the mental health field had been pointed out earlier in one of the Joint Commission studies (Albee, 1959), even if every qualified mental health professional in the country had gone to work for the mental health centers, the supply would have been inadequate to staff the proposed number of facilities. Equally important, few professionals had been trained in the kind of operational patterns and techniques that would be required in this program, and an immediate training need in both quantity and quality was created. The problem was complicated by the fact that there were few, if any, existing structures to provide this training and a meager body of knowledge on which to base it. Moreover, expanding training programs tended to absorb many of the professionals newly trained in this field, leaving few available for employment in the centers. The majority of mental health center staff personnel had been trained in other patterns of service, and had to learn, or relearn, their skills on the job. One major impact of the community mental health center program has been an entirely new and different approach to the development and deployment of mental health manpower. Mental health programs sought to make more widely effective use of professionals through briefer, crisis-oriented therapy, greater use of group therapy, and cooperation with other mental health resources in the community. Increasing use of nonprofessionals in mental health programs also developed (Gartner, 1971; Pearl and Riessman, 1965; Reiff and Riessman, 1965; Rioch *et al.*, 1963).

Psychologists and Social Programs

In response to these developments, a group of psychologists convened at Swampscott, Massachusetts, in 1965 (Bennett *et al.*, 1965) to consider for the first time the training of psychologists for roles in the community. Psychologists had not been trained specifically to know anything about the community, how to work with other community agencies, or how to intervene to change social conditions. To the extent that this knowledge existed among psychologists, it was the product of individual professional experience. Professional psychological training had been oriented toward working in an office, relatively isolated from the community, regarding the patient's problems as entirely a product of his own personality, and considering other conditions as things to which the patient had to adapt. Psychologists at the Swampscott conference began to call themselves *community* psychologists, whereas formerly they might have been called clinical or social psychologists. The developments that grew out of this movement constituted not only a change in location, but a change in ideology and in orientations toward what constituted adequate help (Hobbs, 1964; Reiff, 1970).

At this same time, there were several other socially oriented programs developing that were not necessarily concerned with problems of mental health. One was the war on poverty; another was represented by the programs to rebuild cities and provide more adequate housing for citizens conducted by the Department of Housing and Urban Development (HUD). Many psychologists were attracted to working with these and other programs, generally dealing with the "problems of the cities," as an appropriate arena for "community psychologists." However, beyond that geographical definition, the surroundings were often unfamiliar, and the role and functions unclear.

The problems with which these programs were concerned were equally complex and unclear. As an example, welfare programs have always generated controversy between public assistance and the work ethic, yet traditionally only a minority of those eligible for welfare benefits actually claim them. In 1960, for instance, it was estimated that about a third of those eligible for welfare were actually receiving benefits (Riessman, Cohen, and Pearl, 1964). Those who support welfare programs are concerned about the material deprivations of those in need of assistance. Those who oppose welfare programs tend to focus on what they see as undesirable psychological characteristics, such as dependency and lack of initiative, which lead to the need for such programs and which appear to be reinforced by welfare benefits. The strategy of the war on poverty of simultaneously reaching more of those eligible for welfare assistance and increasing the range of eligibility (Rein, 1969) created an increased number of recipients, which had the effect of making "the welfare problem" look bigger than it had appeared to be before, when in fact these actions may only have been making more visible a problem that existed already but was not fully recognized.

There is a lesson here as well for mental health services. If we increase the number of mental health services in a community, we are likely to find more patients. The community psychologist has to understand something about how communities work in this respect. It doesn't mean that there are more people suffering; it does mean that there are more people who will seek help if it is available. Any new service that is introduced usually attracts more than enough clients, which speaks to the level of perceived need for services in the community. In the mental health field, this is made possible because of the large gap between the number of people who actually use services and the number of people who have serious psychiatric impairments and/or feel that they have problems that are relevant for help (Gurin, Veroff, and Feld, 1960). It is clear, then, that one could continue to provide services and probably never exhaust the supply of clients.

The service situation is not unlike that of the gasoline station attendant who was trying to fill the tank of a large luxury car with the motor running. After a while, the attendant had to ask the driver to shut off the motor because it was getting ahead of the gas pump. Many of the social action programs were seen as attempts to "shut off the motor" and slow down the rate of social handicaps, including psychological impairments. Accordingly, community psychologists began to consider other roles besides the provision of services. Being untrained for this role, and with few precedents to follow, community psychologists' functions began to become diffused into a number of different programs and activities. The incentives to become involved in various activities far exceeded the role definitions for effective functioning in these activities.

To the extent that there was a common rationale behind these activities, it was that the strengthening of the quality of community life could have a beneficial mental health effect, either by reducing sources of stress in the social environment or by increasing the personal competencies and social resources that could aid in resisting the effects of stress (Hollister, 1963). There was a renewed interest in the effects of social conditions (Duhl, 1963; Riessman, Cohen, and Pearl, 1964), environmental characteristics (Kates and Wohlwill, 1966), and early socialization experiences (Hunt, 1968) on the individual, but little or no research demonstrating that these programs had the effect of reducing rates of mental illness.

Some psychologists urged attention to the complexities of community structures and processes as a focus of community psychologists' work (Kelly, 1966, 1968; Klein, 1968). They recognized that adaptational requirements varied in different community settings, and they advocated study of these processes as a basis for developing effective preventive programs. This approach called for different kinds of commitments and competencies than those that were characteristic of most psychologists (Kelly, 1970), but this distinction was mostly lost in the enthusiasm and fervor that predominated during the 1960s, and the long-term perspective of such an approach was contrary to the "action now!" spirit of the times. Psychologists should have known better, but it was quite easy to assume that mental health betterment was social betterment and vice versa in the heady atmosphere of rapid program development characteristic of this period.

Sylvia Scribner (1968) identified four kinds of community psychology roles in the middle 1960s. These were: (1) social movement psychologists, who were identified with political and social movements seeking major change; (2) social action psychologists, who were concerned with professional participation in social programs, usually federally funded, without commitment to a political movement; (3) new clinical psychologists, who were seeking to move beyond the techniques of individual psychotherapy and into new locations to provide professional service; and (4) social engineers, who were concerned with the design of social systems as such, without particular focus on the behavior of individuals.

Clearly, these roles go beyond a concern with mental health, but Scribner concluded by cautioning that while these roles were diverse, they shared a common need for knowledge about the effects of social systems on individuals. Having gone beyond concern with mental health, the role *functions* for community psychologists were anything but clear.

In a series of conferences, members of the Division of Community Psychology of the American Psychological Association sought to achieve greater clarity through exchanges and analyses of examples and principles of community psychologists at work. Conferences were held in Austin, Texas, in 1967 (Iscoe and Spielberger, 1970), in Chicago in 1968 (Division 27 of American Psychological Association, 1971), and again in Austin in 1971 (Mann, 1971). Out of these meetings there emerged the beginnings of a set of consensual values, principles, and concepts, though considerable diversity remained.

At the first Austin conference, Levine proposed a set of postulates that characterize the assumptions of many community psychologists:

> 1. A problem arises in a setting or in a situation; some factor in the situation in which the problem manifests itself causes, triggers, exacerbates, or maintains the problem.

2. A problem arises in a situation because of some element in the social setting that blocks effective problem-solving behavior on the part of those charged with carrying out the functions and achieving the goals of the setting.

3. Help, to be effective, has to be located strategically to the manifestation of the problem, preferably in the very situation in which the problem manifests itself.

4. The goals or the values of the helping agent or the helping service must be consistent with the goals or the values of the setting in which the problem is manifested.

5. The form of help should have potential for being established on a systematic basis using the natural resources of the setting or through introducing resources that can become institutionalized as part of the setting. (Levine, 1970, pp. 72–76)

The set of principles and assumptions that Levine enumerated illustrate the common perspective that community psychologists have for viewing problems as the result of person-setting interactions, and their mutual interest in promoting more effective settings for human behavior. However, at this same time, a recognition of differences among community psychologists also began to emerge.

Rosenblum (1968) described two different role functions for the community mental health center psychologist and the community psychologist, based primarily on the differences in the modes of operation and the goals of their work settings. The former was necessarily more concerned with the development of new service systems and being a part of the services that were provided. This requirement dictated that a certain amount of the community mental health center psychologist's functions had to be concerned with the past and current personal problems of clients. Rosenblum saw the community psychologist as a "participant-conceptualizer," a term coined at the Swampscott conference, concerned with broader aspects of community problems.

This distinction between two types of community psychologists reflected the progression of the field at that time; two of Scribner's kinds of community psychologists, the social movement psychologists and the social engineers, were not a significant number of those who identified with community psychology. To the extent that psychologists were involved in political movements, it was more as individuals than as part of an organized body of psychologists, and those concerned with social engineering did not comprise a large or recognizable group within community psychology. The numerically larger group of community psychologists, those concerned with social action programs and community mental health, were necessarily interested in political movements and with environmental problems, but not as a primary focus of their activity. Despite the distinction drawn by Rosenblum, it was conceptually difficult to specify where, if at all, the line might be drawn between community mental health and community psychology.

Part of this obscurity lies in the vagueness, and perhaps inappropriateness, of the term mental health. As any textbook in abnormal psychology or the psychology of adjustment reveals, definitions of mental health are numerous, complex, and imprecise. Psychologists in community mental health sought to move away from a medically oriented concept of mental health as the absence of mental illness toward a more constructive, growth-oriented concept of "positive mental health." However, this movement away from a seemingly precise idea of mental illness to its opposite opens a Pandora's box of philosophical and conceptual problems in which the notion of health and its medical connotations are of virtually no help. In reviewing this development, Knudson (1963) concluded that psychologists should abandon attempts to rationalize their efforts within the philosophically meaningless and pragmatically limiting language of the obverse of the medical model. Instead he suggested that psychologists define precisely the kinds of human social problems with which they were concerned and study them in their own right. He enumerated several significant problems of social living that were challenging the adaptive capacities of people in modern society and were relevant for psychological study and intervention.

This need was emphasized dramatically by the eruption of numerous incidents of rioting, demonstrations, and disruptive mass behavior in the middle and late 1960s, beginning with racially oriented riots in Watts, California; Detroit, Michigan; and Washington, D.C.; and followed by widespread student demonstrations and antiwar protests. As a group, community psychologists were not prepared to respond to these developments. They had not developed the relevant knowledge and expertise, nor were they publicly visible as appropriate resources. A few psychologists happened to be strategically located through their association with other social action programs so that they were called upon to participate in resolving some of these confrontations (Mann and Iscoe, 1971; Mottola, 1970; Ochberg and Trickett, 1970; Schellow, 1971), and other psychologists began to be called upon after these events to help create social climates that could prevent recurrences of such events (Sikes and Cleveland, 1968; Lipsitt and Steinbruner, 1969; Bartlett, 1972) by improving relationships between community members and public institutions, most notably the police.

These activities clearly went beyond the realm of mental health to a concern with larger social processes, but they raised urgent questions about the appropriate role, the relevant bodies of knowledge, and effective techniques of intervention for the psychologists involved in them. Quite obviously, these activities had ideological implications as well.

Despite the diversity of these activities, the first Austin conference addressed itself primarily to community psychology as community mental health (Iscoe and Spielberger, 1970), being concerned chiefly with distinguishing this approach from traditional clinical psychology in both practices and locations. However, at this conference, Reiff (1970) sounded a slightly different theme. He criticized further the appropriateness of applying the medically oriented concept of mental health to social problems. While recognizing mental health as a significant problem in itself, which could not be denied by changing the language or concepts used to describe it, Reiff also pointed to the need for an understanding of social forces and their psychological effects, and of conceptions of social interventions, as relevant bodies of knowledge for community psychology. He noted that this knowledge could not be derived adequately from conventional clinical concepts in psychology, or even from an entirely interpersonal conception of social forces. Among other needs, Reiff called for a renewed interest in the psychology of mass movements, and in the psychological effects of social forces in changing and raising the hopes and expectations of individuals.

Reiff was also sensitive to the ideological issues involved. In an earlier paper he had called attention to this concern as one that was separate from, but critically important to, the development of new technologies (Reiff, 1966). At the Chicago conference he addressed this issue in detail with respect both to ideological positions within psychology and between psychologists and the community. In a historical survey, he noted that psychology's participation in the shaping and conduct of public policy had been uneven. His analysis revealed that psychologists as a body actively supported professional participation in public policy matters during wartime but shied away from pressing internal social concerns during times of peace.

These different positions of organized psychology could be traced to the fact that there was little internal controversy over the course to be followed during World Wars I and II, but much controversy and division within society in regard to domestic social issues. At such times, psychologists, as well as anyone else, were placed in a position where value judgments would have to be made publicly, an area into which scientists were supposed, fallaciously, not to venture.

Reiff drew an important distinction between the participation of the professional and the citizen in public affairs. He pointed out that unlike the ordinary citizen, the professional's value-oriented decisions are necessarily constrained by knowledge and empirical data, so that they are not entirely determined by values. Where there is no empirical basis for a decision, there is no role for the professional as a professional, and to make professional decisions under such conditions could be irresponsible. As Reiff put it:

> We are certainly not in a position to offer our services . . . to anybody, any place, and on any problem under the sun, to extend the imperialistic flag of psychology over all of society. What is required is to make explicit the basis for our participation in each specific instance. (1971, p. 49)

These same conditions apply, of course, to any professional or scientific group, but it is important to note that where there is a relevant knowledge base to an important social question, professional decision making is both highly appropriate and not exclusively a matter of ideology.

Further insurance against the imposition of the values of professionals was contained in the increasingly prevalent principle, if not always the practice, of citizen involvement in the planning and conduct of new social programs. This principle was enunciated early on for psychologists by Smith and Hobbs (1966) in an American Psychological Association position paper on community mental health programs, and was made a part of Community Action Programs of the Office of Economic Opportunity and the Model Cities programs. This position was made explicit in the principles that Bloom (1971) enunciated at the Chicago conference to guide programs of prevention in mental health.

Again, the Chicago conference concluded with an emphasis on mental health, specifically on primary preventive programs. In a summary statement, Glidewell put forth the thrust of the conference:

> Psychologists involved in community mental health should place the highest priority upon collaborative, self-modifying, social interventions to prevent disorders by facilitating the accomplishment of developmental tasks, especially in children. (1971, p. 143)

He went on to make the point that an early detection and treatment strategy does not constitute a means of population-wide prevention in mental health, using both theoretical grounds and empirical data. He advocated the implementation of several primary prevention strategies, on an experimental basis, which were grounded in previous research findings.

These recommendations emerged in a fertile intellectual climate. Another Joint Commission, this one on the mental health of children, had been established by Congress following the assassination of President Kennedy, in part because it was discovered that Lee Harvey Oswald, who was accused of the assassination, had been diagnosed as mentally ill as a child, but was not treated. If the previous Joint Commission found that mental health services for adults were inadequate, this one's findings indicated that the absence of mental health services for children was a national disgrace. This time, the commission recommendations placed strong emphasis on primary prevention and a system of advocacy for the needs of children. They pointed out that progress in primary prevention could clearly be achieved by improving the nutrition of both expectant mothers and of children, by eliminating poverty, and by improving the climate of social responsibility toward children (Joint Commission on the Mental Health of Children, 1970).

But if the intellectual climate was ripe for such developments, the political and practical climate was not. Although an Office of Child Development was established in the Department of Health, Education, and Welfare, directed by psychologist Edward Zigler, legislation calling for improved comprehensive child care was passed by Congress and vetoed by President Richard Nixon. Increasing amounts of federal funds and public energies were being consumed by the war in Vietnam, and policy concerns and funds were increasingly directed toward problems of crime, alcoholism, and drug abuse. While each of these problems had clearly demonstrated social bases, the overriding concern with public programs was in the establishment of mechanisms to treat, and thereby fix responsibility on, the individual offender, drinker, or addict.

Meantime, the community mental health program, which had inspired high hopes, was advancing at less than a snail's pace. Of the two thousand community mental health centers anticipated in the original legislation, fewer than five hundred had been built by mid-1971. In order for federal funds to become available, separate bills must be passed by Congress to authorize the expenditures and to appropriate the funds. The amount of funds actually disbursed depends further on the apportionment of appropriated funds by the executive branch to various budget categories. From 1964 to 1968, \$200 million were authorized, \$180 million were appropriated, and \$135 million were apportioned to the program. In fiscal year 1968, none of the appropriated funds for mental health centers were allowed to be spent because they were not apportioned. Federal expenditures for community mental health centers from 1964 to 1968 averaged slightly less than 5 percent of the *annual* state expenditures for state mental hospitals (Glasscote, Sussex, Cummings, and Smith, 1969).

Those community mental health centers that did come into being represented a significant expansion in treatment programs in many communities. Psychiatric admissions to state and county hospitals had been increasing at a rate of 2.1 percent per year from 1946 to 1954. After the introduction of major tranquilizing drugs on a large scale in 1955, these admission rates began a steady decline. State and county hospital patient populations dropped 24 percent from 558,922 in 1955 to 426,009 in 1967 (NIMH, 1969). The number of patients in state and county hospitals diagnosed as schizophrenic declined from 259,491 in 1962 to 133,000 in 1972 (Mosher, Gunderson, and Keith, 1974). Community mental health centers provided an alternative to admission to state and county hospitals in those communities that developed a full range of treatment services. But providing such services is not the same as a reduction in the rates of mental health problems.

Because of the large discrepancies between what mental health centers were originally hoped to be and what they actually are, and no doubt because of the additional discrepancy between the number of centers envisioned originally and the small number that actually came into being, the community mental health centers have fallen far short of their original conception. It should be noted that there is considerable variability among these centers, with some of them making genuine attempts to deliver new forms of service, and others doing the same old business under a new name. Few centers have developed any significant prevention programs, and demonstrated effectiveness of primary preventive efforts are very hard to find. It had become clear to many community psychologists that while the community mental health centers represented an important base for some community psychologists, they were far from a sufficient setting for the commitments and functions that community psychologists had conceptualized.

This commitment was forcefully articulated by Kelly in his presidential address to the Division of Community Psychology of the American Psychological Association:

> For me, the social revolutions in our society mark the end of the professional as *the* policy-maker! . . . One thing I am convinced of is that our frame of reference must shift, and our training programs should be redesigned so that the settings for the personal development of the community psychologist are viable, coherent, and of the highest quality. One way to create a richer and more valid enterprise is by teaching the community psychologist to identify with *all* the people in his community and to become involved in the creation of *new* community resources. (Kelly, 1970, p. 529; italics in original)

The concern with the creation of "new community resources" is an important part of the developmental emphasis within community psychology. At the same time, the failure of the community mental health centers to move toward such a goal is evidenced, as well as by any other indication, by the fact that most of them had failed to develop the local financial support that had been envisioned to replace federal funds in the original legislation. When federal financial support evaporated because grant periods had expired, or because of federal administrative impoundment of funds, most of the mental health centers were faced with curtailment of programs, if not threatened with extinction. The kind of resource creation envisioned by community psychologists such as Kelly went beyond the survival of existing community services, yet many community mental health centers were hard pressed to achieve even that limited goal.

The second Austin conference was charged with articulating different models within community psychology, and the preconference papers submitted by the participants reflected a diversity of approaches, concepts, and roles for community psychologists. Just as there is economic wisdom in the diversification of investments, it was recognized that diversity within community psychology was to be valued. In an age of increasing specialization that creates forces for narrow and limited role definitions, the community psychologist had been defined since the Swampscott conference as a generalist. At this Austin meeting it was recognized that a single community psychologist could not be all things to all people, but that the field had to encompass a number of different activities, each of which represented valid ways of helping communities. The position of the participants at this conference could be encapsulated in the statement that community psychology is concerned with participating in planning for social change; with organizing and implementing planned changes; with designing and conducting programs of service to provide for the human needs generated by social changes; and with the development of community resources and processes to deal with the future implications of social changes. It was recognized that these are activities that involve the efforts of persons from several different fields, and that community psychologists should give a high priority to cooperation and collaboration with the community and with other disciplines. On their part, community psychologists can contribute competencies in three clusters of activities: (1) research on the identification and analysis of community problems, surveys of community attitudes, and the evaluation of proposals for community programs, including the conduct and assessment of pilot projects; (2) participation in the design, delivery, and evaluation of community human services; and (3) active professional participation in social action programs of community development, including the design of community social settings that minimize adaptive difficulties and enhance the development of personal competencies within those settings. One example of a high point of this latter kind of activity might be working to create a requirement for, and participating in the preparation of, social environmental impact statements that precede the implementation of technological and social developments, similar to the statements concerning the physical environment that are now required in many instances.

At this conference the community development aspect of community psychology "was seen as discontinuous with clinical psychology and community mental health, requiring different designs for training and for generating knowledge, calling for different criteria of success, and providing different satisfactions from work, roles, and settings" (Mann, 1971). Much of the knowledge on which such activities would be based does not exist, at least in organized form, but the conference participants were able to outline the kinds of knowledge that would be required. They generated three major topics that would provide the focus for a body of knowledge in community psychology:

1. Analyses of social processes. This topic includes discussion of knowledge of past and current social institutions, social movements, and the interaction between economic, social, and political processes. This topic stresses the value of creating knowledge about how historical constraints and large social forces affect a specific community.

2. Study of interactions in a specific social system. This topic emphasizes a more current and intensive analysis of a specific social system or group of systems involved in a change program. Here the focus is on understanding how a specific organization affects individuals and how the organization adapts to change.

3. Design of social interventions. While this is identified as a discrete topic, the design of interventions should be an integral part of the analysis of social forces and the assessment of a particular organization. This point emphasizes that determining the specific level and media for change must derive from previous sources of data.

The body of knowledge for community psychology may thus be outlined into three major topics corresponding to the conceptual analyses that community psychologists employ in doing their work. Within each topic there are three different time orientations, and there is continuous interplay between topics and time levels. The specific content for the dimensions of this outline are presented in Table 1.

From this perspective, it is possible to propose some maxims for the professional activities of the community psychologist. First, to put it plainly, the community psychologist must know what he or she is doing, both conceptually and empirically, in historical, contemporary, and future contexts. Second, while the community psychologist is an agent of change, he or she is more a modifier than an instigator of change processes that are fomented by larger social

Table 1. Conceptual Outline for a Body of Knowledge in Community Psychology

TIME FOCUS	TOPIC FOCUS		
	Developmental Context: Analyses of Social Processes	*Interactions in a Specific Social Setting*	*Design of Social Interventions*
Evolutionary	Dynamic history of social change. History of social institutions and social movements.	Effectiveness of social institutions and social processes. Effectiveness of specific organizations over time.	Defining media, channels, and modalities of interventions. Defining levels of interventions.
Contemporary	Assessment of specific social systems. Effects of alternative interventions upon social systems, institutions, and forces.	Personal and organizational effectiveness in specific settings.	Creating resources and organizing for interventions.
Future	Analysis of alternative contingent futures.	Anticipated processes for creating alternative interventions for people and organizations.	Defining accountabilities for interventions with regard to systems, resources, and future social institutions.

SOURCE: Adapted from Mann (1971).

processes. Third, he or she is a collaborative participant in community events, with accountabilities to present and future coworkers and community constituencies.

While this historical excursion has been necessary to trace the development of community psychology in its social context, it is to be hoped that such exercises can contribute more than a mere beginning definition of a field. Within the body of knowledge outlined here, historical understandings are an important element; but history does not always serve men well. Historical understandings are clearly not sufficient to the challenge of the future, but if humanity is to prevail, if it is to master its future, one of the ingredients of that success will have to be for it to become the master, rather than the slave, of its past. Community psychology stands on the side of affirming this possibility.

References

ALBEE, G. W. *Mental Health Manpower Trends.* New York: Basic Books, 1959.

BARTLETT, D. P. *Human Relations Training for Police in Nashville: History, Analysis, and Prospects.* Nashville, Tenn.: Center for Community Studies, George Peabody College for Teachers, 1972.

BENNETT, C. C., ANDERSON, L. S., COOPER, S., HASSOL, L., KLEIN, D.C., AND ROSENBAUM, G. (Eds.). *Community Psychology: A Report of the Boston Conference on the Education of Psychologists for Community Mental Health.* Boston: Boston University Press, 1966.

BLOOM, B. L. Strategies for the prevention of mental disorders. In Division 27 of the American Psychological Association, *Issues in Community Psychology and Preventive Mental Health.* New York: Behavioral Publications, 1971.

CAPLAN, G. (Ed.). *Prevention of Mental Disorders in Children.* New York: Basic Books, 1961.

CAPLAN, G. *Principles of Preventive Psychiatry.* New York: Basic Books, 1964.

DIVISION 27 OF THE AMERICAN PSYCHOLOGICAL ASSOCIATION. *Issues in Community Psychology and Preventive Mental Health.* New York: Behavioral Publications, 1971.

DUHL, L. J. (Ed.). *The Urban Condition.* New York: Basic Books, 1963.

FARIS, R. E., AND DUNHAM, H. W. *Mental Disorders in Urban Areas.* Chicago: University of Chicago Press, 1939.

FREEMAN, H. E., AND SIMMONS, O. G. Mental patients in the community: Family settings and performance levels. *American Sociological Review*, 1958, *23*, 147–154.

FRIED, M. Social problems and psychopathology. In L. J. Duhl (Ed.), *Urban America and the Planning of Mental Health Services.* New York: Group for the Advancement of Psychiatry, 1964.

GARTNER, A. *Paraprofessionals and their Performance.* New York: Praeger, 1971.

GLASSCOTE, M. A., SUSSEX, J. N., CUMMING, E., AND SMITH, L. H. *The Community Mental Health Center: An Interim Appraisal.* Washington, D. C.: Joint Information Service, 1969.

GLIDEWELL, J. C. Priorities for psychologists in community mental health. In Division 27 of the American Psychological Association, *Issues in Community Psychology and Preventive Mental Health.* New York: Behavioral Publications, 1971.

GOFFMAN, E. *Asylums: Essays on the Social Situation of Mental Patients and Other Inmates.* Garden City, N.Y.: Doubleday, Anchor Books, 1961.

GURIN, G., VEROFF, J., AND FELD, S. *Americans View Their Mental Health.* New York: Basic Books, 1960.

HOBBS, N. Mental health's third revolution. *American Journal of Orthopsychiatry*, 1964, *34*, 822–833.

HOLLINGSHEAD, A. B., AND REDLICH, F. C. *Social Class and Mental Illness.* New York: Wiley, 1958.

HOLLISTER, W. (Chmn.). Symposium on *Primary Prevention: Modification, Mediation, and Utilization of Stress.* American Orthopsychiatric Association, Washington, D. C., 1963.

HUNT, J. MCV. Toward the prevention of incompetence. In J. W. Carter (Ed.), *Research Contributions from Psychology to Community Mental Health.* New York: Behavioral Publications, 1968.

ISCOE, I., AND SPIELBERGER, C. D. (Eds.). *Community Psychology: Perspectives in Training and Research.* New York: Appleton-Century-Crofts, 1970.

JOINT COMMISSION ON MENTAL ILLNESS AND HEALTH. *Action for Mental Health.* New York: Basic Books, 1961.

JOINT COMMISSION ON MENTAL HEALTH OF CHILDREN. *Crisis in Child Mental Health.* New York: Harper & Row, 1970.

KATES, R. W., AND WOHLWILL, J. F. (Eds.). Man's response to the physical environment. *Journal of Social Issues*, 1966, *22*, no. 4.

KENNEDY, J. F. *Message from the President of the United States Relative to Mental Illness and Mental Retardation*, 88th Congress, First Session, U.S. House of Representatives Document No. 58. Washington,

D. C.: U.S. Government Printing Office, 1963.

KELLY, J. G. Ecological constraints on mental health services. *American Psychologist*, 1966, *21*, 535–539.

KELLY, J. G. Towards an ecological conception of preventive interventions. In J. W. Carter (Ed.), *Research Contributions from Psychology to Commumity Mental Health.* New York: Behavioral Publications, 1968.

KELLY, J. G. Antidotes for arrogance: Training for community psychology. *American Psychologist*, 1970, *25*, 524–531.

KLEIN, D. C. *Community Dynamics and Mental Health.* New York: Wiley, 1968.

KNUDSON, A. New perspectives regarding positive mental health. *American Psychologist*, 1963, *18*, 300–306.

LEVINE, M. Some postulates of practice in community psychology and their implications for training. In I. Iscoe and C. D. Spielberger (Eds.), *Community Psychology: Perspectives in Training and Research.* New York: Appleton-Century-Crofts, 1970.

LIPSITT, P. D., AND STEINBRUNER, M. An experiment in police-community relations: A small group approach. *Community Mental Health Journal*, 1969, *5*, 172–179.

MANN, P. A. Mid-winter conference of the Division of Community Psychology, American Psychological Association. Division of Community Psychology, *Newsletter*, 1971, *5*, no. 3.

MANN, P. A., AND ISCOE, I. Mass behavior and community organization: Reflections on a peaceful demonstration. *American Psychologist*, 1971, *26*, 108–113.

MOSHER, L. R., GUNDERSON, J. G., AND KEITH, S. J. (Eds.). *Schizophrenia Bulletin*, 1974, no. 10, p. 8.

MOTTOLA, W. C. Impact of a desegregating school system. Presented at symposium: *The Social Impact of Consultation.* American Psychological Association, Miami Beach, Florida, 1970.

NATIONAL INSTITUTE OF MENTAL HEALTH. *Patients in State and County Mental Hospitals, 1967.* Chevy Chase, Md.: U. S. Department of Health, Education, and Welfare, Public Health Service Publication 1921, 1969.

OCHBERG, F. M., AND TRICKETT, E. Administrative responses to a racial conflict in a high school. *Community Mental Health Journal*, 1970, *6*, 470–482.

PEARL, A., AND RIESSMAN, F. *New Careers for the Poor.* New York: Free Press, 1965.

PLOG, S. C. Urbanization, psychological disorders, and the heritage of social psychiatry. In S. C. Plog and R. B. Edgerton (Eds.), *Changing Perspectives in Mental Illness.* New York: Holt, Rinehart & Winston, 1970.

REIFF, R. Mental health manpower and institutional change. *American Psychologist,* 1966, *21,* 540–548.

REIFF, R. The need for a body of knowledge in community psychology. In I. Iscoe and C. D. Spielberger (Eds.), *Community Psychology: Perspectives in Training and Research.* New York: Appleton-Century-Crofts, 1970.

REIFF, R. Community psychology and public policy. In Division 27 of the American Psychological Association, *Issues in Community Psychology and Preventive Mental Health.* New York: Behavioral Publications, 1971.

REIFF, R., AND RIESSMAN, F. The indigenous non-professional. *Community Mental Health Journal,* Monograph Series, no. 1, 1965.

REIN, M. Choice and change in the American welfare system. *Annals of the American Academy of Political and Social Science,* 1969, *385,* September, 89–111.

RIESSMAN, F., COHEN, J., AND PEARL, A. *Mental Health of the Poor.* New York: Free Press, 1964.

RIOCH, M. J., ELKES, C., FLINT, A. A., USDANSKY, B. S., NEWMAN, R. G., AND SILBER, E. National Institute of Mental Health pilot study in training mental health counselors. *American Journal of Orthopsychiatry,* 1963, *33,* 678–689.

ROSSI, A. M. Some pre–World War II antecedents of community mental health theory and practice. *Mental Hygiene,* 1962, *46,* 78–98.

ROSENBLUM, G. The new role of the clinical psychologist in the community mental health center. *Community Mental Health Journal,* 1968, *4,* 403–410.

SCHELLOW, R. Active participation in police decision making. American Psychological Association, Washington, D. C., 1971.

SCHWARTZ, D. A. Community mental health in 1972: An assessment. In H. H. Barten and L. Bellak (Eds.), *Progress in Community Mental Health,* vol. 2. New York: Grune & Stratton, 1972.

SCRIBNER, S. What is community psychology made of? Division of Community Psychology, *Newsletter,* 1968, *2,* 4–6.

SIKES, M., AND CLEVELAND, S. Human relations training for police and community. *American Psychologist,* 1968, *23,* 766–769.

SMITH, M. B., AND HOBBS, N. The community and the community mental health center. *American Psychologist*, 1966, *21*, 499–509.

STANTON, A. H., AND SCHWARTZ, M. S. *The Mental Hospital: A Study of Institutional Participation in Psychiatric Illness and Treatment*. New York: Basic Books, 1954.

YARROW, M. R., CLAUSEN, J. A., AND ROBBINS, P. R. The social meaning of mental illness, *Journal of Social Issues*, 1955, *11*, no. 4, 33–48.

YOLLES, S. F. Past, present and 1980: Trend projections. In L. Bellak and H. H. Barten (Eds.), *Progress in Community Mental Health*, vol. 1. New York: Grune & Stratton, 1969.

2. Concepts of Community and Their Implications for Community Psychology

Interest in the community was stimulated during the 1960s by a number of governmental programs that had the term "community" in their title. Most notable among these were the Community Action Program of the Office of Economic Opportunity and the Community Mental Health Centers program. The early excitement, probably as much as the demonstrable achievements of these programs, has led to the term "community" becoming almost a shibboleth. People talk about working "with the community" or "in the community" or "for the community," phrases that are reminiscent of Lincoln's Gettysburg Address. In the 1970s, interest has developed in community corrections programs, community health care, etc.

It might be said that the term community is in danger of becoming one of those magic words that are invoked in place of, rather than as an indication of, a well-conceived plan of theories, techniques, and procedures. If this is so, it may be because people have been more hopeful than thoughtful in developing the programs to which the term community becomes attached. It is sometimes difficult to do otherwise for two reasons. One is that the pressing nature of many current problems is felt to be so urgent that there is a greater instigation to action than to reflection; and there is no mistaking that the majority of persons involved in these undertakings are action people. The second reason may be that the kind of thinking required for such a conceptual plan is singularly difficult. If it is so hard to define "community," then it is equally hard to define the "with whom," the "in where," and the "for whom" of many social programs.

Evidence that a field of thought does not develop its conceptual storehouse overnight is indicated by developments in the community mental health field. The first legislation authorizing the construction of community mental health centers was passed in 1963 (Public Law 88-164). The original plan called for financial support for a three-year period to cover two-thirds of construction costs (Glasscote, Sanders, Forstenzer, and Foley, 1964). In 1965, Public Law 89-105 provided similar assistance for staffing community mental health centers (Brand, 1968), which was to extend over a five-year period. In 1967, both construction and staffing grant periods were extended to 1970 (Yolles, 1969). However, the programs required the preparation of mental health plans by each state and the writing of regulations by the National Institute of Mental Health to govern the preparation of grant applications and the disbursement of funds, difficult tasks that have barely kept abreast of the legislative and executive changes in the program (Glasscote, Sussex, Cumming, and Smith, 1969).

Such a climate provides little opportunity or incentive for the development of imaginative programming. By the time conceptualizations in the field had begun to develop, the future funding of the programs had encountered serious obstacles. The federal administration had impounded funds appropriated for the centers, and funding bills have faced presidential vetoes each time they were passed in the 1970s.

There were some ideas about community mental health center programs that had predated the original legislation, as reviewed in Chapter 1, but much of it was largely the extension of previous practices to new settings. Some conceptual approaches to the community with implications for mental health programs emerged during the latter half of the 1960s, but the majority of this work consisted of descriptions of programs with little attention to concepts of the community. It was not until the 1970s that a significant number of publications on the operation of community mental health centers, which included consideration of community processes, had been produced by the National Institute of Mental Health. These developments will be reviewed in more detail in subsequent chapters. It is clear, however, that the legislated need for action, backed up by financial necessity, outraced the thinking in the field about the community. Almost certainly, many of the community mental health programs could have benefited immensely from better conceptual models than those that were available when the movement in this direction began, and many such programs can still benefit from a clearer framework of the community and its implications for social intervention.

Definitions of Community

What is a community? A term so familiar to us all is surprisingly difficult to define precisely, and a little reflection indicates that the term has several meanings. The Random House Dictionary (Stein 1969) gives seven definitions of community:

1. A social group of any size whose members reside in a specific locality, share government, and have a common cultural and historical heritage.
2. A social group sharing common characteristics or interests and perceived or perceiving itself as distinct in some respect from the larger society within which it exists.
3. *Eccles.* A group of men or women leading a common life according to a rule.
4. *Ecol.* An assemblage of plant and animal populations occupying a given area.
5. Joint possession.
6. Similar character; agreement; identity (of interests).
7. The community (the public, society).

Most people would recognize a community if they saw one, yet these definitions indicate that while there are some general properties that can be used to define communities, they do not necessarily apply to all meanings of the term. The things denoted by "community" are things that are shared, or common, such as geography, government, culture, or personal characteristics; but not all of these things are shared by all members of "a community." Once we define a community, say by specifying a locale, we include some persons and exclude others who might share some other defining property of "community"; such as persons having common racial, religious, or cultural characteristics; or persons sharing common interests.

The federal programs referred to above contain either express or implied definitions of community. For the Community Action Program, people meeting the government guidelines for defining a level of poverty comprise a community of interest, or constituency, to whom the programs are directed. For the community mental health programs, and for many of the other "community" programs, the community is an area or location. Thus, each community mental health center was to serve a "catchment area" of from seventy-five thousand to two hundred thousand population. In a largely implied sense, it could be said that these programs involved the last of the dictionary definitions of community cited above as well; that is, the community as society, the public.

These definitions, each in a different way, overlook the fact that social programs are embedded in the contexts represented by the several other definitions given by the dictionary. If one were to think about these definitions in terms of the sociological concept of reference groups, it is clear that the various "communities" that relate to these programs are both overlapping and, at times, antagonistic. A community is more than an area or population; it is also a set of social, political, economic, and governmental processes. Such considerations make it imperative to attend to the functional as well as the structural properties of a community, and to explicate the different meanings the concept of community may have in regard to particular programs.

Historically, sociologists have been the leading scholars of the field of community studies. Louis Wirth (1956) defines "community" and "society" as being different varieties of the more general concept of "social group." One traditional distinction between these two kinds of social groups is to assign to each separate properties that are essential to social functioning. One of these properties is the concept of symbiosis, familiar to students of biology, which is perhaps more clearly understood in human social terms as interdependence. The interdependent aspects of social life have been used as one of the defining characteristics of "communities." The other property, traditionally used to define "society," is that of consensus. As Wirth puts it:

> A territorial base, distribution in space of men, institutions, and activities, close living together on the basis of kinship and organic interdependence, and a common life based upon the mutual correspondence of interests tend to characterize a community. Society, on the other hand, has come to refer more to the willed and contrac-

tual relationships between men, which, it has been assumed, are less directly affected than their organic relationships by their distribution in space. (1956, p. 10)

Wirth goes on to note that every community may be considered a society, but not every society would qualify as a community. While a society has some of the ingredients of a community, the historical importance of territorial limits in the definition of community has to do with the processes of communication and common experience, which are more likely to be shared by residents of a given locale than by persons more widely dispersed. A more fundamental distinction is drawn by Toennies (1957) using the sociological concepts of *Gemeinschaft* and *Gesellschaft*. While these concepts refer respectively to the definitions that Wirth gives for community and society, they also have an important historical distinction. Toennies saw the commitment to a common good that was an inherent property of the *Gemeinshaft* form of social organization as something that was based on a tradition of common folkways and mores, of a deeply felt sense of obligation to participate in the life of the community, and that was found only in the smaller, simpler forms of social organization. Psychologists would say that this form of social organization was based on mutual identification of the participants with each other. In Toennies's view, the more complex organization of the large city and the state was not based on these elements, but on a more tenuous set of agreed-upon conventions and mutual fear of reprisal for violating those conventions. This *Gesellschaft* form of social organization he likened to a state of latent war, one that threatened to destroy the stronger psychological linkages of *Gemeinschaft*. His concept of the *Gesellschaft* corresponds to the "willed and contractual relationships" that Wirth uses to define society.

Historically, the distinction between these two forms of social organization that has the most important significance for present-day concerns dates from the end of the feudal systems of the Middle Ages and the beginning of the individualism of the Protestant Reformation. Rexroth (1974) notes that during the Middle Ages there were clearly defined reciprocal obligations between serfs and landowners, and, indeed, land ownership entailed its own obligations to those who lived on and worked the land. The dissolution of this system, accompanied by the liquidation of the assets of the churches of the time, which supported an elaborate set of charitable organizations, ushered in a new system in which the fate of the individual was not based on assumed reciprocal obligations but on whatever bargains and contractual relationships the individual could strike for himself. Naturally, those with few resources, the poor, were in the least favorable bargaining position and did not establish contractual relationships with the society.

As mutual obligations were dethroned in the name of individualism, social supports were also removed to be replaced by whatever economic supports the individual could command. Goodwin (1974) feels that the change from a system of reciprocal obligation to one based on the monetary value attached to exchanges between people began an era that, together with increasing technology and specialization of work, has produced increasing alienation. Under the old system, obligation was an all-or-none matter. Under a system of monetary values, obligations were things to be negotiated as to the degree of obligation, and those in the best bargaining position would necessarily come off such a process with greater advantages. One could scarcely imagine a medieval baron searching for "an obligation loophole"; either the obligations were fulfilled or they were not, and if not, the baron ran the risk of having those who were obligated to him, from above and below, default or revolt. While there were, no doubt, malevolent barons who did default on their obligations, the important point is that the obligations were there as part of the system, a point that was not open to debate. In present-day society those obligations are not part of the system and are very much open to debate, both as to principle and as to their monetary amount.

Thus, while modern means of communication and travel increase the likelihood that persons dispersed over larger areas than those usually associated with the concept of community will share some common experiences and traditions, societal systems based on willed contractual relationships cannot share the implicit psychological sense of reciprocal obligation that comes from the *Gemeinschaft* experience of community living. At the same time, these technological advances of communication and travel increase the geographical range of interdependencies to which persons in different communities are tied, complicating the relationships among those residing in a common territorially defined community.

Within these separate definitions of community and society, it must be recognized that there are different implications for action. There is, for example, a long-standing debate in American society between local and federal initiatives. To some extent this debate reflects the conflict between *Gemeinschaft* and *Gesellschaft*; at least that is often the rationale given by those on the local level for opposing federal programs. This argument would be more convincing, however, if the old form of reciprocal obligation existed in those communities. In its absence, as exemplified by continued resistance to equal-rights initiatives in education and employment, the argument must be seen in its true light as a debate over the form of *Gesellschaft* that will exist in a given community.

During the 1960s, there was apparent widespread social support for national social programs—as witness the legislation enacted—and this support was backed up by legal actions that resulted in judicial decisions seeking to promote greater realization of the promises of the Constitution with regard to individual rights. The public visibility given to the gulf between social principle and social reality for many citizens awakened a national consciousness that sought to bring the benefits of an affluent society to all of its citizens.

The legislative programs enacted under this state of consciousness were termed "Great Society" programs, and while many of them used the term "community" in either their title or their concepts, they were clearly the embodiment of social policy at the societal rather than at the community level (Levitan, 1969; Moynihan, 1969). Indeed, there is little to indicate that this distinction was given more than passing attention in the rapid development of these programs (Marris and Rein, 1967).

However, it seemed that no sooner were these programs erected than disenchantment and misgiving began to set in, particularly with regard to the more controversial programs. This process was aided in large measure by the interposition of a controversial, undeclared, and divisive war, but the seeds of the reaction could be foreseen in the process of the civil rights struggle. The civil rights movement was, among other things, clearly a contest between national and local initiatives, and as such generated considerable local resistance in those communities that had opposed the establishment of official practices of equality. Despite this resistance, measurable progress was made during the 1960s in the implementation of specific programs and in changes in public behavior. While some changes in interracial attitudes took place during this period (Pettigrew, 1969), there is reason to believe that behavioral changes regarding equality were based more on respect for the law and perceived social norms against discriminatory behavior than on enduring changes in attitudes (Dreger and Miller, 1969).

It might be expected that prolonged maintenance of behavioral changes could eventually lead to changes in attitudes; but, at least until such changes occur, normative support alone is a fragile base for developing lasting change unless it is backed up by relatively enduring commitments (Cohen, 1964). As the civil rights movement began to broaden to an economic movement, as represented by the famous Poor People's March on Washington (Hunter, 1968), the affirmative-action plans to require equality of employment in federally financed projects, and other explicit efforts to implement quota systems and establish equality of condition rather than equality of opportunity (Moynihan, 1971; Executive Order 11246), politicians found that an issue had developed which they could exploit by raising questions about "forced integration." To be sure, these developments were complex and had many varied bases, but this reaction against progress in civil rights could not have occurred, and indeed occurred less often, where communities felt a sense of ownership of their commitment to equality, that is, as a reciprocal obligation, and did not see integrationist goals as something imposed from the outside.

This development illustrates that where tension exists between national, that is, societal, goals, and local, or community, goals, progress will be slow, if not aborted. This is, of course, an issue of long standing, going back to the founding of the Republic, and it is reflected in the various provisions of the Constitution allocating powers to federal and local governments. It can be observed then that as communication, contact (through travel and mobility), and interdependencies become more nationalized, imposing more of the properties traditionally associated with communities on a societal level, and vice versa, there arises a pressing need to make visible and explicit those features of community life that can become obscured in social complexity: the common commitments and reciprocal obligations that accompany any set of interdependencies but have ceased to occupy a prominent position in our conscious perception of the social system. The challenge to community psychology is nothing less than the illumination of these facts of community life and the encouragement of the participation of citizens in these processes. The alienation and divisiveness of contemporary social life require a perpetuation and a strengthening of those *Gemeinschaft*-like elements of a psychological sense of community.

The Relevance of Psychology to Community Studies

Historically, psychology has been concerned with the study of the individual and with intrapsychic phenomena. To the extent that psychologists ventured beyond the outer skin of their subject of study, it was in the area of social psychology, which was concerned primarily with the effects of others (the group) on individual behavior. Recent research developments have indicated that the intrapsychic perspective is insufficient even for the study of the individual. Studies of the stability of personality characteristics over time (Child, 1963) and of the predictability of behavior from personal traits (Mischel, 1968) have demonstrated the limitations of an entirely intrapsychic approach. The role of the situation has come to be recognized as important in understanding behavior (Barker, 1968; Fried, 1968; Katz, 1967; Wicker, 1969).

At another level of psychological enterprise it has become increasingly apparent that social and community conditions are heavily implicated in the applied concerns of psychologists, not only as effectors of the behavior of subjects of psychological study (Barker and Gump, 1964; Fried, 1964; Leighton *et al.*, 1963) but also as a modulator of the activities of psychologists and other social agents as well (Levine and Levine, 1970). Out of these developments, psychologists who first began to define themselves as community psychologists (Bennet *et al.*, 1965) have broadened their perspective to include a concern with community processes. This change in orientation does not imply, however, a lack of concern with the individual. Indeed, the Swampscott conference, at which community psychology was first articulated, focused on the relationship between the individual and social systems.

Within this perspective, community psychologists are interested in both individuals and communities in two different yet complementary ways. In one sense there is a focus on the individual as an *agent* of community life, and on the community as an arena or *setting* in which individual behavior occurs, is socialized, and is fostered and constrained. In another sense, the focus is on the individual as an *object* of community life, and on the community as a *medium* for actuating changes in the quality of individual experience.

Much of the writing in the field of community psychology has addressed itself to this relationship between the individual and social systems, sometimes emphasizing one more than the other. It is probably accurate to say that psychologists' knowledge of the individual is more extensive than their knowledge of the processes by which individuals and social systems articulate. Moreover, it has been traditional to oppose the two levels of explanation as if they were mutually exclusive; that is, to argue whether individual or collective explanations of behavior are preferable (cf. Bendix, 1952; Katz and Kahn, 1964, Ch. 13; Wrong, 1961). In philosophy this procedure is known as reductionism, and its purpose is to simplify the explanation of phenomena by assuming a single frame of reference.

This procedure also has a social history force behind it, however. The divisions of labor for acquiring knowledge represented by the departmental structures of universities have usually included departments of psychology and departments of sociology. These divisions are known as disciplines, and signify the marking off of intellectual territories for one group or another. At some point in history these distinctions were probably both rational and convenient; but consider what happens when, as would appear to be the case today, the problem areas and the challenges to knowledge no longer fit these distinctions. The scholarly investigator can attempt to explain the object of concern—say, a significant social problem—by claiming that it is the result of processes with which his or her discipline is identified. A scholar in another discipline can make the same claim for his territorialized concepts. Thus, for example, problems of drug abuse may be said to be the result of personal inadequacies or peculiarities by psychologists and psychiatrists; sociologists, however, may claim that such problems are the result of alienating social conditions. Clearly, it is possible for both of these positions to be "right" in the sense that these are necessary factors; but continuing inquiry along these lines is more likely to increase the detailed knowledge of each discipline than it is to reach an explanation sufficient to lead to some practical resolution of the problem. In fact, there are many persons in each of these areas of study, and in others, who are not inhibited by these artificial distinctions between areas of "proper" investigation. Still, the presence of this force toward intradisciplinary purism tends to make coherent study of some social phenomena difficult by impeding *inter*disciplinary cooperation and raising arguments of dubious relevance. To judge the quality of a line of inquiry according to its conformity with the subject of study for a particular discipline tends to encourage the same sort of overspecialization from which society already suffers. But if community psychology is to develop as a scholarly field to which the usual expectations of psychological subject matter do not entirely apply, then it is incumbent on that field to develop a set of explicit criteria by which its work is to be judged. Crossing disciplinary boundaries does not mean being subjected to the standards for inquiry for both psychology and some other field; neither does it mean being free from any standards at all.

Probably more so than in the physical sciences—because social science studies have implications for social organization and government programming—reductionism regarding the validity of social science findings occurs also in the political ideologies advanced by one or another political party. Although there is a preponderant national ideology of emphasis on individualism, there are differing political views, for example, on the role of government and society in protecting and promoting conditions of individual life. Besides public rhetoric, public funds to support research, education, and social programs are differentially allocated according to prevailing ideologies, and thus effect significantly the kinds of scholarly and professional activities that are promoted and rewarded. For example, during the administration of the Democratic party in the 1960s, one response to the riots that occurred in many urban areas was to provide funding for studies of the social causes of riots; while during the Republican administration of the 1970s, one response to the riots on college campuses was to provide funding for studies on how to control riots. Although all sciences are subject to this force of political ideology, the social sciences are effected to a greater degree. If the result of social science inquiry is at variance with a political ideology, the politicians find it in their interest not only to dispute the result, but to discredit the science as well. Conversely, a social science finding that is consonant with prevailing ideology may be accepted too uncritically. In either case, society is the loser. Politicians tend to reduce questions to one or another kind of explanation in line with their ideology in order to make an issue and to represent themselves as an embodiment of one side of that issue. This tends to create a mentality of social problem solving that supports single monolithic solutions to complex issues. The social conditions in which people live and the problems they confront are not organized that way, and the social science that commits itself to such a reductionistic viewpoint is necessarily involved in a political game that is subject to dramatic ups and downs, and which probably averages out to mediocrity. Community psychology will be well advised to heed the admonition of Philip Green (1971) to avoid the pragmatic and politically prudent standards of the policymaker and public administrator:

> Unhappily, this concern with what "is" and neglect of what may be, could be, or will be, makes the creation of explanatory or critical social theory impossible; with such a focus one can never do more than predict that tomorrow will be like today, with a few minor changes. Such typical instances of realism as the exercise of prudent foresight about next year's elections are no more an adequate substitute for social theory than the calm conviction that the sun will rise tomorrow is an adequate substitute for astrophysics. There are plentiful pressures, as it is, to produce a present-ridden social theory: witness the failure of mainstream social science to foresee *any* of the major crises that now threaten the stability of the United States. One cannot help but trace at least some part of this failure to the coincidence of perspectives between American social scientists and our governing elites; to honor in any sense—as policy-oriented research necessarily does—the wisdom of the "practical man" is therefore but to institutionalize that unfortunate coincidence. (Green, 1971, p. 15)

If community psychology is to develop independent and appropriate standards for its work, then, they cannot come from past or present social policy alone, but must emanate from a conceptual approach to the problems that it addresses independently of social policy. Since social policy in the past seems not to have been concerned with the community as such, but rather with societal processes, the development of such standards based on an examination of community processes is indeed possible.

Accordingly, the reader will find here more emphasis on community processes, and on individual-community interactions, than on the individual as such. This is not accidental, nor does it signify social reductionism. On the contrary, a deliberate effort has been made to reorganize and balance knowledge in such a way that it will have more implications for individual living in community systems. Political systems require opposing views and act on the basis of compromise. The point of view presented here is not, hopefully, a compromise, but an integration of the different levels of explanation found in traditional social inquiry. Accordingly, in addition to addressing a set of problems in a new way with the hope of generating new solutions, community psychology is necessarily involved in legitimizing new kinds of inquiry and in establishing new criteria for the acquisition of knowledge and the organization of scholarly activities. It is necessarily concerned with political processes as a subject of study and with establishing new criteria for public social programming, a concern that is clearly political, but which is conceptually a sub-area of a broader human social concern.

These remarks do not mean that the object of this field of study is to create a new, all-inclusive, super-monolithic system of knowledge and social programming. That is the very kind of "oneness" that community psychology hopes to counteract. A crude criterion for community psychology as a collective enterprise might well be the number of diverse programs it can stimulate to deal with problems in different settings. A more refined criterion would be the extent to which it can generate understandings of individual and social problems and establish guidelines for constructing from among alternative approaches those programs that are effective in particular settings in accomplishing particular goals that vary from setting to setting.

Social Process and Social Science

It is obvious from the foregoing that the development of a community psychology must consider jointly the perceptions individuals have of their communities, the concepts of community life social scientists bring to bear on social problems, and the political ideologies that those empowered to organize social programs impose on their efforts. It is necessary to recognize further that these three factors are seldom in agreement, and that the degree of compatibility and tension among these factors changes over time. This state of affairs cannot be judged good or bad; rather it is taken as a given, as a reality with which all of these forces must be concerned over and above their own positions. There is an extensive literature on the relationship between social science and social policy, much of which is summarized in Lyons (1971), including an extensive bibliography to the major works on the subject. Less well covered in existing literature is the relationship between the perceptions of individuals of their community and either social science or social policy, and that area is of major concern for community psychology.

At different periods of time it is possible to find more social emphasis given to one of these forces than to others, and at any given time there exist opposing views regarding each of these forces. Few Americans have never entertained the wishful fantasy of a completely unfettered social life, of escape to some isolated, ruggedly self-reliant existence. Yet we quickly realize our interdependence with others to maintain our social existence. The ideal of the ruggedly individualistic frontier people, an ideal that is still with us, is tempered by the realization that sooner or later that form of life had to rely on some form of social organization, a well-organized band of citizens or a sheriff who was a good shot, in order to survive. Despite the lure of fantasy, the *laissez faire* philosophy on which these nostalgic dreams are based has its limitations. In our contemporary complex society, adherents to this philosophy may more often than not mean that they want strict regulation for others and *laissez faire* for themselves.

Since the 1960s, the individualistic orientation toward community and social policy has taken a number of forms. On the one hand, there are those who seek greater participation in social decision making in order to achieve some influence over their own destinies. University students organized to demand participation in academic decision making; poor and minority-group members have striven for more equitable representation and for control of institutions that affect their own lives. While consumerism is presently a strong force in society, it remains to be seen whether it will have any significant or lasting impact on economic decisions, or whether it will remain at a fairly token level as a complaint department far down the ladder of the economic system. Further, it is too early to determine if the focus on marketing consumerism will distract this force from participation in more significant governmental policy decisions. On the other hand, there are those who by ideology or passivity support a nonpolicy of nonparticipation. Finally, a subvariety of individualism with regard to social policy may be found among those who "dropped out" of participation in social institutions to pursue alternative forms of social organization in an effort to be less dependent on existing social structures. This movement led to the formation of communal living arrangements and minority separatist organizations.

There remain, of course, large numbers of individuals who may favor one or another of these sentiments at different times, but who generally attempt to adapt to the prevailing social conditions. They may grumble and complain, but they may also experience social and community pride at times. Some of them care deeply about their community and their society and participate actively in organizations of various kinds that have as their aim the improvement of social life. Seldom do they join organized political movements. They may not feel a sense of social efficacy, but neither do they expect that they should have such influence.

The first two positions outlined above both emphasize the importance of the individual, but they differ in their views on the distribution of social power and influence. In fact, social life involves an inherent compromise between individual and collective claims; power, or influence, is a necessary part of that form of life. It is out of an effort to distribute, modulate, and manage that power that political systems develop and in turn sustain themselves. The last group mentioned above, those who are not consistently committed to a particular ideology, constitute a critical ingredient in the political process. As they attempt to adapt to changing conditions of economics, prevailing social philosophies, and emergent social problems, their attitudes toward political positions regarding the form of social policy change, and as they do they effect the posture of political leaders.

Social programs have always been subject to these forces. In analyzing the development of attitudes and programs concerned with mental illness, White observed:

> Science could advance but little until suitable institutions were created, and institutions could not be created until public opinion was ready to support them. It was no accident that mental hospitals came simultaneously with the American and French revolutions. They sprang from the same growing sense of human dignity and social responsibility. (1956, p. 6)

The influence of these forces on developments in the mental health field is an especially illustrative one, since mental illness has clearly been viewed historically as a personal trouble. Yet, in the appropriate social climate, the summation of such personal troubles can become a social issue. From White's observation we can hypothesize that personal troubles can become a social issue when a sense of social responsibility is activated. It can be hypothesized further that a sense of social responsibility can be maintained at a more stable level by mobilizing and strengthening the sense of community of which we spoke earlier.

Levine and Levine (1970) conducted an extensive historical survey of social programs from which they concluded that the form of helping services varies in a cyclical fashion with the political and social forces of the times. They found that in the latter part of the nineteenth century and the beginning of the twentieth there was an atmosphere of social reform and the development of numerous community-oriented programs, both accompanied by large numbers of immigrants seeking integration into American society. Community centers were developed which served both as a focus of local social life and as a basis for seeking changes in social policy. Their descriptions of numerous social innovations of that earlier period are strikingly similar to some of the developments of the 1960s, a period which they note was also accompanied by immigration: the increased migration of southern blacks into northern cities. However, they also point out that these earlier movements ignored, or in some cases opposed, the existing political structures, and that local politicians often regarded them as naively idealistic. Following World War I the reform atmosphere changed to one of reactionary conservatism during the 1920s, and with this change of political atmosphere, enthusiasm for social innovation diminished. Now, from the vantage point of the present, we may view some of the same developments occurring in the 1970s in reaction to the movements of the 1960s.

The Levines' analysis demonstrates that larger social forces influence the sense of social responsibility that ebbs and flows during these cyclical periods. The existence of these forces and their effects on the psychological sense of community pose an important but relatively unexamined area for psychological inquiry. A nonpsychological explanation of this cyclical pattern can be obtained from Boulding's analysis of social-change phenomena using Hegelian dialectics. According to this view, a social innovation—or thesis, as it is called in the language of dialectics—contains within itself some contradiction. This contradiction tends to create an antithesis, or opposing reaction, as the thesis develops. Following the zenith of the thesis, the antithesis becomes ascendant. The antithesis also contains a contradiction, and its decline is followed by a synthesis. Boulding describes the synthesis as a reinstatement of the thesis (1970, p. 39) but goes on to say that in a dynamic system the synthesis contains elements of both in an integrative fashion. As he notes, whether the synthesis is due solely to the cyclical activity or also to some cumulative process is an unsettled question. The process tends to repeat itself indefinitely.

Probably the most often cited example of this process is in the Marxist doctrine concerning the contradictions of capitalism, in which cycles of revolution and reaction follow each other inevitably. A more familiar example in American society might be represented by the rise of Roosevelt's New Deal, followed by the socially quiescent years of the Eisenhower administration during the 1950s, followed in turn by Johnson's administration of the Great Society programs, which he himself saw as an effort to complete the work begun under Roosevelt (Kearns, 1976). From the preceding discussion it would seem that since all social movements or programs represent a compromise between individual and social concerns, there is always room for contradiction within them. Thus, this dialectical cycle may well be an inherent property of social life.

But, as Boulding notes, this cyclical nature of social change is not the only feature of social life. The cycle does not merely return to its previous point of social functioning with the passage of time. There is also a cumulative process of development in social functioning, which Boulding attributes to learning. Its manifestations are found in the acquisition of technology and in changes in the socialization practices administered to the young. Thus, social change can be viewed as a combination of these two processes. The former, dialectical, process is more familiarly seen in what are referred to as revolutionary changes; the latter is more akin to an evolutionary process. The peaks and valleys of cycles of the more rapid revolutionary changes can be imagined describing their arcs across a graph, but the cumulative effect of evolutionary changes that take place during a given period of cyclical activity raise the baseline of social functioning, so that the resulting combined graphic representation of this process is tilted upward. Accordingly, while dialectical processes may represent embodiments of past ideologies, policies, and practices, which give rise to the observation that things are constantly changing while remaining the same, these processes occur in a changing evolutionary context, so that the conditions they confront are never exactly identical.

These concepts are more descriptive than explanatory, however. Left unexplained are the relationship between revolutionary and evolutionary change processes and, for our purposes, the relationship between these societal processes and the promotion of reciprocal obligations—the psychological sense of community. For the present, we must be content to recognize that these larger social forces influence social life profoundly; but we must also realize that such an understanding is an insufficient base for the development of a psychology of the community.

The proposal that psychology may contribute to the improvement of community life also requires that we examine the relationship between the perceptions that individuals have of their communities and their perceptions of social science. This notion, too, is not without a history of fluctuating popularlity. A central conflict is that between common-sense knowlege and the knowledge of social science.

Bennis, Benne, and Chin (1969, pp. 29–30) describe how Lester Ward's proposals for the application of technology to the improvement of social institutions were reacted against by his sociological colleagues. They quote William Graham Sumner's assertion of a *laissez faire* society as an ideal that excluded the meddling of social scientists. In more recent times, B. F. Skinner's (1971) proposals for a technologically managed society have generated considerable reaction from supporters and detractors in both social science and politics. One is tempted to say that it is the "meddlesome" nature of these proposals that contributes to their rejection; that is, no one asked the writers to propose them. However, the history of a number of presidential commissions created during the 1960s to study pressing social problems does not show a significant record of actual implementation of their recommendations, even though they were asked to make them. Clearly, the stance of political leaders toward these recommendations has depended upon how the recommendations looked to their most visible constituents, and it must be concluded that social science does not substitute for the political process. What may very well determine the utilization of scientific knowledge is the breadth of shared need for solutions, and the consonance of proposed remedies with prevailing social values.

There is also the problem that if social science is perceived as dignifying with scientific language what everyone already knows, it has little perceived value. The physical sciences are not subject to this problem to the degree to which the social sciences are. Boulding has stated the problem in these words:

> If we want to navigate a satellite or produce a new drug or a new hybrid, or even explode a nuclear weapon, we do not call in the old wives. In social systems the old wives, or at least their husbands, are called in all the time. Creating a peaceful world, abolishing slums, solving the race problem, or overcoming crime and so on, are not regarded as suitable subjects for scientific technology but are regarded

> as fields where a pure heart and a little common sense will do all that is really necessary. Either we have no really explicit concept of social systems at all, or we regard knowledge about social systems as something which can be achieved in the ordinary business of life. In the case of simple social systems, this is true. In the case of complex systems, unfortunately, it is totally false, and many of our failures and difficulties arise from this fact. (Boulding, 1967, p. 881)

These considerations speak to the gulf of knowledge and understanding that often exists between the scientific community and the rest of society. This gulf is not merely one of years of education, or command of terminology, concepts, and techniques, but it is also a social-psychological one. Many scientists and citizens are simply not in tune with each other's thoughts, experiences, and values. Under these conditions, when a significant social crisis arises that requires the joint efforts of scientific knowledge and popular support, concerted effort is inordinately difficult. It was in recognition of the need to reduce the social gap between scientists and citizens that George Miller (1969) urged psychologists, in a presidential address to the American Psychological Association, to "give psychology away to the people" as a means of promoting human welfare. This does not mean that science should be tailored to find what people want to find; indeed, much of science is based on questioning accepted beliefs. It does mean framing questions for investigation in terms of what people perceive as their needs, and, when planning programs that apply scientific knowledge to problems, devising solutions that will be effective and supportable in terms of the public's sense of accountability.

Skinner's (1971) assumption that members of a society should opt for a social organization based on behavioral technology because it is in their best interest overlooks what every cultural anthropologist, and every politician for that matter, knows: that people do not always act in their self-interest with the efficiency that some abstract conceptualization of social organization might prescribe. Of course, Skinner's proposals also beg the question of which self-interest people will elect to pursue, and brings into bold relief the fact that society serves multiple and sometimes competing interests. Merely deciding to implement such a scheme, in the sense in which the notion of decision making is ordinarily used, is a revolutionary proposal; that is, it is in the realm of a dialectical thesis and tends to generate reaction. According to the two-factor description of social change that Boulding discussed, important, lasting social developments are more likely to result from evolutionary, nondialectical processes than from revolutionary movements.

Boulding finds nondialectical philosophies more closely identified with cooperation and a sense of community and feels that dialectical processes are ultimately destructive. At various times social scientists have characterized human beings as essentially competitive or essentially cooperative, according to the predominant character of the times in which they were writing. In fact, both conflict and cooperation are characteristic of human social organization, with one or the other being predominant at different times (Coser, 1972). If Boulding is right that evolutionary development tends to change, and reduce, the impact of dialectical processes, then this assumption has important implications for efforts at deliberate social change. The fostering and development of these processes would have to follow hierarchical, developmental stages in which certain processes of social development must be completed before others can be implemented; this process would have to include the resolution of conflict as part of the developmental task. Such a process could not be successfully imposed but would have to follow as differences between individuals, groups, and communities are reconciled and overcome through common experience. The experiences of community psychologists during the 1960s have reinforced for them the principle that cooperation with community members, through personal and working relationships, is critical to social progress in a number of different contexts (Bloom, 1971; Mann and Iscoe, 1971; Mann, 1973). Unfortunately, these relationships are too often sought out hurriedly in times of rapid change or crisis, and ignored during noncrisis periods. As Mann and Iscoe point out, however, it is critical to develop these relationships during noncrisis periods in order that such cooperative relationships may serve the resolution of social crises, which in turn can promote evolutionary development.

In this context, cooperative relationships with citizens become not just an important technical aid, but a standard for the community psychology enterprise. It is as easy for the psychologist to withdraw to a technologically preoccupied, specialized, and individualistic enterprise as it is for any other citizen in our society. For the community psychologist such a direction invites failure. In a way, we have been caught with our sense of community down. Under these conditions, the manipulation of economic and political systems is insufficient. One important contribution to overcoming the social-organizational manifestation of what Alvin Toffler (1970) has called "future shock" is the cultivation of cooperative relationships between citizens and community psychologists.

Planning and Human Relations

Numerous technological schemes were developed during the 1960s to promote management and planning. Among the most popular was systems analysis (von Bertalanffy, 1956). This concept was first applied on a large scale as a device for procurement and development of the space program. Its demonstrated success as a planning device has led to its being applied to numerous organizational problems. As a technique, systems analysis is content-free and, theoretically, can be applied to any system. In 1972, a proposal was made that physicists who were facing unemployment because of a reduction in funds for the space program should be employed in planning social programs for the cities because of their knowledge of systems analysis. Naturally, this suggestion generated a reaction on the grounds that planners should also have some knowledge of the problems with which they were dealing.

The fear of highly technical, impersonal planning and programming is one basis for reluctance to embrace social programming. There is a general ambivalence toward technology, which has characterized reactions to practically every new mechanical device that has been invented, from the steam engine to the automobile to the airplane. During the 1950s and into the 1960s, considerable apprehension was generated over the prospect that automation and computer technology would displace huge numbers of workers from their jobs. In the late 1960s and 1970s, this ambivalence was focused on the ecological crisis by "environmentalists," and against the impersonalization of an overtechnologized society by popular writers (Reich, 1970; Roszak, 1969).

Yet it is clear that each of these reactions takes place against a baseline of increasing technological capability, illustrating the two processes described by Boulding. The cycles of thesis and antithesis concerning technology describe their arcs along a rising baseline of technological evolution. The important question to be raised for community psychology is not whether to oppose technology, but whether provisions for human social concerns are keeping pace with this curve.

Among the most widespread applications of psychology has been the use of human relations concepts in problems of organization and management (Bennis, 1969; Katz and Kahn, 1964; McGregor, 1960). The emphasis in this approach is on the improvement of human relations among members of an organization as a means of increasing organizational functioning. Improved communications and greater participation in decision making are sought through this means in order to counteract the depersonalized and mechanized feeling that tends to develop in bureaucratic organizations. The experiences of these psychologists have also demonstrated the importance of shared perceptions of problems and expectations for solutions among the participants in these change efforts (Glidewell, 1959). This approach, known as organizational development, contains many of the humanly oriented ingredients that are clearly necessary for the development of social programs on a community level.

However, the transfer of organizational development concepts into the field of community psychology requires careful reflection. Members of bureaucratic organizations take certain constraints on their assigned roles for granted. The goals of organizations can be clearly defined and measured more easily than is true for communities or societies, and the participants can anticipate some fairly direct change in their sense of efficacy and in the payoff of increased organizational effectiveness as a result of these programs. At another level, the organizations in which these programs have been conducted are relatively freestanding private enterprises, and the psychologists providing the service are typically outside, entrepreneurially based consultants. These organizations face a fairly predictable market for changes in their output and are relatively free to adapt means oriented toward market-defined ends.

Communities and community institutions do not enjoy these freedoms. Both their establishment and their purpose are frequently multiply determined. Their dependence on the political process makes them less flexible to respond to changing conditions, and, at the same time, less able to engage in long-term planning. In the marketplace, organizations are also free to fail, which means they can take calculated risks. The freedom of communities to engage in risk taking is greatly limited, and the goal for community institutions becomes more often maintenance and survival than development and effectiveness. Community institutions are not free to fail, but the development of their effectiveness is frequently constrained.

Viewed in quasieconomic terms, it would be difficult to specify the nature and quality of the products of communities, the market for those products, and the goals of community institutions, except in superficial ways. These considerations do not negate the need to improve the quality and effectiveness of communities, but they do specify some important differences from other forms of human organization, and they highlight the need for an approach based on an understanding of community processes.

Implications of Community Processes for Community Psychology

Many of the programs discussed in this chapter have been *societal*, rather than community, programs. While rather elaborate efforts have been made to promote community participation in planning such programs as community mental health centers, model cities, and community action programs, the goals of these programs have been societal goals which may or may not be shared by the local communities, and their development has been inspired by federal financial incentives. This is not to say that most communities do not need such programs, or that many of the problems faced by certain cities are not shared by many others. Nor is the point of making this distinction to argue the issue of local versus national control. Far more important is the fact that nationally defined programs tailored to be spread across a wide range of communities must necessarily be tailored toward the most conservative end of the social progress spectrum.

At one extreme, one is reminded of a line from the old "Lum and Abner" radio program, which was focused on life in a backward "hillbilly" community. One of the inhabitants said, "The state highway department brought us a stop sign the other day, but we ain't figured out what to do with it yet, since we ain't got no crossroads here." At another extreme, the availability of funds and the imperatives of the need to spend money during a given fiscal period may lead to the implementation of projects that require more time for careful thought and planning than is available. A dramatic example of this problem was portrayed when, in the summer of 1972, a part of the Pruitt-Igo housing development in St. Louis, constructed during the 1960s, was deliberately destroyed by dynamite because the design of the project had proven not only to be ineffective in improving the quality of life for the residents, but had actually contributed to an increase in the rate of crime and other social problems.

Mere retreat to local initiative, however, would be to abdicate to our traditionally reflexive political heritage, one that does not have a distinguished history of solving the kinds of problems faced today. The evolutionary baseline of progress is at a point where numerous problems are societal in scope, while others are of a community nature. A more effective approach would seem to be to eliminate the debate over federal versus local *programs*, and to begin to define *problems* as more or less societal in scope, or more or less community-based in extensity, and then to tailor programs by beginning with this distinction.

At the same time, it must be remembered that communities, as well as states and regions, vary in their stages of evolutionary development; the level of concern, the *psychological* readiness to engage in certain types of social programs, and the degree and quality of community organization into which programs would be thrust and on which they would be dependent, vary accordingly (Hauser, 1969). In the face of this reality, it would be shortsighted to propose uniform social programs across communities; it would be equally shortsighted to advance a single model of community psychology that would be concerned with a diversity of problems and settings.

In the following chapters we will consider in more detail functional characteristics of communities, general social and psychological principles of change and their implications for individuals, and the criteria that will be employed in the remainder of the book. Following that, we will examine four models of community psychology that have been employed, and we will attempt to draw from them implications for studying community problems, developing intervention strategies, and evaluating the success of these efforts.

The state of the art is such that, while it would be desirable to present a buffet of completely prepared offerings, we will have to be content with a perusal of what is more analogous to a salad bar and attempt to create something that is socially both nutritious and palatable. It is the writer's hope that the work of organizing this material will be such as to guard against the reader's eye being larger than the stomach, and that by doing so, the field of community psychology will be well fed, but still sufficiently hungry to pursue actively future goals.

References

BARKER, R. G. *Ecological Psychology.* Stanford: Stanford University Press, 1968.

BARKER, R. G., AND GUMP, P. *Big School, Small School.* Stanford: Stanford University Press, 1964.

BENNETT, C. C., ANDERSON, L. S., COOPER, S., HASSOL, L., KLEIN, D. C., AND ROSENBLUM, G. (Eds.). *Community Psychology: A Report of the Boston Conference on the Education of Psychologists for Community Mental Health.* Boston: Boston University Press, 1966.

BENDIX, R. Compliant behavior and individual personality. *American Journal of Sociology,* 1952, *58,* 292–303.

BENNIS, W. G. *Organizational Development: Its Nature, Origins, and Prospects.* Reading, Mass.: Addison-Wesley, 1969.

BENNIS, W. G., BENNE, K. D., AND CHIN, R. (Eds.). *The Planning of Change.* New York: Holt, Rinehart & Winston, 1969.

BERTALANFFY, L. v. General system theory. *General Systems,* 1956, *1,* 1–10.

BLOOM, B. Strategies for the prevention of mental disorders. In Division of Community Psychology, American Psychological Association, *Issues in Community Psychology and Preventive Mental Health.* New York: Behavioral Publications, 1971.

BOULDING, K. E. Dare we take the social sciences seriously? *American Psychologist,* 1967, *22,* 879–887.

BOULDING, K. E. *A Primer on Social Dynamics.* New York: Free Press, 1970.

BRAND, J. L. The United States: A historical perspective. In R. N. Williams and L. D. Ozarin (Eds.), *Community Mental Health: An International Perspective.* San Francisco: Jossey-Bass, 1968.

CHILD, I. L. Problems of personality and some relations to anthropology and sociology. In S. Koch (Ed.), *Psychology: A Study of a Science,* vol. 5. New York: McGraw-Hill, 1963.

COHEN, A. R. *Attitude Change and Social Influence.* New York: Basic Books, 1964.

COSER, L. A. (Ed.). Collective violence and civil conflict. *Journal of Social Issues,* 1972, *28,* no. 1.

DREGER, R. M., AND MILLER, K. S. Comparative psychological studies of Negroes and whites in the United States: 1959–1965, *Psychological Bulletin*, Monograph Supplement, 1968, *70*, no. 3, part 2.

FRIED, M. Social problems and psychopathology. In L. J. Duhl (Ed.), *Urban America and the Planning of Mental Health Services.* New York: Group for the Advancement of Psychiatry, 1964.

FRIED, M. Evaluation and the relativity of reality. In L. M. Roberts, N. S. Greenfield, and M. H. Miller (Eds.), *Comprehensive Mental Health: The Challenge of Evaluation.* Madison: University of Wisconsin Press, 1968.

GLASSCOTE, R., SANDERS, D., FORSTENZER, H. M., AND FOLEY, A. R. *The Community Mental Health Center.* Washington, D. C.: Joint Information Service, 1964.

GLIDEWELL, J. C. The entry problem in consultation. *Journal of Social Issues*, 1959, *15*, no. 2, 51–59.

GOODWIN, R. N. *The American Condition.* Garden City, N.Y.: Doubleday, 1974

GREEN, P. The obligations of American social scientists. *Annals of the American Academy of Political and Social Science*, 1971, *394*, March, 13–27.

HAUSER, P. M. The chaotic society: Product of the social morphological revolution. *American Sociological Review*, 1969, *34*, 1–18.

HUNTER, C. A. On the case in Resurrection City. *transAction*, October 1968.

KATZ, D. Group process and social integration: A systems analysis of two movements of social protest. *Journal of Social Issues*, 1967, *23*, no. 1, 3–22.

KATZ, D., AND KAHN, R. *The Social Psychology of Organizations.* New York: Wiley, 1964.

KEARNS, D. Who *was* Lyndon Baines Johnson? Part II. *The Atlantic Monthly*, June 1976, 65–90.

LEIGHTON, D. C., HARDING, J. S., MACKLIN, D. B., MACMILLAN, A. M., AND LEIGHTON, A. H. *The Character of Danger.* New York: Basic Books, 1963.

LEVINE, M., AND LEVINE, A. *A Social History of Helping Services.* New York: Appleton-Century-Crofts, 1970.

LEVITAN, S. A. *The Great Society's Poor Law.* Baltimore: Johns Hopkins Press, 1969.

LYONS, G. M. (Ed.). Social science and the federal government. *Annals of the American Academy of Political and Social Science*, 1971, *394*, March, 1–128.

MANN, P. A. *Psychological Consultation with a Police Department.* Springfield, Ill.: Charles C. Thomas, 1973.

MANN, P. A., AND ISCOE, I. Mass behavior and community organization: Reflections on a peaceful demonstration. *American Psychologist*, 1971, *26*, 108–113.

MCGREGOR, D. N. *The Human Side of Enterprise.* New York: McGraw-Hill, 1960.

MILLER, G. A. Psychology as a means of promoting human welfare. *American Psychologist*, 1969, *24*, 1063–1075.

MISCHEL, W. *Personality and Assessment.* New York: Wiley, 1968.

MOYNIHAN, D. P. *Maximum Feasible Misunderstanding.* New York: Free Press, 1969.

MOYNIHAN, D. P. (Ed.). *Toward a National Urban Policy.* New York: Basic Books, 1970.

PETTIGREW, T. Racially separate or together? *Journal of Social Issues*, 1969, *25*, 43–69.

REICH, C. A. *The Greening of America.* New York: Random House, 1970.

REXROTH, K. *Communalism: From Its Origins to the Twentieth Century.* New York: Seabury, 1974.

ROSZAK, T. *The Making of a Counter Culture.* Garden City, N.Y.: Doubleday, 1969.

SKINNER, B. F. *Beyond Freedom and Dignity.* New York: Knopf, 1971.

STEIN, J. (Ed.). *The Random House Dictionary of the English Language.* New York: Random House, 1969.

TOENNIES, F. *Community and Society: Gemeinschaft and Gesellschaft.* Translated and edited by C. P. Loomis. East Lansing: Michigan State University Press, 1957.

TOFFLER, A. *Future Shock.* New York: Random House, 1970.

WHITE, R. W. *The Abnormal Personality.* New York: Ronald Press, 1956.

WICKER, A. W. Attitudes versus actions: The relationship of verbal and overt behavioral responses to attitude objects. *Journal of Social Issues*, 1969, *25*, 41–78.

WIRTH, L. *Community Life and Social Policy.* Chicago: University of Chicago Press, 1956.

WRONG, D. H. The oversocialized conception of man in modern sociology. *American Sociological Review*, 1961, *26*, 183–193.

YOLLES, S. F. Past, present, and 1980: Trend projections. In L. Bellak and H. H. Barten (Eds.), *Progress in Community Mental Health*, vol. 1. New York: Grune & Stratton, 1969.

3. Community Processes and Orientations Toward Change

From a psychological standpoint, communities are social systems that serve to meet human needs. Individuals are seldom conscious of the community as a social system in their everyday lives, and they go about their usual activities with little awareness that at least some of their behavior contributes to the social processes by which the community operates. The ideology of our society is individualistic, and we prefer to see the community system as supportive of, but subordinate to, our individual interests. This supportive role is demonstrated by the fact that we are more likely to think about the community as a social system at times when we are frustrated, when social problems of one kind or another become so visible as to cause alarm, or when the behavior of others seems to intrude unjustifiably on our individual interests. In short, we are more likely to be aware of the community when it fails to meet some of our needs.

In the ideal case, the behavior of individuals in satisfying their needs and in carrying out community processes is the same behavior. The arrangement whereby the satisfaction or frustration of one person's needs is related to the satisfaction or frustration of the needs of others is what is meant by the concept of interdependence. In actuality, perfect congruence between individual needs and social functioning does not exist, and the conflict between individual and community needs is always present—sometimes in latent forms, and at other times in more manifest conditions.

The contradictory threads of individualism and community are intertwined in our history. A nation of immigrants, probably no recent society is as well suited as American society to reflect these forces or, perhaps more correctly, to experiment with them as part of its own development. A romanticized history of rugged individualism enjoys great popularity, and the early settlers and pioneering immigrants necessarily embodied that independent spirit of which many Americans even today are zealously proud. Many citizens feel that to champion individualism is to honor the important parts of the country's history.

Yet one's view of history can be quite selective. The notion of freedom, so important to our ideology, could be said to apply to groups as well as to individuals. Religious freedom, for example, provides that groups are free to practice their own religions. The immigrants tended to come in groups and to settle in national clusters. Each thrust into the wilderness was soon followed by the development of a community which served needs for companionship, security, and economic efficiency. Some of the pioneering settlements were developed from the beginning with a communal purpose, often based on a utopian plan. Examples include New Harmony, Indiana, the Amana colonies in Iowa, and Oneida, New York, to mention just a few of the better known among several such communities (cf. Nordhoff, 1960; Rexroth, 1974; Robertson, 1970; Wittke, 1964).

The Puritans of Massachusetts, for example, while seeking religious freedom for themselves as a group, could not be considered to have placed a high value on the freedom of the individual. Rexroth (1974) notes that commitment to a common ideal, most often a religious one, was a critical ingredient of the successful communities among these ventures. But that common commitment necessarily placed restrictions, although voluntary ones, upon individuals. Much of the early out-migration from these communities seems to have resulted from a perceived lack of individual freedom on the part of those who moved on. In time, those communities that failed to adapt to this tension frequently declined in their social structure, some of them failing altogether.

In our contemporary society, despite our emphasis on individualism, it is striking that social isolation and alienation are strong contributing factors to mental and emotional difficulties, even in the midst of dense population. Studies based on treated psychiatric cases indicate consistently that persons who are single, divorced, or separated are overrepresented in the treatment population compared to married persons (Fried, 1964; NIMH, 1971; Malzberg, 1959; Ryan, 1969). While these studies are open to alternative interpretations, a number of other studies support the social isolation hypothesis. Recovery from mental illness is more likely when the patient has interpersonal relationships available in the community (Freeman and Simmons, 1963; Wagenfeld, Turner, and Labreche, 1967). Also, Langner and Michael (1963) report that single, separated, and divorced persons in their untreated sample had higher rates of impairment than did married persons.

On a group level, studies of psychiatric combat casualties (Kardiner and Spiegel, 1947) found that men were able to tolerate the realistic fear generated in combat situations so long as they were able to maintain their sense of relatedness to their group. Under conditions where the individual perceived the group as potentially protecting and mutually supporting, such fear could have an invigorating and bracing effect. Traumatic effects were more likely to occur if the individual's reliance on the protective relationship to the group became questionable. Shaw (1971) has summarized a number of studies of groups in different settings, the results of which can be taken to support the conclusion that highly cohesive groups, compared to less cohesive groups, produce more interaction, more accomplishment of goals that the groups set for themselves, and more satisfactions for their members.

On a societal level, Durkheim's (1951) theory of anomie led him to the finding that suicide rates and alienating social conditions were related. Other studies conducted in this general framework have found rates of psychiatric symptoms to be related to personal alienation and estrangement (Kleiner and Parker, 1969; Langner and Michael, 1963; Reinhardt and Gray, 1972) and social disorganization in communities (Leighton *et al.*, 1963).

However, the conflicting nature of the individual and social orientations presents itself in the fact that the same social forces that produce the beneficial effects of cohesiveness also produce strong pressures for conformity and dependency (Shaw, 1971). Social pressure can be a stifling force when carried to extremes, and social rejection or exclusion can have damaging effects on the individual (Goffman, 1963). It is well, then, to recognize that the effects of individualism and collectivism are dual and that these two levels of interpretation are reciprocal, rather than taking the view that emphasis on one level is preferable to emphasis on the other.

Traditionally, psychology has been concerned with individual phenomena—that is, processes that are internal to the behaving individual—and tends to hold social processes constant; while sociology has studied variations in social processes while holding the individual constant. Social psychologists have attempted to bridge these two areas of study in their work. If we are to develop an integrated psychological understanding of human behavior in which both levels of inquiry are to be given appropriate importance, it is necessary to become sophisticated in discourse at each of these levels. Otherwise, simplified assumptions about either level may do violence to the facts (Smelser, 1967).

In the field of social psychology, considerably more empirical knowledge has been collected about the effects of groups and interpersonal relationships on individual behavior than has been collected concerning the effects of communities on behavior. In the field of sociology, studies are more often oriented toward societal processes than toward community processes as such. The study of community psychology, to explore the area between these two levels, is relatively undeveloped. However, the specification of this level is important for reasons other than mere orderliness of scholarship. Since community psychology is both a domain of inquiry and a sphere of action, attributes of the "participant-conceptualizer" role, selection of the community level has important strategic implications as well.

As we noted in Chapter 2, communities and societies share many common attributes, but the two distinguishing characteristics that single out the community as an important level of study are the closer interdependence and the opportunity for closer social interaction among the members than is true of societies. Consensus on any level is based on shared perceptions and expectations. Even in interpersonal relationships there exists some distortion of interpersonal perception. Close interaction provides an opportunity to correct these distortions (Mann, 1971), while the absence of close interaction may actually contribute to distortions (Lemert, 1962). At the societal level, consensus is frequently based on perceptions of the positions of abstract groups whose members are assumed to believe certain things or prefer certain action, rather than on personal interactions. One example of such a perception is the so-called silent majority, whose members' beliefs and opinions cannot be confronted in reality, but to whom politicians have attributed certain beliefs and opinions nevertheless. On the community level, such groups can be made real through interaction, and their perceptions and expectations can be assessed and possibly influenced. The same can be said for any social stereotype. On the other hand, while the interpersonal and group levels provide even greater opportunities for this kind of close interaction, they are not tied to the political and economic characteristics of social structure in the stronger sense that communities represent. Groups do not reach the level of the nonpsychological sources of need satisfaction, such as community planning and zoning, employment, and recreation, which are provided at the community level. Accordingly, while interpersonal and group processes are an important aspect of community life, they are insufficient to an understanding of, or access to, the relationship between community structure and individual behavior.

In order to develop a psychology of the community it is necessary to have an understanding of community structure and function. In this chapter we will examine some of the common features of communities, which will allow us to establish a set of criteria against which to judge the various models of community psychology that will be examined in the following chapters. In discussing these principles of community structure and function we will pay particular attention to two qualities: the stability of community processes, and the ways in which communities change.

Community Social Systems

The term social system implies an entity in which there is some maintenance of structure over time, and in which the various parts of the system maintain some ongoing relationship to each other. In order for any entity to be recognized as such, it must possess some continuity over time. When we speak of a community as a social system, we are referring to a system of social processes; we might also refer to a family, an organized social group, or a nation as a social system. By definition, then, communities as social systems must possess some ongoing processes, and it is the ongoing nature of these processes that define the term stability. We can see readily that if it were not for the stability of these processes, life would indeed be chaotic. One of the main functions of a community, or any social system, is to reduce some of the chaos that would otherwise occur in completely unsystematized relationships.

At the same time, it is easy to recognize that conditions change both within social systems and in their surrounding environment, so that the operations of a social system must also change over time.

The only exception to this rule would be a completely closed system in which no changes of input are received. Communities, however, are open systems; they are open to changing conditions or inputs from their environments. In the abstract, a community system must serve to reconcile the conflict between needs for stability and needs for change. The reconciliation effort is based on a complex set of processes that involves virtually every citizen. An examination of some of the elements of these processes is our concern here.

The social system of the community is composed of smaller subsystems of interpersonal relationships and social groups on one level and formal organizations on a slightly more complex level. The community as a system must articulate with these processes, providing a suprasystem of relationships among groups and organizations. The community articulates with the level of social interaction among members of the community when the structure of its processes facilitates need satisfaction. The concept of the community reaches the level of social systems when these processes are carried out relatively independently of individual actors; that is, if a given set of individuals were replaced by another set in the same situation, the process would remain pretty much the same.

The link between interpersonal behavior and the functioning of community social systems is the concept of institutionalization. When an individual internalizes the expectations of a social system, these expectations become the standards by which the individual and others evaluate that person (Parsons, 1951). By contrast, when there is an absence of shared expectations and commitments, a condition of anomie exists. The person who does not share in the set of social expectations or who is not integrated into a role or social position is said to be alienated from the system. Similarly, a social system in which expectations are not fulfilled is alienating. When this condition exists for a large number of people who should be integrated into social positions that are important for the social system, that system is characterized by a low degree of institutionalization and is consequently unstable. For example, Gamson (1968) presents data from a sample of countries that, though limited in number, show a strong positive relationship between the percentage of alienated citizens and the frequency of disruptive events such as riots, assassinations, demonstrations, and general strikes.

Katz and Kahn (1966) differentiate between social systems and groups on the basis that groups are marked by face-to-face contact of members and interpersonal resolution of differences, while social systems operate on contacts between subsystems, and differences are resolved by compromise. Ordinarily we think of the social system level as being more complex and including larger numbers of people than the group or interpersonal level. Thus, while group and interpersonal behavior can be governed by consensus of individuals, this is not always practical at the social system level (Katz, 1967). Sometimes intrasystem differences cannot be resolved completely before it is necessary for the system to act as an organized entity. Once this action becomes necessary, the system must act *as if* these internal differences had been resolved and speak with one voice. In speaking of community functions, then, it is well to bear in mind that what is represented is a set of relationships between individuals and among groups and organizations that we speak of as the community for the sake of abstract convenience. While these processes are independent of any given individual, group, or organization, they are nevertheless the result of these other levels of functioning acting together. It is important to note that the operations of groups and organizations acting together as part of the community system involve different considerations than would be the case if one were interested only in the operations of groups or organizations in their own right. It is, therefore, necessary to specify the level at which one is concerned with community processes at any particular time.

Community Functions

Sociologists, such as Sanders (1966), use the term community "process" to refer to patterned sequences of social interaction occurring between people with some regularity, and the term community "function" to refer to operations of the community as a social system. All community functions are based upon and carried out through community processes, but, of course, not all patterns of social interaction are necessarily related to performing community functions. The difference turns in part on the degree of organization and regulation that is imposed by the community on social interaction in order to guarantee the performance of community functions.

For example, the social interaction of men and women is a product of individual personalities, but the reproduction and raising of offspring is seen as a function of a social institution, the family, which has important implications for community functioning. Accordingly, the interaction of men and women, particularly in sexual behavior, is regulated both by law and by established rituals and customs. The prescribed patterns of interaction sequences serve community functions, yet there is much interaction between men and women that is not related to these functions. Whether men and women should receive equal treatment under the law in matters of employment, marriage and divorce, and other areas; the age at which persons are legally permitted to marry; the grounds for divorce; all are issues that are frequently debated on the grounds of their implications for community functions. These concerns illustrate in only one area the kinds of issues that are involved in community processes, and the importance attached to them.

Sanders lists ten community operations that are essential elements of the community's functions. Some of these functions serve to maintain the community as a social system. These are:

- recruitment of new members
- socialization
- communication
- social control
- integration through adjustment

Other functions serve the individuation of members within the system. These are:

- allocation of goods and services
- differentiation and status allocation
- allocation of prestige
- allocation of power
- social mobility

By dividing these ten functions into two groups we are emphasizing the issue we referred to earlier: the inherent tension between individual and social claims. In this sense, the community functions as a social system both to maintain itself and to distribute its social benefits to its members; but in reality it is the members of the community, interacting through community processes, who accomplish these functions.

It might be added that the integration or coordination of maintenance and individuation functions is itself an important maintenance function for the community. Social systems that are nearly exclusively maintenance oriented, such as dictatorships, and those that are nearly totally oriented toward individuation, such as anarchies, each have their own problems. In a complex society it is natural and easy to perceive the maintenance functions as being the work of "them," of some remote "establishment" or elite group. This tendency may be increased in an open society where people are free to have a sense of nonparticipation in social affairs. However, observation of a more simple society illustrates that the two functions are performed by the same people. The difference is that in a complex society there is more delegation of authority for maintenance functions to specialized social institutions than in simple societies, and there is more opportunity to assume that the responsibility is delegated also.

Having reviewed these functions of community life, we may say that the relationship between individuation functions and maintenance functions in a social system are in a constant state of flux—a dynamic equilibrium, as distinct from a static condition. This condition of dynamic equilibrium is based on the several levels of community processes that we have reviewed: variations in individual needs and in patterns of social interaction; changing inputs to organized groups and consequent changes in their relationships to each other; differences in socialization patterns and the internalization of social norms with resultant variations in institutionalization and alienation; and the open nature of social systems and their need to operate on the basis of compromise, with the result that social differences are incompletely resolved and perfect consensus (shared expectations and commitments) is seldom reached.

Given this list of possibilities for change-oriented forces in community social systems, one may wonder at the stability such systems show over time. The social cement that seems to bind such systems together with whatever stability they possess comes largely from the interdependent nature of human social life, and the conscious awareness of that interdependence in a sense of community purpose. In examining this topic we will begin a consideration of community dynamics and change mechanisms.

Community Purpose

Throughout plant and animal life the community is a fundamental form of social organization. Such arrangements seem to serve the "purpose" of survival of the species at a biological level. At a social level, the purposes of community living become numerous and complex. What happens in community life may or may not be the result of any purpose, but, unlike plants and other animals, the members of human communities are capable of holding consciously determined goals for their collective living.

Goal setting frequently accompanies examinations of the "state of the community," and gives deliberate meaning to community living. Establishing community purposes or goals is one kind of community process that may serve the maintenance functions of the community. Assessment of community functions, and the establishment of purposes, operates most regularly immediately preceding elections of community officeholders, on occasions of community celebrations, and around critical decision-making issues that effect large numbers of community members. The latter instance occurs frequently in connection with some pressing need for change—for example, in response to sagging economies or an increase in social problems, which may serve to significantly raise the community's consciousness of itself and cause it to take stock of its effectiveness.

The purposes of individual actors in these processes are basically their own; they may conflict with or they may mesh with and complement those of others. At the same time there are many people in a community who have visions of what the community aspires to be. Events such as those mentioned above tend to raise the salience of such conceptions among community members. When there is a degree of consensus on these aspirations, we may speak of a community having a purpose. The social-psychological purpose of a community is made up of the goals that community members set for their collective efforts, while the functions of the community are the achievements of community processes in fulfilling these goals. Both community purposes and functions may change over time. This is the aspect of community life to which the term community dynamics refers.

Community Dynamics

There are two key concepts that refer to the dynamics of a community. These are *equilibrium* and *integration*. Equilibrium refers to the state of balance among the social forces in a community. This concept assumes, of course, that at least some of these forces are in opposition to each other. We have already noted that there may be conflict among individual purposes, and between individual and collective purposes. The conflicts are not in perfect balance, however, and the actions that these conflicts produce continually rearrange the equilibrium among these conflicting forces. In Kurt Lewin's (1951) field theory, social forces are assumed to be arranged in what he terms a "quasi-stationary equilibrium." Such an equilibrium tends toward balance, but it is constantly in flux rather than static.

The integration of a social system has two references (Parsons, 1951, p. 36). One is the functional interrelationship of components within a social system, that is, coordination among its working parts or processes as we are using the term here. The other is the distinctiveness of the social system within its environment, that is, its identity or integrity as a system in relation to other systems. Thus, Parsons identifies two fundamentally important processes of integration: the inner workings of the system, and the maintenance of its boundaries with other systems.

The dynamics of a community operate on several levels at once, and they represent changing states of equilibrium over time. As noted in Chapter 2, if we define a community as an interdependent population sharing common territory and interests, then some processes must exist to reconcile conflicting interests and maintain common concerns if that community is to persist as a social system over time. Consider the problem of equal educational opportunity. Solving this problem requires articulation and reconciliation of the legal processes of the community with the processes of education, residential distribution, ethnic and racial group identities, politics, and economic subsistence. It is a problem that tests the internal integration of the community social system.

In another sense, suppose we consider a community as a geographical location. Consider a community that has depended upon an agricultural economy that is no longer adequate to support its population. If the community "succeeds" in attracting a large manufacturing concern that is part of a larger international conglomerate to bolster its economy, it is conceivable that this development may alter community processes so that they are oriented more toward the interests of the conglomerate and less toward the needs of the local residents. In this instance, a problem in boundary maintenance would be created that would test the capacity of the community to maintain its identity as an integrated social system in relationship to other social systems.

Equilibrium, then, is a defining characteristic of a social system. A community may be high or low in internal integration and still have the same degree of equilibrium. A community with a high degree of integration has a higher ratio of complementarity to conflict than one with a low degree of integration. If we assume that complementarity is a cohesive force, and that conflict is a divisive force, then a community system with a high degree of internal integration would seem to have also a high degree of integrity in relation to surrounding social systems, and a community with a low degree of internal integration would have more problems of a boundary-maintenance nature. Perhaps this serves to explain at the level of a social system why civil disturbances in communities with low internal integration are frequently blamed on "outside agitators." This observation can be made whether or not outside agitators are in fact involved; indeed, systems with low internal integration would seem to be more vulnerable to outside intervention, but they are also less capable of managing conflict that may arise from internal stimuli.

More than from other factors, differences in degrees of internal community integration result from differences in shared expectations and commitments, the same characteristics that we mentioned earlier as affecting degrees of institutionalization-alienation. At the level of the social system, however, we are talking about shared expectations and commitments among subsystems, even though these expectations and commitments may also be shared among individuals. The history of the behavior of United States society toward the problem of poverty during the 1960s and early 1970s can serve as an illustration of this point.

It may be said that equality of economic opportunity is a shared expectation among Americans. Yet the writings of social analysts, such as Michael Harrington's *The Other America* (1962), brought to the attention of society the gap that existed between these expectations and their fulfillment for many citizens. Governmental response to the recognition of this gap was a commitment to the war on poverty that implied the expectation that poverty would be eliminated. After all, the United States had never lost a war.

Within the Office of Economic Opportunity programs the phrase "maximum feasible participation" was articulated at first as if it too was based on the same degree of shared expectations as the war on poverty. Accounts of the thinking of the framers of this concept suggest that its shared meaning was taken for granted to the point that they did not bother to discuss it (Rubin, 1969); yet the lengthy and heated controversy that arose surrounding this concept can be traced directly to a failure of shared expectations concerning its meaning (Moynihan, 1969). As Rubin puts it, "When the law was passed, the black leaders of the ghettos were ready to participate; indeed, they threw the full weight of their organized power into the demand that they be permitted to do so fully" (1969, pp. 17–18).

The chronicle of disruptive and discouraging interactions, on several levels, which has followed the life cycle of the Community Action Programs, punctuated periodically by legislation to restrict the participation of poor people, to reduce levels of funding, and finally to dismantle the programs, was infused with virtually every conceivable charge and countercharge, prejudice and accusation of prejudice, that could be dredged up. It seems amply justifiable to say that what began with a confusion about value orientations was transformed into a perceived failure of motivational orientations, that is, a questioning of the commitment to fulfill what was assumed to be a shared expectation.

The dynamic interplay by these two levels of integration (stability) in social interaction is illustrated by the residue of doubt that still remains concerning the motivational commitment of society to fulfill its stated goals. The ability—indeed, the willingness—of society to engage in social interaction toward shared goals is thus heavily influenced by our perceptions of the motivational commitments of others, a commodity referred to as "trust." It is this dimension of the concept of community that James Q. Wilson (1968) fears may be lost in modern American cities. The expectations that people have of other people and of social institutions are powerful influences on the likelihood that purposive social interaction will be maintained over time. Particularly in institutionalized social interaction, the ability to predict the actions of others on the basis of expectations is an important contributor to a sense of personal and social stability, to a feeling of security. In turn, the established shared expectations constitute an important source of resistance to change in the purposes of social interaction, and lasting changes can probably not be achieved without developing new shared expectations. Both Marris and Rein (1967) and Moynihan (1969) have been critical of the omission of any requirement for community development prior to the initiation of Community Action Programs as a serious limitation on the chances for success of the community action strategy. The essense of such a developmental process would have been the development of new shared expectations.

On the other hand, it seems clear that one of the considerations in the implementation of the CAP programs was a distrust at the federal level of state and local decision-making processes, and the introduction of relatively autonomous agencies into the community structure was done at least in part on the assumption that they would have more freedom of action. This strategy brings into bold relief the topic of social influence processes, a topic of such key importance in community functioning that no discussion of community processes would be complete without it.

Social Influence

Social influence processes have two reference points, according to Gamson (1968). Traditionally, influence refers to the actions of individuals within the system, concerned with who gets what, when, and how. Another focus of influence processes is social control, that is, the collective uses of power to regulate conflict within the system. Gamson's analysis of influence and power groups within social systems divides the actors into partisans—those who seek to increase or protect their own allocations; and authorities—those who seek to maintain the social system.

Gamson assumes that partisans' influence efforts are dependent upon their perception of fair treatment by authorities, and their estimates of the costs and benefits of attempting influence. Authorities, on the other hand, are constrained to at least create the impression of fairness. When authorities are perceived as unfair, and particularly when they are seen as taking a partisan role, they increase the risk of attempts by partisans to exert influence and, consequently, their own need to increase forces of social control. An application of this framework to the actions of partisans and authorities in a community conflict situation is presented in Mann and Iscoe (1971).

French and Raven (1959) distinguish five types of social power. These are:

1. Reward power. Here the basis of power is the ability of one person, A, to reward another, B. If B sees A as the mediator of rewards that B can obtain, the chances of B's changing behavior according to A's influence are increased. Reward power also increases the attraction of B toward A, which increases A's power, as will be noted below.

2. Coercive power. Coercive power depends on A's ability to punish B if B fails to conform to the influence attempt. This type of power is limited to those behaviors that are punishable by A, and tend to decrease the attraction of B toward A. Accordingly, this type of power is only effective if A is also able to constrain B's activities to those areas where the punishment is salient.

3. Legitimate power. Legitimate power exists when B acknowledges A's right to influence him, and his obligation to accept the influence. In social systems such influence is associated with certain social positions; in groups it is associated with certain social roles. Legitimate power associated with a position is usually specified in the form of laws or social norms, including the legitimate use of reward or coercive powers. However, the range of power is limited, and attempts to exert legitimate power beyond these defined limits may result in a loss of power within the legitimate range.

4. Referent power. This type of power is based on B's liking for A and desire to emulate A, but it is not the same as conformity to obtain praise (reward power) or to avoid ridicule (coercive power). It is because B comes to judge and value his own behavior according to A's standards. This concept is the same as identification in personality development. Over time, referent power may develop from reward power through the increasing attraction of B toward A. "Charismatic" leaders exercise this type of power, and the use of celebrity endorsements in advertising attempts to capitalize on it, but it is also an important genuine source of influence in family and interpersonal relationships.

5. Expert power. Expert power depends upon B's attributing superior knowledge or information to A, and B's trust that A will act truthfully. The range of expert power is limited to the area of expertness, and, as with legitimate power, attempts to extend influence outside this area may diminish the original expert power.

Ultimately, conflicts within a social system are resolved through laws and elections, but there is considerably more resolution of real or potential conflict through the exercise of these influence attempts in everyday social interaction. One meaning of freedom in Western society is the ability to exercise and resist various types of influence. In describing each of the types of power above, care has been taken to indicate also the limitations on such power, on the implicit assumption that different types of influence attempts generate different types of resistance to change. French and Raven note that, in general, the more legitimate the influence, and the more influence attempts increase attraction, the less the resistance that is generated; conversely, less legitimate influence attempts and those that decrease attraction tend to create more resistance.

Most readers will be familiar with the visibility, at least by reputation, of the organized attempts to influence legislation that we call "lobbying," and of the actions of interest groups in trying to promote their own causes in state legislatures and in Congress. At the same time, the fact that less than a majority of the registered voters usually exercise their franchise in elections speaks to the low salience of participation in political affairs for most citizens. This condition, of course, creates a popular power vacuum that provides increased opportunities for organized influence efforts.

On the other hand, one seldom sees or hears of "lobbying" of the sort associated with state and national legislative bodies at the community level, yet students of community decision making have demonstrated that few significant community decisions are made solely by elected officials (Hunter, 1953). Each community has its own "power structure," a pyramidally shaped hierarchy of influential citizens who mold community policy. Persons at the top of such structures are frequently those who control an accumulation of reward and coercive powers and have demonstrated their competence in its use to influence community action. They frequently exercise some measure of legitimate and reference power over those immediately below them in the power structure, but are usually not highly visible to most community members in the exercise of power.

Communities vary in the extent to which their power structures tend to represent individuals or organizations, but individuals frequently have behind them the backing of organizational resources. Although important organizations sometimes resort to bald-faced coercive means to influence community policy, such as when a business leader threatens that a certain policy will lead to a reduction in his work force and a loss to the economy of the community, it is clearly in the interest of the cohesiveness of the power structure to act in ways that promote cohesiveness in the community, such as through the use of influence attempts that promote attraction and liking and minimize resistance and conflict. It would seem particularly important from French and Raven's analysis that such influence efforts work through legitimate channels, in appearance, reality, or both, so as to avoid the risk of loss of legitimate power.

Hunter (1953) correctly questions the legitimacy of such invisible forces in a democratic society; yet, as Gamson (1968, pp. 23–28) points out, the visible exercise of influence by a perceived illegitimate source creates a power vacuum that invites resistance and conflict. In a democracy, such power structures are theoretically a special case of delegated authority, made possible by the nonparticipation of large numbers of citizens in organized political processes. The theoretical correctness of Hunter's criticism lies in the fact that citizens are largely unaware of, or at least unresponsive to, this implicit delegation of authority, and democratic ideals require the participation of an informed citizenry. Whether an informed and responsive citizenry would make any difference is an empirical as well as an ideological question. Such questions, however, deal largely with the maintenance functions of the social system, while the individual community member is more frequently concerned with his fate in the community's individuation processes.

It is in the allocation of the benefits of community life that such power structures pose the most delicate questions for individuals. Benign power structures may enhance the quality of life for many citizens, but they are unmistakably vulnerable to the maintenance of competitive inequalities, that is, to limiting or blocking equal access and equal opportunity to participation in community affairs, by virtue of the fact that some of the power structure's influence efforts are devoted to maintaining a favored position for those in power.

Moreover, depending upon the effectiveness of corrective processes in the community as a whole, such systems create the possibility of the development of undeserving elites, such as those cited by the physicist Gabor (1972) as the basis for the downfall of several societies.

This review of social power brings into relief a point that has not received as much attention as it deserves in discussions of community programs. That question is what sort of social influence structure is implied in consideration of the development of community programs? The previous discussion of the war on poverty pointed out that, to some, increased participation means increased influence for the participants, while to others it means increased social control.

It should be clear from our discussion that increased participation does result in increased social control from the standpoint of maintenance of the social system, although this type of maintenance does not necessarily preclude change in the system as some would believe. On the other hand, increased influence in the hands of participants is another problem. Clearly, some partisans see this as a form of changing the influence structure of the community, perhaps through the lens of their faith that such changes will result in policies in line with their own values and beliefs. Others apparently make the same assumption and fear that changes will result that are not consistent with their goals.

Aside from considerations of vested interests, the real problem for the community is the degree to which authority can be distributed among large numbers of people for making programmatic decisions so as to both enhance their sense of effectiveness and still maintain an effective social system. This is a complex question to which we will return in a later chapter. We turn now to a summary of the discussion and to a set of criteria that will be used in evaluating the models of community psychology to be reviewed in the following chapters.

Psychological Approaches to Community Processes

We have reviewed community processes on the levels of interpersonal relations, groups and organizations, and social systems. Central to these processes is the concept of shared expectations and interdependent functioning. The process becomes more formalized as we move from interpersonal relations to social systems, and the level of analysis changes from groups composed of social roles and governed by social norms to the analysis of the interaction among community institutions. As a social system the community performs several functions, which we have grouped into maintenance and individuation functions. An important topic in this process is the role of social power and influence, both from the standpoint of the individual actors within the system and the authorities charged with system maintenance.

The continuity and equilibrium among these processes creates stability in the system over time, promoted by the interdependent nature of community life and reinforced from time to time by community awareness of problems and goal-setting processes. The stability of these processes is based also on shared expectations, social norms, and laws. The structure of these community processes comprise built-in or systemic resistance to change.

Yet each of these processes is subject to errors or variation. One type of variation produces alienation or social exclusion; the other produces partisan competition for enhanced individual allocations. Both have the potential for change in the system if they exist in sufficient numbers and may activate social control mechanisms; that is, the result is increased use of influence processes within the social system. The use of influence tends to increase resistance above that present in the form of systemic resistance, although some types of influence create more resistance than others. A third factor, changes in external inputs, may also activate these processes and produce change.

These community processes are the context in which models of community psychology are applied. This discussion has leaned heavily on sociological and social-psychological concepts in order to create a context in which the models of community psychology can be evaluated, while keeping that context relatively free of elements of the models to be reviewed. The term "models" as used here requires further discussion. In an analytic sense, "model" refers to a way of representing the structure and function of the entity that is the subject of study—in this case, the community. A model is not a theory, but rather a precursor of theory, which it is hoped will be helpful in providing a framework for generating systematic statements about the relationships among structures and functions that might eventually comprise a theory. In this case, we will examine four models of community psychology according to the assumptions that each makes about community processes and human behavior, and the typical research and types of interventions that each model generates.

These models all have in common the fact that they are utilized by persons who identify themselves as community psychologists, and that they are applied to community problems. However, they do not deal with the same types of problems or the same levels of community processes. Each has developed in a somewhat unique historical context, based on somewhat different theoretical assumptions. They are not alternatives for each other in this sense, but they are alternative approaches in the context of community problems. Thus, in order to provide some basis for comparison, it is necessary to generate criteria against which their respective assumptions, research, and interventions can be judged on conceptual grounds. The following criteria have been abstracted from this discussion of community processes and will provide a basis for evaluating each of the models.

1. Conceptualization of ongoing community processes. This criterion asks how the model presents an understanding of the workings of the community. It is further concerned with how knowledge about the community is generated, what assumptions about human behavior are made, and the extent to which these

assumptions are subject to empirical tests.

2. Value assumptions. This criterion is concerned with how the model generates goals and purposes for community action. How does the model assume that statements of community and program goals are generated? What ideological assumptions are explicit or implicit in the model and how are these shared in the community?

3. Conceptions of change processes. How does the model regard stability, resistance, and change in community systems? What intervention strategies are employed in the model? What provision does the model make for unanticipated secondary consequences of intervention?

4. Role of participation. What are the mechanisms for participation of change agents and community members in the change process? In what community settings does the model operate?

5. Role of accountability. What are the mechanisms for accountability of change agents and community members and to whom are they accountable? What provision is made for developing shared expectations on results?

6. Survival value. What are the life expectancies of the change processes, programs, and settings involved in the model? What are the evolutionary stages in the change process? How are succession of personnel and programs provided for in the model, including training and knowledge-generating bases?

References

DURKHEIM, E. *Suicide.* Translated by J. A. Spaulding and G. Simpson. New York: Free Press, 1951.

FREEMAN, H. E., AND SIMMONS, O. G. Mental patients in the community: Family settings and performance levels. *American Sociological Review*, 1958, *23*, 147–154.

FRENCH, J. R. P., JR., AND RAVEN, B. The bases of social power. In D. Cartwright (Ed.), *Studies in Social Power.* Ann Arbor: Institute for Social Research, University of Michigan, 1959.

FRIED, M. Social problems and psychopathology. In L. J. Duhl (Ed.), *Urban America and the Planning of Mental Health Services.* New York: Group for the Advancement of Psychiatry, 1964.

GABOR, D. *The Mature Society.* New York: Praeger, 1972.

GAMSON, W. A. *Power and Discontent.* Homewood, Ill.: Dorsey, 1968.

GOFFMAN, E. *Stigma: Notes on the Management of Spoiled Identity.* Englewood Cliffs, N. J.: Prentice-Hall, 1963.

HARRINGTON, M. *The Other America.* New York: Macmillan, 1962.

HUNTER, F. *Community Power Structure.* Chapel Hill: University of North Carolina Press, 1956.

KATZ, D. Group process and social integration: A systems analysis of two movements of social protest. *Journal of Social Issues*, 1967, *23*, 3–22.

KATZ, D., AND KAHN, R. *The Social Psychology of Organizations.* New York: Wiley, 1966.

KARDINER, A., AND SPIEGEL, H. *War Stress and Neurotic Illness.* New York: Hoeber, 1947.

KLEINER, R. J., AND PARKER, S. Social mobility, anomie, and mental disorder. In S. C. Plog and R. B. Edgerton (Eds.), *Changing Perspectives in Mental Illness.* New York: Holt, Rinehart & Winston, 1969.

LANGNER, T. S., AND MICHAEL, S. T. *Life Stress and Mental Health.* New York: Free Press, 1963.

LEIGHTON, D. C., HARDING, J. S., MACKLIN, D. B., MACMILLAN, A. M., AND LEIGHTON, A. H. *The Character of Danger.* New York: Basic Books, 1963.

LEMERT, E. M. Paranoia and the dynamics of exclusion. *Sociometry*, 1962, *25*, 2–20.

LEWIN, K. *Field Theory in Social Science.* New York: Harper & Row, 1951.

MALZBERG, B. A. Statistical study of first admissions with psychoneurosis in New York State, 1949–1951. *American Journal of Psychiatry*, 1959, *116*, 152–157.

MANN, P. A. Effects of anxiety and defensive style on some aspects of friendship. *Journal of Personality and Social Psychology*, 1971, *18*, 55–61.

MANN, P. A., AND ISCOE, I. Mass behavior and community organization: Reflections on a peaceful demonstration. *American Psychologist*, 1971, *26*, 108–113.

MARRIS, P., AND REIN, M. *Dilemmas of Social Reform.* Chicago: Atherton, 1967.

MOYNIHAN, D. P. *Maximum Feasible Misunderstanding.* New York: Free Press, 1969.

NATIONAL INSTITUTE OF MENTAL HEALTH. Socioeconomic characteristics of admissions to outpatient psychiatric services—1969. DHEW Publication, no. (HSM) 72-9045. Washington, D.C.: U.S. Government Printing Office, 1971.

NORDHOFF, C. *The Communistic Societies of the United States.* New York: Hillary House, 1960. (Originally published, 1875.)

PARSONS, T. *The Social System.* New York: Free Press, 1951.

REINHARDT, A. M., AND GRAY, R. M. Anomia, socioeconomic status, and mental disturbance. *Community Mental Health Journal*, 1972, *8*, 109–119.

REXROTH, K. *Communalism: From its Origins to the Twentieth Century.* New York: Seabury, 1974.

ROBERTSON, C. N. (Ed.). *Oneida Community: An Autobiography.* Syracuse, N. Y.: Syracuse University Press, 1970.

RUBIN, L. B. Maximum feasible participation: The origins, implications, and present status. *Annals of the American Academy of Political and Social Science*, September 1969, *385*, 14–29.

RYAN, W. *Distress in the City.* Cleveland: The Press of Case Western Reserve University, 1969.

SANDERS, I. T. *The Community.* 2nd ed. New York: Ronald Press, 1966.

SHAW, M. E. *Group Dynamics: The Psychology of Small Group Behavior.* New York: McGraw-Hill, 1971.

SMELSER, N. J. Sociology and the other social sciences. In P. F. Lazarsfeld, W. H. Sewell, and H. L. Wilensky (Eds.), *The Uses of Sociology.* New York: Basic Books, 1967.

WAGENFELD, M. O., TURNER, R. J., AND LABRECHE, G. Social relations and community tenure in schizophrenia. *Archives of General Psychiatry*, 1967, *17*, 428–434.

WILSON, J. Q. The urban unease: Community vs. city. *The Public Interest*, Summer 1968.

WITTKE, C. *We Who Built America.* Cleveland: The Press of Case Western Reserve University, 1964.

Part II
Examination of the Models

4. The Mental Health Model

The mental health model of community psychology has its roots in the community mental health center movement, the history of which has been traced in Chapter 1. The community mental health center legislation—and the various plans and regulations developed for its implementation—is largely a logistical plan based on a geographical conception of the community. The community mental health center is supposed to serve a "catchment area" composed of from seventy-five thousand to two hundred thousand people. The mental health model is an attempt to conceptualize a strategy for influencing human behavior, largely within the setting of the community mental health center.

The concept of the community mental health center is an attempt to provide greater coverage and impact of mental health services to a given area. The term "coverage" refers to bringing mental health services to a greater number of people. The term "impact" refers to the effectiveness of the service in dealing with mental health problems. The presence of a community mental health center that meets the criteria of required services will provide increased coverage of a population if the services are utilized. The mental health model attempts to address the question of impact of mental health services on mental health problems.

In the context of the community, the mental health model differs from the traditional clinical model in a number of ways, some of which have to do with the assumptions the model makes, some of which have to do with the technologies employed, and others of which have to do with the goals that are sought. The primary characteristics of the mental health model of community psychology are best seen through an examination of the assumptions on which it is based.

Assumptions

When the Joint Commission on Mental Illness and Health published its final report, it was clear that they believed that the problem of mental illness could and should be controlled. Their recommendation was to vastly expand the treatment facilities available to the population, and to advocate early treatment as a means of prevention (Joint Commission, 1961). While this was a bold assertion in its own right, it was not nearly bold enough for some who argued that no disease that occurs in the numbers indicated in the commission's own studies had ever been controlled by treatment (Sanford, 1955; Dubois, 1961). These writers argued that the experience of public health efforts has consistently shown prevention to be more effective than treatment in the control of disease.

This controversy raised also the question of whether problems of mental health are "mental illnesses" analogous to physical illnesses (Szasz, 1961), and it gave rise to different conceptions of such problems. These are topics that in themselves have already consumed much more space than can be devoted to them here. The arguments involve more than the "true nature" of mental health problems; they also have implications for ideologies, strategies in the delivery of services, and technologies for treating the problems. While there are some forms of mental illness that have demonstrable biological bases, the majority of the evidence does not support the contention that most cases of "mental illness" are based on physical disease. Rather, the terms "disease" and "illness" are seen as metaphors that represent the current way of viewing such problems, just as in earlier days such conditions were viewed alternatively as demonic possession or moral deficiency according to the predominant mode of thinking during that period of history (Sarbin, 1969). Those who pursue this argument see the development of efforts at prevention as a revolution in the mental health field (Hobbs, 1964) that should lead to a new way of viewing these problems.

These controversies have not been resolved in the field of mental health, and it is clear that in the more than ten years since its inception, community mental health centers have been overwhelmingly more involved in treatment than in prevention. While the mental health model to be presented here is not synonymous with everything that occurs in community mental health centers, it borrows heavily from concepts in clinical mental health fields, as well as from the public health field. Thus, the first important assumption of the mental health model is its emphasis on prevention.

1. CONCEPTS OF PREVENTION

In order to understand the approach to prevention, it is necessary first to define some of the terms used in public health to study and control disease problems. These terms come from epidemiology, the study of disease rates in populations. The term *incidence* refers to the number of new cases of a disease that occur in a specified population during a given period of time. Thus, incidence rates are conventionally expressed by the following formula:

$$\text{Incidence} = \frac{\text{Number of new cases}}{\text{100,000 population}} / \text{Year}$$

The term *prevalence* refers to the number of existing cases of a disease, both new and old, in a population during a given period of time. Prevalence rates are expressed by the formula:

$$\text{Prevalence} = \frac{\text{Number of new cases + old cases}}{\text{100,000 population}} / \text{Year}$$

Note that part of the formula for prevalence rates is made up of the formula for incidence rates, in that new cases appear in both. Thus, any decrease in the incidence rate also decreases the prevalence rate, by definition, but a decrease in the prevalence rate does not necessarily decrease the incidence rate. For example, treatment programs may reduce the number of old cases and thus reduce prevalence rates, but treatment cannot reduce the incidence rate.

In the concept of prevalence, the rate is composed of both new and old cases. Variation in the number of old cases in existence when incidence is constant is a reflection of the chronicity of the disease. Even a disease that has a low incidence rate can develop a high prevalence rate if there is no effective treatment for it. The foregoing, however, holds true only for nonfatal diseases, for if a disease produces fairly rapid fatality, prevalence will not increase if there is no effective treatment. Similarly, where there is effective treatment, even a high-incidence disease will not generate prevalence rates much higher than the incidence.

Finally, it is necessary to distinguish between disease rates based on treated and "true" cases. Treated incidence or prevalence rates are based on the number of cases that are actually treated. Such figures in the field of mental health may tell us, as Bloom (1968) has pointed out, nothing more than the epidemiology of psychiatric treatment. True incidence or prevalence rates include both treated and untreated cases of a disease and obviously provide a more accurate picture. Such statistics are very hard to obtain, since it is difficult to identify untreated cases systematically.

In public health terminology, prevention is aimed at three different levels. Primary prevention seeks to reduce the incidence of disease and is the type of prevention most people think about when the term prevention is used. Bloom (1968) describes three general strategies employed in primary prevention. In the first, the intervention may be planned to affect the population as a whole, as in the sanitation of public water supplies. This is a population-wide approach. The second, called a milestone approach, involves contact with members of the population at some specified point in time, such as requiring immunization against certain diseases prior to school entrance. The third type of primary preventive intervention consists of specific measures directed toward some population group that is especially vulnerable to the disease or its effects. This is called a high-risk-group approach, and is exemplified by encouraging elderly citizens to obtain influenza vaccination prior to an expected epidemic, or by safety measures taken to protect workers in certain hazardous industries. The important distinguishing feature of primary prevention is that the preventive intervention occurs prior to the occurrence of the disease in those individuals in whom it is to be prevented.

Secondary prevention is based on the assumption that early identification and treatment of a disease will decrease its severity and chronicity. Secondary prevention, then, seeks to reduce prevalence rates by reducing the number of old cases that exist. Obvious requirements are diseases that can be detected early and effective treatment. Secondary prevention does not seek to reduce incidence and, by definition, requires the occurrence of the disease in some individuals before preventive steps can be taken. This is the type of prevention advocated by the Joint Commission report (1961) mentioned earlier, and one can see the increase in the availability of services (increased coverage) as an attempt to make secondary prevention possible. Secondary prevention is a treatment-based strategy. Successful secondary prevention, however, requires more than the mere availability of services. There must also be an increase in utilization of services, and the services must in fact be effective in reducing severity and chronicity.

Tertiary prevention is the most difficult of the types of prevention to understand as prevention, and points up the importance of understanding what is being prevented. Tertiary prevention also seeks to reduce the prevalence rate by preventing relapses among recovered cases of a disease. It is essentially a rehabilitation strategy, and is most clearly seen in efforts to help to reintegrate former state mental-hospital patients into the community, such as in the form of halfway houses (Raush and Raush, 1968) and aftercare clinics. Again, this effort is directed at old cases.

2. CONCEPTS OF POSITIVE MENTAL HEALTH

A large part of the burden of efforts to foster primary prevention falls on the need for a definition of mental health that is more than the absence of mental illness. However, the search for a suitable definition has consumed the attention of numerous writers with little notable impact on the field of mental health activities. One part of the studies of the Joint Commission was an attempt by Jahoda (1958) to identify such definitions. Jahoda's list included the following characteristics: autonomy, integration, growth and self-actualization, positive attitudes toward the self, perception of reality, and environmental mastery. While Jahoda's list is perhaps the most widely cited, there are numerous others as well. These various sets of criteria for positive mental health all contain in one form or another some conception of growth and development, of autonomy or individuality, and of relatedness to one's environment, including other people.

Any such listing of characteristics is bound to generate a philosophical discussion in which exceptions to the various characteristics are cited. Such exceptions usually involve taking an example of an extreme of one of the dimensions or characteristics cited and raising the question of whether such an extreme is mentally healthy. For example, in regard to autonomy, is a recluse mentally healthy? Or is an individual who is so related to his environment that he cannot take individual action mentally healthy?

Besides perhaps illustrating a dislike for extremes, such discussions are not particularly useful. They tend to distort the original meanings of the terms involved by their application to cover any unusual situation. They tend to generate *ad hoc* qualifiers that eventually become thought of as part of the original criteria, such as a statement that moderate degrees of these characteristics are mentally healthy becoming translated into the notion that moderation itself is mentally healthy. However, a large difficulty with such concepts is that they are frequently based on logical opposites of characteristics of mental illness (White, 1952). As White noted, "When one adds up the qualities, derived from this process of extrapolation, the resulting portrait bears little resemblance to any actual life" (1952). Such extrapolated traits are the sort of thing to which Newbrough (1964) refers as the use of mental health as a euphemism for mental illness and reflects the fact that many of our assumptions about positive mental health are in fact based on studies of the mentally ill.

However, White (1952) cites a more fundamental problem, and that is the limited usefulness of the health metaphor. Since the medical concept of health is the absence of disease, White argues that to go beyond such a statement to speak of positive mental health is to go beyond the concept "health" as a metaphor. Once this is done, one is no longer talking about health, but about something else. Suppose, for example, one of your friends is an extremely popular and effective leader. You would probably not speak of him as "healthy," although he might well be healthy, too. Rather you would be concerned to find something more descriptive about his behavior or personality.

Many writers have repeatedly emphasized that concepts such as those referred to by the term "positive mental health" are fundamentally value concepts (Sarbin, 1969; Smith, 1950, 1959, 1961). The various difficulties noted above may well be due in large part to a need for some scientifically based concepts to guide people's lives in a time when older values are felt to be no longer useful (White, 1952). There is nothing inherently wrong in doing so, of course, but such efforts should be clearly labeled as studies of values, even though they may be scientific. But, again, the recognition of the importance of values underscores another dimension to such concepts, viz, their relativity to particular environments.

Throughout the writings of workers who tend to follow what is here called the mental health model, two clusters of characteristics of positive mental health tend to be emphasized. The first is the development of competence or coping abilities (Phillips, 1967); the second is a sense of social relatedness (Sarbin, 1968). While these clusters may be referred to by a number of terms, they all seem to be related to the fact that the major findings of epidemiological studies of mental illness tend to center around social class and social isolation as major contributors to higher rates of mental illness. The picture is actually not that simple, as we shall see in a later discussion, but this linkage is critical in the assumptions that underlie the preventive efforts in the mental health model. Stated simply, it is that if these factors, social class and social isolation, are associated with increased rates of mental illness, then the fostering and development of competence, coping skills, and social relatedness will decrease rates of mental illness.

Two points should be noted here. One is the assumption in this propositional statement that differences in social class reflect differences in competency and coping abilities that account for the epidemiological relationships. This is not an assumption that can be taken lightly, and we will examine its complexity and validity later. Another point of note is that programs of prevention are not expected to be perfect. That is, they need not eliminate every source of risk or eliminate every case of mental illness in order to be worthwhile. Mental illnesses are, according to the overwhelming weight of the evidence, complexly determined processes. If only one of the determining factors is reduced or eliminated, substantial reduction in rates of the problem can be obtained (Bloom, 1965; Sanford, 1972).

3. THE SOCIAL-ENVIRONMENTAL CONTEXT

Although some representation of the social environment is found in most theories of personality, the predominant tendency in the mental health field has been to locate the source of the difficulty within the individual. This sort of personality reductionism is strategically important in the treatment of the individual case, since the treating mental health professional's interventions are generally limited to working with the individual patient and, in some cases, the family.

However, the growth of epidemiological evidence implicating environmental factors in mental illness has risen in the last several years to the point where it commands serious attention. While the role of intrapsychic trauma was important in Freud's psychoanalytic theory, and studies of psychological casualties during wartime emphasized the mediation of stress through group cohesiveness (Kardiner and Spiegel, 1947), the role of social factors associated with everyday living commanded little attention until recent years. Plog (1969) cites numerous examples of nineteenth-century epidemiological thinking associating mental illness with social conditions. While the methods were somewhat crude by present standards, it is striking to compare the conclusions that Plog reviews with those of present-day epidemiological studies. The fact that such findings have not gained more attention and have not generated more research is probably a reflection of the phenomenon described by White, which was mentioned in Chapter 2; namely, that they fell into a climate in which the predominant values and technologies were not prepared to utilize them.

Attention to the social-environmental context in the mental health model emphasizes the view that mental health and mental health problems are a product of the relationship between the individual and the environment. Such a view does not depreciate the role of personality, but rather increases the salience of social factors, which have almost necessarily tended to become obscured in clinical practice. This view requires both a longitudinal and a cross-sectional perspective on social factors, with a resultant emphasis on changing salience of different social factors in the development of both the individual and the community.

The three basic assumptions underlying this model—control of mental health problems through prevention, conceptions of positive mental health, and increased salience of the social-environmental context—are embedded in the typical research and typical interventions of this model. We move now to a consideration of typical interventions, following which we will consider the research that is typical of the mental health model.

Typical Interventions

There are two major types of interventions that are characteristic of the mental health model: crisis intervention and mental health consultation. Programs of prevention in public health assume that disease occurs as a function of both the susceptibility of individuals and the presence of stressful or noxious factors in the environment. Thus, some programs of prevention are designed to strengthen the resistance of individuals to disease through diet, immunization, etc., while others are aimed at reducing the environmental risk factors, such as impure water or air pollution. In the field of mental health the parallels are the development of individual coping skills and the reduction of environmental stresses.

CRISIS INTERVENTION

The notion of crisis intervention is based on concepts of crisis from several different sources. Social and political crises occur frequently enough that we recognize them readily. Miller and Iscoe (1963) review the observations of several writers on such crises, and note that while crises are perceived as threatening and potentially dangerous upsets in social equilibrium, they also contain powerful incentives for change and the opportunity for growth. On an individual level, Rapoport (1962) cites an unpublished paper by Lindeman and Caplan that defines crisis as the state of an individual reacting to a hazardous situation.

Much of the theory and technique of crisis intervention dates back to Lindeman's (1944) work with grief reactions to bereavement and to Erikson's (1953) concept of "normal" crises in personality development. In the abstract, these writers view a crisis as a demanding problem-solving situation, which may arise out of acute disruptive experiences in people's lives, such as disaster situations or loss of loved ones, or which may occur in normal development as changing demands are encountered when the individual moves from one stage of development to another or makes a major transition in life situation. Caplan (1955, 1958) defines a crisis as a period of emotional upset that he feels endures for from one to six weeks. Such crises are brought about by changes in environmental forces and the individual's reaction to them. It is important to understand that not all environmental changes produce crises; crisis is dependent upon the individual's experience of changes. Caplan assumes that crisis states are not emotional illnesses, but that emotional illnesses are always preceded by some past period of crisis that changed the individual's equilibrium in the direction of ill health. Chief among the characteristics of the crisis state are feelings of tension, emotional unpleasantness, and disorganized problem-solving behavior. These in turn may create a lethargy resembling depressed states. However, these states of crisis are always resolved one way or another.

The goal of crisis intervention is to aid in the resolution of crises toward growth and development, toward a higher level of functioning that improves the individual's ability to cope with subsequent crisis situations. While a number of techniques may be employed in particular crisis situations, they have two major goals: the mobilization of cognitive resources, such as improved consideration of alternatives, talking through the crisis situation and gaining alternative perspectives on it, and improved reality testing on the gains and consequences of various alternatives; and the mobilization of social resources, such as friends, family, and help-giving agencies.

Crises may be arranged on a continuum of normally occurring events, such as school entrance, school transition, marriage and parenthood, to more severe situations involving stress or loss, such as divorce, loss of a job, or bereavement (McGee, 1968). Similarly, vulnerability to crisis may be varied according to personal susceptibility, particular social groupings, or life situations. Bereavement, for example, may not be the crisis for individuals living in situations of extended family membership, where other friends and relatives are close at hand, that it would be for individuals living in relative isolation from such resources.

Anthony (1972) reports two surveys of symptoms of emotional disturbances in children, one of which found a high rate of transient, crisis-related symptoms, and the other of which found relatively high rates of children with disturbances that were not transient but already established emotional disorders. This distinction is critical for the type of prevention that is possible with the two types of cases. If one assumes that the successful resolution of crisis situations, normal or otherwise, will decrease the likelihood of later emotional difficulties, then intervention could have a primary prevention effect. In the presence of already established disorders, the effects of crisis intervention will be toward secondary prevention.

Besides their strategic importance from a preventive standpoint, Caplan (1964) assumes that persons in crisis are more accessible to help-giving efforts and more amenable to change because of the disequilibrium that exists in such states. The particular importance of this assumption is that crisis intervention may be able to achieve gains that would take much longer under noncrisis situations. Halpern (1973) constructed a paper-and-pencil "crisis test" comprised of sixty items describing behavior and feelings associated with the crisis state. The test was administered to groups of people in four different crisis situations: divorce, newly admitted mental hospitalization, bereavement, and students in personal crisis. For each group a comparable noncrisis control group was also tested. The crisis groups in each situation scored higher than the comparable noncrisis group, although the hospitalized mental patients did not score as high as the other groups, a result that is consistent with Caplan's views on the relationship between crisis and emotional illness cited earlier. Halpern also found a negative correlation between the crisis score and the *K*-scale of the Minnesota Multiphasic Personality Inventory, a measure of defensiveness, suggesting that persons in crisis are less defensive.

However, a study by Gerber (1969) tests the accessibility hypothesis more straightforwardly. He reports on a program in which persons who had recently lost a family member through death were offered professional assistance in working through their bereavement. Eighteen out of twenty families, or 90 percent, accepted the offer, a surprising result to the researchers, and twenty four of twenty six family members involved in the service rated the brief psychotherapy that they received as either "helpful" or "very helpful." The question of actual effectiveness of crisis intervention, however, requires more extensive consideration.

Two considerations bear on secondary prevention efforts through crisis intervention with established disorders. One is the assumption that persons in crisis are more amenable to change so that significant improvement can be obtained in a brief period of intervention. The other is the effectiveness of successful crisis intervention in reducing the likelihood of subsequent disorder.

While crisis intervention as a widely used technique has only been practiced for a relatively brief period of time, a few studies have appeared that have attempted to assess the outcome of these efforts. Jacobson *et al.*, (1965) report improvement rates that compare favorably with conventional treatment rates in patients treated during an intensive three-day stay in a hospital setting. Langsley and Kaplan (1968) studied a sample of seventy five patients treated through family crisis intervention and not hospitalized and a control sample of seventy five hospitalized patients. While 100 percent of the control sample was hospitalized, none of the crisis intervention subjects were hospitalized. On a six-month follow-up, 17 percent of the crisis intervention sample had been hospitalized but 21 percent of the control sample had been rehospitalized. Besides a considerable saving in hospital days and expense, 83 percent of the crisis intervention sample escaped the stigma and other implications associated with hospitalization.

There are few reports in the literature on the effectiveness of recent crisis intervention programs with children. However, Eisenberg and Gruenberg (1961) noted in a review of earlier secondary prevention efforts with children that psychogenic disorders associated with early maternal deprivation are reversible upon prompt intervention, and that school phobia, a form of separation anxiety in elementary school children, responds favorably to prompt intervention, but that neither of these conditions responds well to later interventions. They report studies of treatment of other childhood emotional disorders where response to treatment is less certain, but where brief therapy of as few as five sessions produces results comparable to or better than more lengthy treatment. Similarly, Phillips and Johnson (1954) and Phillips (1970), using symptom remission as a criterion, report results favoring brief treatment over more extended conventional methods with children.

The Joint Commission on Mental Health of Children (1969) estimated that 20 percent or more of school children display transient symptoms of emotional distress associated with crises. A caution needs to be observed, however, with special reference to intervention in normal crises with children. If the crisis is viewed as normal, then the symptoms of behavior are not those of mental illness. Yet a child exhibiting signs of such crisis-based emotional disturbance is very much more likely than an adult to elicit the response of several "interventionists"—parents, teachers, perhaps even friends. The spontaneous occurrence of these phenomena make it quite difficult to make predictions among children as to future difficulties on the basis of treatment or no-treatment criteria.

An important consideration for the preventive impact of crisis intervention with children is what Lewis (1965) calls the continuity hypothesis. In reviewing studies of whether children who show emotional disturbance will manifest mental health problems as adults, Lewis finds only mild support for the hypothesis. If adult mental health problems are defined as relatively mild, nonincapacitating symptoms, continuities tend to exist, but if the criterion is mental hospitalization as an adult, then continuity tends not to hold. Three studies that followed up children who were treated at child guidance clinics (Michael, Morris, and Soroker, 1957; O'Neal and Robins, 1958; Sindberg, 1970) who were matched with various control groups, indicate that treatment as a child is effective in preventing hospitalization as an adult. These studies deal with treatment techniques that were not necessarily crisis intervention oriented, so that the evidence for the effectiveness of crisis intervention is only analogous.

Most such studies have not separated cases as to severity, which might lead to different results. Anthony (1972) notes, for example, that most screening devices for emotional disturbance in children cannot discriminate well between transient "crisis" disturbances and established emotional disorders in children. Thus, if both transient and more enduring symptoms are used as the basis of predicting adult mental health status, one would not expect to find much continuity.

We must conclude that the data on the preventive impact of crisis intervention is too sparse to have demonstrated any very general findings. As is true with all treatment studies, adequate control samples are critical and may be more difficult to obtain for crisis intervention than for other techniques. It seems likely that crisis intervention will prove more effective with some conditions than others, but data on this question are not yet available.

Crisis intervention does appear to be effective in preventing hospitalization for adults, and evidence from other studies suggests it may be for children as well. This finding is significant not only in terms of the social-psychological consequences of hospitalization, but also in terms of the cost. Such an effect of reducing severity and chronicity would have an impact on reducing prevalence rates.

One limiting factor that we have noted is that the crisis intervention approach does not systematically attempt to modify the host or environment, but seeks to increase coping skills in individuals. It may be, particularly in children, that other social institutions are in a more advantageous position to do this systematically than is the mental health professional. This consideration leads us to the other typical intervention of this model—mental health consultation.

MENTAL HEALTH CONSULTATION

Mental health consultation is an indirect intervention. Unlike crisis intervention or traditional forms of mental health treatment, the mental health professional who functions as a consultant does not meet with the patient or client directly, but attempts to influence intermediaries who do have direct contact with the client or patient. These intermediaries are referred to as "caregivers" and are defined as persons who are in a strategic and significant "natural" relationships with the potential recipients of the effects of consultation, the clients. Such caregivers may be teachers, ministers, nonpsychiatric physicians, nurses, policemen, and others who may have an ongoing relationship with "persons-at-risk" of mental health problems, but whose work with such persons is not explicitly of a mental health nature.

As a strategy, mental health consultation is derived from three considerations, First, mental health consultation employs a mental health professional functioning as a consultant who may consult with several caregivers. These caregivers in turn have several clients. From a manpower standpoint, the effects of the mental health professional's work is spread over more persons than would be the case if each of these people had to be seen individually for treatment. Thus, one consideration in mental health consultation is an economy of manpower (Caplan, 1959, 1970).

A second consideration is the recognition of the fact that the majority of people turn to a natural caregiver, rather than to a mental health professional, in times of mental and emotional difficulty. Large-scale surveys, such as those conducted by Gurin, Veroff, and Feld (1960) and Elinson, Padilla, and Perkins (1967), have found that among people who admit they have had a problem for which they felt they should seek help, fewer than 20 percent of them indicated they would seek help from a mental health professional. This consideration is one of accessibility or relevance of help.

A third consideration, which derives in part from the second, is that persons in a natural care-giving role are more likely to be available, both psychologically and physically, during times of crisis, than is the mental health professional. Policemen, for example, have long been aware that they are a logical helping resource for many people, if for no other reason than that they are open for business twenty four hours a day. Liberman (1969) interviewed a sample of people who had used the police for help with a mental health problem, and found that these people regarded the police as a natural helping resource that they would use again in similar circumstances. Some caregivers, by virtue of their role, are simply in contact more often or for more extended periods of time with potential clients than are mental health professionals. Teachers would be one example of this category. Accordingly, this third consideration is a factor of availability or psychological presence.

The second and third considerations listed above are important to understanding the strategy of prevention in mental health consultation. Unlike direct treatment strategies, mental health consultation provides a basis for modifying the social-psychological environment represented by those in caregiver positions in such a way that the positive mental health of potential clients can be enhanced. It is assumed that the individual's relationships with key persons in his environment, including natural caregivers, have important implications for personality development. While these relationships are of continuous social importance, they are of special significance during periods of crisis in normal growth and development. At these times, this network of relationships forms what Caplan (1974) calls "support systems," which are instrumental in resolving crises in the direction of growth. It is in this way that mental health consultation can be conceptualized as having a primary preventive impact. However, mental health consultation does not necessarily have this type of preventive impact. The various possible preventive outcomes will be discussed further in the context of mental health consultation theory.

Types of Consultation

The concept of consultation has a long history with varied meanings. It may mean the calling in of a specialist to give an expert opinion, such as is done frequently in medicine, engineering, and other fields. Recently, education has been using the term consultant to refer to persons who are expert in particular areas of curriculum, such as mathematics, language arts, etc. A few years ago such persons were called supervisors. Consultation has other possible meanings that are important to distinguish from the sense in which the term is used here.

The term mental health consultation refers to a specific mental health method in which a consultant meets with a consultee or group of consultees for the purpose of resolving problems that the consultee has in performing some care-giving function for a group of clients. The scope of mental health consultation is limited to the work-role-related problems of the consultee, and the purpose of mental health consultation is to improve the care-giving functions of the consultees relevant to the mental health of their clients.

Mental health consultation differs from psychotherapy in that the consultant limits the scope of the relationship to work-role-related problems of the consultee, rather than broader and more historical concerns that might be the concern of a client or patient in psychotherapy. Moreover, in psychotherapy, there is an explicit request for personal help from the patient, and a contract is usually specified between the patient and therapist as to the work that will be done by each bearing on the patient's problem. In consultation the focus is on the client's, rather than on the consultee's, problem.

Consultation differs from administration in that the consultant does not provide leadership or policy in carrying out the work of the consultee. Consultation also differs from supervision in that the consultant, who is usually from a different professional field than that of the consultee, does not take responsibility for evaluating the consultee's job performance or generating expectations for the consultee's work in the consultee's field (Rhodes, 1960; Bindman, 1966). Accordingly, the consultee is free to initiate consultation on problems defined by the consultee, and to accept or reject the consultant's point of view. Finally, consultation differs from collaboration in that the consultant does not participate in carrying out action that may result from the consultation.

There are a variety of other types of consultation that have many similarities to mental health consultation. However, these types of consultation belong more specifically to other models that will be considered later in this book. We will limit our consideration here to the method of mental health consultation developed primarily by Gerald Caplan and his associates.

MENTAL HEALTH CONSULTATION THEORY

Caplan's approach to mental health consultation assumes that the consultant and consultee are both professionals who are interacting for the purpose of resolving some problem that the consultee presents. Implicit in his model is the assumption that the consultee is potentially capable of providing appropriate and effective service to the client, but is temporarily unable to do so for one of several reasons. It is clear from his writing that Caplan believes the most important aspect of the consultee's helping role is a close emotional relationship between consultee and client. As Caplan puts it:

> This type of consultation does not have the goal of increasing the consultee's knowledge about emotional life or mental health. It does have the goal of increasing his professional skill. Its one goal is to allow the

> consultee to make maximum use of his professional skill undisturbed and unhampered by the various unresolved problems in his own personality.
>
> The technique aims at maintaining or increasing the psychological closeness of the consultee and his client by helping the consultee to become more comfortable in this human relationship. (1959, p. 128)

Caplan further believes that the teaching of techniques tends to increase, rather than decrease, the emotional distance between consultee and client and conflicts with the goals he hopes to achieve in consultation. As we shall see, Caplan places considerable emphasis on attempting to reduce factors that interfere with adequate helping behavior on the part of the consultee.

Caplan recognizes a variety of kinds of consultation (1963). *Client-centered case consultation* involves the attempt to find a solution to dealing with a professional case. The focus is on the most effective means of helping the client. *Consultee-centered case consultation* refers to consultation in which the focus of attention is on the consultee's problems in trying to help a particular client, rather than on the client as such. This is a type of consultation to which Caplan has devoted the major part of his thinking on consultation, and it will receive more detailed examination momentarily. *Program-centered administrative consultation* is a type of consultation in which the focus is on some aspect of a program and involves resolving problems with or making recommendations for policies, planning, or conduct of specific programs. *Consultee-centered administrative consultation* again focuses on the consultee, or a group of consultees, in helping them to deal with problems they are having in the planning or conduct of a program of services. Notice that while the latter two types deal with administrative concerns, the consultant does not take an administrative role. The consultee-centered type of consultation focuses on specific problems that the consultee manifests in attempting to deal with a case or a program and is based on further theorizing that is important to understanding this model of consultation.

Consultee Problems

Caplan (1963, 1970) has identified four major consultee problems. These are (1) lack of knowledge, (2) lack of skill, (3) lack of confidence, and (4) lack of objectivity. For problems of lack of knowledge and skill, Caplan recommends that the consultant help the consultee to improve in these respective areas. However, he points out that it is important that the consultant understand the appropriate professional behavior and expectations for the consultee's own field and not try to turn the consultee into a mental health professional. When problems of this sort occur frequently, a staff development training program is a more efficient solution than is consultation. Problems of confidence should be handled by nonspecific ego support, according to Caplan.

The problem of objectivity is one to which Caplan has devoted considerable attention. His view is that such problems result from some conflict in the consultee's own past history, often of a kind similar to the problems of the client, which interferes with the consultee's ability to get close to the client and to be professionally helpful. Caplan designates such problems "theme interference."

In Caplan's terms, a theme for the consultee takes the form of a syllogism with an "initial category" linked to an "inevitable outcome" by the theme in the consultee's mind. Such a theme might take the following form:

> "This child comes from a broken home."
> (Initial category)
> "All children from broken homes become juvenile delinquents."
> (Theme)
> "Therefore, this child will become a juvenile delinquent."
> (Inevitable outcome)

One possible way of changing the consultee's perception of such a case might be to show the consultee that a particular client is an exception to the initial category. However, Caplan objects that such a procedure simply establishes this client as an exception and does nothing to reduce the theme. Instead, Caplan recommends that the consultant explore material related to the case in considerable detail with the consultee, interspersed with anecdotes and examples, for the purpose of helping the consultee discover evidence for exceptions to the inevitable outcome. In this way, he feels that the theme interference will be reduced.

However, aside from these technical considerations, an important question about consultation is the consultee's motivation for seeking out the consultant. As we shall see, this is a complex question. As with any help-seeking behavior, seeking out the consultant is affected by many factors. Caplan (1959, 1963) assumes that consultees seek consultation because they are in a state of crisis. This assumption allows the use of several of the other assumptions we noted before in discussing crisis intervention: increased openness to change, opportunities for growth, and increased accessibility to help. The person who is to be the consultee, however, must be aware of the availability and relevance of the consultant before seeking this resource during times of crisis. The importance of the consultant's developing a relationship with potential consultees is emphasized by Caplan in a process he calls "creating proximity" (1959). This process of spending time becoming acquainted with the consultee and the consultee's social system is also important in enabling the consultant to become familiar with the working patterns in the consultee's professional setting and developing hypotheses about appropriate helping behavior for persons in that field. This process also helps the consultant to avoid imposing solutions that might be relevant for a mental health professional but inappropriate for someone in the consultee's situation. It is further assumed that reduction of theme interference will have a carry-over effect to other clients with similar problems.

A number of Caplan's concepts have been tested. Benjamin (1967) examined the assumption that consultees in crisis are more receptive to consultation. Using a crisis group, defined by high emotionality and low confidence in coping with the situation, he found that they did not differ from a comparison group in receptivity to consultation. The crisis group was more receptive than those low in emotionality and low in confidence, but less receptive than those high in emotionality and high in confidence. Thus, his results provide partial support for the crisis assumption. Emotionality and confidence seem to be important separate factors in influencing receptivity to consultation, although both are a part of the crisis state.

Richman (1970) tested the existence of theme interference. He reasoned that if there were such a thing as a theme as a characteristic of individuals who might be in a consultee role, then such individuals should be consistent in picking out a certain class of behavior problem as being more serious than other kinds of problems in a forced-choice situation. He constructed a series of behavioral descriptions and paired them so that each description was presented once with every other description. His subjects, who were advanced undergraduate education majors, were asked to choose the more serious behavioral problem in each pair. His results supported the theme interference hypothesis.

Mann (1973) examined the effect of shared expectations on the consultation process. This is one aspect of the relationship between consultant and consultee that Caplan emphasizes, and it is importantly related to the consultant's providing information that is consonant with the consultee's work role. The results demonstrated that teacher consultees who reported that the consultant's behavior was consistent with their expectations also rated consultation as being more helpful and reported more positive changes in the children about whom they sought help than did teachers who saw the consultant's behavior as discrepant from their expectations.

Caplan (1970) presents some data on the effectiveness of the theme interference technique. Independent raters judged the change in objectivity of consultees from the beginning to the end of consultation. Both specific and nonspecific theme interference reduction techniques showed significantly more increases in objectivity, compared to unlinking (showing the client to be an exception to the initial category), education (communicating mental health information), support-reassurance, or where none of these was used.

EXAMPLES OF MENTAL HEALTH CONSULTATION

A number of varied mental health consultation projects have been conducted in which some effort was made to evaluate results. Many of these studies have used graduate students learning consultation as the consultants, and therefore it is difficult to say that any negative results reflect on the method itself. Cutler and McNeil (1966) and Pierce-Jones, Iscoe, and Cunningham (1968) employed student consultants in large-scale consultation projects with teachers in several different schools. Cutler and McNeil found changes in attitudes that were more favorable, while Pierce-Jones, Iscoe, and Cunningham found no significant differences in attitudes between teachers in schools that received consultation and those in control schools. In fact, in the latter study, teachers' attitudes in both consultation and control schools appeared to be somewhat less favorable from a mental health standpoint at the end of the project, a factor that suggests that some social or cultural influence may have been operating that wiped out any effect that consultation might have had.

In the Cutler and McNeil study, some positive changes, relative to control groups, were also found in the children of teachers who received consultation. Trione (1967) used school psychologists as consultants to teachers and found that teachers' attitudes improved and the students' achievement levels improved, relative to appropriate control groups. On the other hand, Berk (1971) attempted a complex analysis of teacher interaction with students in a consultation program and found no significant differences between before- and after-consultation conditions.

These studies using teachers as consultees present a number of conceptual and methodological difficulties. Besides those already mentioned concerning the training and experience of the consultants, it is not clear whether the instruments and observations employed are appropriate. Research projects of this type are necessarily set up to administer a common set of measures to all consultees—and sometimes to clients—involved in the overall project. Yet, as Caplan's model indicates, mental health consultation may have a number of different goals insofar as the consultee is concerned, depending upon the type of problem presented. For example, a study that employs teacher attitude measures necessarily assumes that attitudes are what consultation should seek to change. But some consultees may present problems of lack of knowledge or skill or confidence that might be improved by consultation and still not reflect in changes on attitude measures. More varied and complex instruments and data-collection procedures than have been employed typically would be required to identify changes according to the goals of particular consultation efforts. A similar difficulty affects trying to measure changes in children's behavior on the assumption that they should all change in the same way.

A further consideration is that, as Caplan's model assumes, one is dealing in these situations with consultees who, it must be assumed, are reasonably well-trained professionals in their fields to begin with. The improvements that might be obtained are limited by a "ceiling effect" such that the more competent the teacher-consultees, the less relative change can be demonstrated. This problem of weak effects has been discussed by Rossi (1969) in the general context of evaluating social programs. This is not to say that consultation has little effect; indeed, relatively small effects may make significant differences in the functioning of individual consultees and clients; rather, the point is that as the general level of social functioning improves, it is increasingly difficult to demonstrate changes using relatively gross or global measures.

For example, studies of consultation programs with policemen provide a different perspective on this problem. Caplan's model of theme interference reduction assumes that the consultee is a well-trained professional whose use of skills ordinarily associated with that profession is helpful to clients' mental health problems. In the case of policemen, however, very little, if any, of their training in the past has been concerned with dealing with mental health problems. Moreover, policemen are typically recruited from socioeconomic backgrounds in which sophistication about such problems is not common (Lipset, 1969). This is not to say that policemen are not, in some cases, capable of being helpful to people in difficulty. But those policemen who do develop such capabilities do so more as a result of individual experience than as a consequence of deliberate efforts to acquire the relevant knowledge and skills. Accordingly, one could not begin with the assumption that problems that policemen might present for consultation would be more the result of theme interference than they would be of a lack of training.

Bard and his co-workers (Bard, 1970; Bard, Zacker, and Rutter, 1972) designed a consultation and training program to assist policemen in intervening in family crisis situations. In addition to a structured training program, the policemen received individual consultation on a regular basis. The project demonstrated that the policemen became more effective in managing family crisis situations, that citizen attitudes toward the police improved, that the trained policemen sustained fewer injuries in such situations, and that they were better able to maintain their objectivity as a result of the project, despite the fact that measured policemen's attitudes did not change.

Mann and his associates (Mann, 1973) conducted a similar program with a police department, using training sessions and individual consultation, along with a series of interagency meetings involving policemen and representatives of a variety of social and mental health agencies. They found that policemen's behavior in handling family crises changed—from relying on legal solutions, such as referral to courts or attorneys, to more reliance on attempts to mediate disputes and make referrals to mental health agencies. They also found that persons referred actually followed through in seeking the service suggested. Similar to the findings of Bard *et al.*, there was no change in measured attitudes of policemen toward a variety of mental health issues.

These studies demonstrate that under certain conditions, attitude changes may not be necessary to improved functioning of consultees where knowledge and skill are significant needs. Mann suggested that these needs seemed to be preponderant among policemen compared to problems of objectivity, and that Caplan's list of problems might be usefully viewed as a hierarchy, so that problems of knowledge, skill, and confidence would be approached first in that order, and, when they were overcome, problems of objectivity might then comprise a larger proportion of the remaining need for improvement.

Mental health consultation is, relatively speaking, an infant technique with much more to be learned about its effectiveness. There are some promising beginning findings, the majority of which are limited to its effects on consultees, but there is relatively little known to date about its effects on clients and virtually nothing is known about its actual impact on prevention. Mental health consultation with caregivers whose clients are children, such as teachers, day-care workers, etc., has the promise of promoting primary prevention to the extent that the social environment of children is improved, sources of stress are reduced, and enhanced coping skills result from this process. Consultation with caregivers whose clients are adults, on the other hand, may have either primary or secondary preventive effects depending upon the situation of the client. Many of the family crisis situations in which policemen are involved, for example, can only be effectively resolved through early treatment and constitute secondary prevention. Other timely interventions by caregivers with adult clients who are not in need of mental health treatment could conceivably have primary preventive effects. However, much more thought, planning, effort, and research are needed before such effects can be demonstrated.

Typical Research

While the preceding review has mentioned a number of different research studies, our purpose here is to present a more systematic perspective on the role of research in the mental health model under consideration. Recall that at the beginning of this chapter some concepts from epidemiology were discussed. The focus of preventive efforts throughout this discussion has been on the reduction of incidence or prevalence rates of mental disorders. We turn now to more detailed consideration of how such estimates may be used in this model, and some of the problems associated with their use. We will consider epidemiological research in three contexts: as a search for leads to etiology of mental disorders; as attempts to establish base rates for mental disorders; and as a means of evaluating programs.

The implications of epidemiological research on possible leads to etiology are most important in that they provide directions for treatment and control of mental disorders. The history of epidemiology shows us that it is not necessary for research to identify the precise or only "cause" of a condition in order for intervention to be successful. As Bloom (1965) has pointed out, it was not necessary even to have a correct etiological theory for pre-germ-theory epidemiologists to discover the linkage between improper environmental sanitation and a number of dread diseases, and to successfully reduce the rates of such diseases by improving sanitation and water purity. Some such elementary observations are necessary in order to begin to construct at least tentative theories. However, application of the epidemiological analogy to mental disorders presents a number of problems.

For example, we have already discussed the limited usefulness of epidemiological studies based on treated cases. Such factors as the availability of treatment services, attitudes toward the use of treatment, and attitudes toward the recognition of such disorders as treatable all may introduce systematic biases into the use of treated cases as an estimate of the true distribution of cases in the population. Nevertheless, the great majority of such research has relied upon studies of treated incidence and prevalence because the data are much more readily obtainable and the problem of defining what constitutes a case is reduced considerably.

Notable among such studies are those of Faris and Dunham (1939) and Hollingshead and Redlich (1958). The former found a concentration of first admissions of hospitalized psychoses, except manic-depressive psychosis, in the central core of Chicago and a decrease in the rate as one went outward from the center. These findings were subsequently associated with poverty, social disorganization, poor housing, and a number of presumably stressful conditions. The latter surveyed all cases in treatment in New Haven, Connecticut, and found that the highest rates of psychosis were associated with lower-class status, while the highest rates of neurosis were associated with middle-class status.

These studies have been variously interpreted to indicate (1) that psychoses are the result of increased stresses in lower social classes (social causation); (2) that psychoses are found in lower social strata because such persons "drift" downward in the social structure, but that such conditions may be caused by some other, possibly genetic, factor (social selection); and (3) that the differences in social class distribution are associated with differing access to treatment, so that (a) lower-class persons are more likely to have to rely on hospitalization where they receive minimal treatment; and (b) lower-class persons are more likely to be diagnosed as psychotic because of their behavior and life-style, while middle-class patients are more likely to be diagnosed as neurotic and treated as outpatients. Each of these explanations may be true to some extent without being mutually exclusive of each other, but it is really not possible to make meaningful inferences about etiology using treated cases unless one makes the difficult assumption that the same factors that contribute to mental illness also influence who will seek or receive treatment.

However, studies of true rates are considerably more difficult and expensive to conduct, and they have their own kinds of problems. Dohrenwend and Dohrenwend (1969, 1972) examined forty four studies of true prevalence. These studies employed various attempts to count untreated as well as treated cases. Some studies used records and/or informants, some used direct interviews with subjects, and some used a combination of these methods. Some studies have included all residents of a particular geographic area, and some have used a representative sample of one thousand or more persons. One of the most ambitious of these studies, the Midtown Manhattan Study, employed questionnaires and psychiatric interviews of subjects (Srole, Langner, Michael, Opler, and Rennie, 1962). From this research, a twenty two-item questionnaire that effectively discriminated between patients and "well" subjects was developed, which has since been employed in several subsequent studies.

The Dohrenwends (1972) discuss some of the problems with this type of research in the context of the variations in rates—from less than 1 percent to more than 60 percent—that are found in these studies. Reviewing a number of factors, including time periods studied and type of geographical area, they find that the age range studied and the definition of what constitutes a case are the largest contributors to this variability. They note that more recent studies tend to find higher rates and to employ more extensive definitions of case criteria.

As to substance, of the various demographic variables examined in these studies, including age, sex, race, and socioeconomic status, only the latter is consistently related to prevalence rates. They find no consistent relationship between neurosis and social class, but schizophrenia and personality disorders consistently have the highest rates in the lowest stratum of society.

The Dohrenwends (1969) designed a study to test the social causation and social selection argument. They employed the twenty two-item Midtown scale and matched interviewers, who were neither psychiatrists nor clinical psychologists, with subjects in ethnicity to minimize the tendency to cross-ethnic defensiveness, which has been noted in other studies. They argued that if one controls for income and education—two typical indices of social class—and then compares relatively advantaged groups, such as Jewish and Irish, with relatively disadvantaged groups, blacks and Puerto Ricans, then higher rates among the disadvantaged groups could not be evidence of social selection, but could be interpreted as a result of increased deprivation and could address the causation-selection issue.

In a sample of over sixteen hundred subjects they found that for comparable levels of education the disadvantaged groups had lower levels of income than the advantaged groups, thus justifying the use of the term. Their results showed a higher rate of symptoms for all ethnic groups at lower income levels than at higher income levels, and a higher rate for Puerto Ricans than for the advantaged groups, but not for blacks compared to advantaged groups. Thus, the results on the crucial selection versus causation question are equivocal. Using other data, the Dohrenwends shed additional light on these findings. They note a tendency for ethnic groups to differ in their response set to these questions, such that Puerto Ricans tend to say yes (yea-saying) more readily to some items and Irish tend to say no (nay-saying) to some items. Thus, in groups of psychiatric patients matched for types of disorders, the Puerto Ricans still obtained higher symptom scores. This raises the question of the meaning of the symptom scores employed in these studies in determining what constitutes a case.

The Dohrenwends point out that the symptom scores tend to increase with stressful situations and to decrease with positive events. Citing the point noted earlier in this chapter concerning crisis situations, they emphasize the need to distinguish between transient symptoms as a response to situational stress and symptoms representative of continuing disorder. Though they show in their study that lower-class and black groups are generally subject to more frequent and more severe stress than middle-class and white groups, they argue that whether the result of these effects is transient or continuing makes an important difference in the kind of intervention one considers. If the effects result in genuine disorders of a relatively enduring kind, then treatment for the specific disorder is indicated. If the result is a relatively transient disruption of functioning, then nonspecific preventive interventions are in order. The research problem is thus clearly defined, but the type of study they envision has yet to be conducted. One can probably safely assume, from the studies on transient situational disturbances reviewed previously, that a sizable proportion of "cases" would be responsive to such preventive interventions, whether one favors social causation or social selection as the explanation of the epidemiological findings.

The question of how much of total prevalence rates might be apportioned into the categories of transient and disordered cases is also important in establishing base rates in evaluating the effects of preventive programs. Recall that the concept of prevalence is composed of both incidence and duration. If we are interested in primary prevention, then presumably we must know not only what is a case, but also when a case becomes a case, in order to know the incidence rate. Yet studies of true incidence rates are virtually impossible to conduct. The Dohrenwends found only one such published study, conducted in Sweden, which has a far more elaborate system of social record keeping than is likely to be tolerated in this country. We are left, then, with the problem of very likely being able at best to obtain data on prevalence.

However, it may be possible under some conditions to infer changes in incidence from changes in prevalence rates, since the former are contained in the latter. If we recall that prevalence rates are composed of incidence and duration, it would be possible to infer changes in incidence if one knew the prevalence rate and the changes that occur in existing cases as to duration. Besides clarifying the ambiguities as to transient and more enduring disorders, which the Dohrenwends have defined, a number of other considerations indicate that a one-time collection of data is of no value in establishing base rates from which to judge the effectiveness of various interventions, nor is mere before-and-after measurement adequate to make such assessments.

While a number of known factors may be controlled in designing such studies, there are likely to be numerous unknown factors that cannot be controlled in this kind of research. Any degree of cyclic trends in prevalence rates, for example, would prevent the valid inference that a before-and-after change was the result of the intervention. Campbell (1969) has shown how erroneous inferences about the effects of an intervention can be drawn from before-and-after measurements on data that have a cyclical nature. After a record high number of traffic fatalities in Connecticut in 1955 a severe enforcement program against speeding was instituted. The following year the number of fatalities declined. The difficulty in interpreting this data is that in previous years the number of traffic deaths had risen and fallen in alternate years with no change in the enforcement procedure. Therefore, was the change in fatalities following the enforcement program a result of the program or merely the usual fluctuation in the figures? Campbell shows how an extended time series design can help to answer this question, in this case by showing that fatalities continued to decline in subsequent years. It is obvious that this particular example suffers also from the use of numbers of deaths, rather than a rate of deaths as a function of the number of drivers or the number of miles driven, which could artificially influence the numbers.

The important point for establishing base rates and evaluating the effects of programs is that time series designs substantially increase the kinds of inferences that can be made about the effects of interventions, as well as to increase the confidence that can be placed in such inferences. According to this type of design, regular periodic true prevalence studies would be conducted on the population in question. Additional studies on the effects of various treatment programs, along with data on spontaneous recovery rates, could be used to estimate changes that could be expected to occur in prevalence rates as a function of changes in duration. Any remaining changes in the prevalence rate over and above those that occur from normal fluctuations in the rates over time would be attributed to changes in incidence.

A second approach to supplement this type of periodic monitoring of prevalence would be a longitudinal study of specific populations, with appropriately matched control groups, that are the recipients of preventive interventions. Some approaches to this type of research were mentioned in the section on crisis intervention. Similar, more restricted monitoring processes could be established for special high-risk populations.

Glidewell (1969) has demonstrated that such longitudinal research with relatively small samples is subject to a number of limitations, but can be conducted satisfactorily if one does not wish to ask too many questions of the data. A particular difficulty in such studies is the loss of subjects over time as a result of geographical mobility, withdrawal from the program, etc. Some of these difficulties could be compensated for to some extent if such studies were conducted in the context of large-scale periodic monitoring processes.

Longitudinal research of this type presents a number of practical problems, as well. The fact is that few such studies have been conducted because of the expense involved, the difficulty of obtaining long-term funding commitments, and the problems of managing changes-in-process among personnel, research procedures, and interventions. The present prospect that such studies will be conducted on anything like the systematic basis outlined here is extremely slim also. There is little evidence to suggest that service delivery systems—for the most part community mental health centers—are in the least bit interested in or able to support such efforts with the commitments to service and shortage of funds that they face already. The orientation of the majority of practitioners in the field is not toward research, and a specific set of personnel charged with responsibility for such studies and free of competing demands would be required to manage such a task. The absence of such an effort, however, severely limits the meaningfulness of attempts to evaluate mental health interventions. This is, of course, not a new state of affairs in mental health. Few studies of the effectiveness of treatment programs have been conducted as a regular part of traditional clinical treatment programs. One critical difference, however, is that treatment programs have been based, at least indirectly, on a fee-for-service basis where it was possible to document the number of patients served, if not the effectiveness of the service. It is considerably more difficult to justify indirect and preventive services on this basis, and, since it is also harder to convince people to support preventive programs in general, the absence of data on effectiveness of such programs is a significant problem.

Typical Settings

The typical setting envisioned for the mental health model is the community mental health center. However, a number of other settings may conduct some or all of the elements of the mental health model. In recent years, for example, a number of crisis intervention services have developed in hospitals, family service agencies, and volunteer telephone counseling services. Nevertheless, the community mental health center remains the most likely and promising setting for this model. How close does the community mental health center come to fulfilling this promise?

One must begin to answer this question with the understanding that it asks not about the performance of the community mental health center in general, but about the development of the mental health model of community psychology in the community mental health center. Despite the advocacy of secondary prevention in the report of the Joint Commission on Mental Illness (1960), the preponderant mode of practice has been the delivery of traditional clinical services in most mental health centers. That element of the model that has probably been utilized most often is crisis intervention. As for consultation, a survey of a representative sample of community mental health centers had this to say: "Consultation appeared to be the least understood of the essential services, both in terms of what it is supposed to consist of and what it is supposed to accomplish" (Glasscote, Sussex, Cumming, and Smith, 1969, p. 27). They found that staff in seven of the eight centers were doing some consultation, primarily of a case variety, and either showed little interest or faith in primary prevention or, in the case of the one center where staff expressed an interest in primary prevention, were constrained from spending time on it by the program director. At the same time, the agencies with which these centers worked, such as schools and courts, expressed a preference for treatment rather than consultation.

This limitation can in many ways be seen as a failure of education on several levels. As community mental health centers were implemented, there were few professionals trained in the mental health model and many trained in the traditional clinical model. In turn, these persons were not in a position to educate the community about something they neither understood nor believed in, and consequently community requests continued to be for more of the same, and so on in a self-perpetuating cycle. That community attitudes are necessarily so oriented can be discounted by the observation that in communities where preventive programs have been implemented, persons in such agencies can be educated toward preventive goals. Accordingly, as much of this limitation on implementation can probably be laid to the shortage of adequately trained manpower as to the limitations in the setting itself. This is, of course, a question that cannot be answered until more trained personnel arrive on the scene. We must also note with seriousness the comment cited above that the program director limited the efforts of the staff in one center to engage in primary prevention activities. This suggests that newly trained personnel must not only arrive, but must in some degree occupy positions of leadership.

Another important question to ask of a setting is its source of funding. As a precedent for federal funding of local mental health activities, the federal legislation and associated allocation of funds was indeed a bold new step. How close has this hope come to being realized? We noted in Chapter 1 that of the two thousand anticipated community mental health centers, less than five hundred were in operation by 1971. Is this the result of communities not wanting such facilities in the face of federal funds? Perhaps so in part, but a look at the actual federal funding performance provides a different perspective.

The process of making funds available through the federal government consists of three steps. Expenditures must first be authorized by Congress, and then appropriated by Congress, and finally the moneys appropriated must be apportioned among federal agencies by the executive branch. Glasscote, Sussex, Cumming, and Smith (1969) reported that of $30 million authorized by Congress for community mental health centers in 1968, only $22 million were actually appropriated and only $15 million were made available to the National Institute of Mental Health by the executive branch through apportionment. This total is slightly less than the state of Washington spent in that year to run its three state mental hospitals. They found that from 1964 to 1968 the amount spent for construction and staffing of centers was $232 million, which is approximately what was required to run the New York State Department of Mental Hygiene for five months. Finally, they estimated that if all the funds authorized for the eleven-year period of 1964 through 1974 were made available (they weren't) the total of $580 million is about what it costs to run the state mental hospitals of New York, California, Massachusetts, Pennsylvania, and Illinois for one year. If one added the total state and local matching funds that were to be added to these federal funds in that period, the total expenditure would still be less than the expenses of public mental hospitals for a one-year period in 1969.

Thus, federal funding has fallen far short of its original mark, and the strategy that community mental health centers could be funded eventually from state and local sources out of the savings of keeping people out of the state hospitals has failed for lack of implementation rather than its correctness. This strategy, incidentally, has understandably never been embraced enthusiastically by state mental hospital personnel who, besides wanting to maintain their employment, have never been adequately funded either in most states. Accordingly, the system that exists currently is financially a dual system with piecemeal expenditures in both areas—hardly the sort of plan that was envisioned originally.

One consequence of this shortcoming in funding is that community mental health centers have been forced to rely increasingly on fees-for-service from patients, which tends to encourage a return to the traditional clinical model and provides diminishing support and incentive for programs of prevention. The community mental health center remains the major feasible setting for such programs, nevertheless, but considerably more progress must occur before that potentiality will be realized.

Assessment of the Model

In reviewing the model in light of the criteria presented in Chapter 3, we find that it conceptualizes community processes in terms of personal (individual) functioning and interpersonal relationships. The community is conceptualized primarily as a geographical area in which the model is concerned with processes of mental health and illness of individuals. It assumes that individuals have tendencies toward health, positive development, and competence, and that the community may serve to hinder or promote those tendencies. Key significance in the community is assigned to those in the role of caregiver and to social support. These assumptions are subject to empirical test, but the model has not developed to the point that these assumptions have been tested to date.

The mental health model assumes some global values that are very likely to be shared in the community: it is better to be out of the hospital than in it; it is better to be well than ill. Beyond this, however, the critical value assumptions have to do with a commitment to prevention. To what extent is prevention a shared value and how does one develop a consensus within the community on this value? The model itself tends to assume that prevention is a shared value, but says nothing about a process for reaching consensus. It is well to recall that the community mental health center movement emanated from the deliberations of national commissions and federal legislation, and provisions were made for local and state participation and planning in the development of centers, but the model itself says nothing about these processes. Thus, the people interested in developing such a program must look elsewhere for guidance on its implementation.

The model assumes that community change processes are a

function of rational decision making, based largely on economic considerations. Thus, as it is discovered that primary and secondary prevention are more economical, the community will change from its reliance on hospitals and extended treatment. This assumption makes two serious omissions. First, it overlooks the political significance of existing patterns of mental health care in the community, the need satisfactions (personal as well as economical) enmeshed in that system, and the expectations that community members have toward what is a significant institution in the community. On the other hand, the original plan for funding such centers only for five years probably placed too much significance on the political process in the Congress, inasmuch as legislation involving longer periods might have been too difficult to pass, and it undervalues the realities of how long it takes for changes in community institutions to occur. As one looks at the current development of settings for this model, this has been a serious deficiency in planning.

On a more general level, nothing in the model addresses changes in the form of community processes themselves. This assumption of stability is inherent in the emphasis on changes in the individual as a consequence of interpersonal processes. The closest one comes to a recognition of social change is the notion of crisis, although crises are not necessarily of this sort; that is, they are defined as personal crises subjectively experienced. Similarly, the model makes no assumptions about unanticipated secondary consequences of intervention, such as the reactions appearing in some places concerning the early release into the community of hospital patients.

Although there are provisions for citizen participation in the conception of mental health centers, again nothing in the mental health model itself deals with this issue. The recognition of the importance of the caregiver role, and the coordinate relationship between consultants and caregivers that is emphasized in mental health consultation, is a limited form of participation, and certainly one in which shared expectations are important, but the sense of participation does not extend beyond this. The respect accorded to the integrity and competence of other professions in mental health consultation theory seems to imply a reciprocal respect for the integrity and competence of the mental health profession, yet the issue of professional prerogatives and community control (Roman, 1969; Schiff, 1972) has surfaced in several communities and is one on which the model is silent.

As already indicated in the section on research, the model makes provision for accountability to the community, but the potential system of demonstrating preventive impacts has not been established. Here we must recognize that the model itself provides potentially for accountability—in fact, it may depend upon it—but the community is not accustomed to either asking for or supporting an adequate accountability system.

Finally, we may ask what provision the model makes for its own life cycle and for the evolution of programs. On the one hand, it is tempting to say that the model is too young to have a sense of history; yet its clinical ancestors have such a history of change. One factor that clearly limits this perspective is the tendency in the model to assume stability of community processes and to emphasize change in individuals. Even if it were conceivable that prevention could eliminate the need for treatment facilities, what new needs might be generated? It is often expressed as a hope that an increase in the positive mental health of individual community members, according to the criteria proposed by several writers, would result in improvements in community life. There is no question that the reduction of social stress, particularly in high-risk environments, and the improvement of self-respect, coping skills, and consideration for others among individuals would make for a more pleasant way of life in many respects. If such goals are attainable, then what would community life be like at that point? Would it mean more of what we already have for everyone? Would individual and social needs change in any way? Would expectations toward social and economic systems change? These are questions that are not asked in this model.

The tendency to focus on individual history and to give less attention to social history is a serious limitation of the mental health model as a model in and of the community. It has failed to anticipate social and political community processes, has not provided sufficiently for the generation of an adequate knowledge and training base, and has not addressed the question of community change at the social level.

In summary, the mental health model has important contributions to make for the individual development of members of the community, but it lacks an adequate conception of the community itself, which has led to a number of difficulties in its further development. These are issues that are being discussed by persons associated with this model, as well as by others. The answers, however, will have to be found in some other model that can provide the conception of the community that is lacking in the mental health model.

References

ANTHONY, E. J. Primary prevention with school children. In H. H. Barten and L. Bellak (Eds.), *Progress in Community Mental Health*, vol. 2. New York: Grune & Stratton, 1972, 131–158.

BARD, M. *Training Police as Specialists in Family Crisis Intervention.* Washington, D.C.: U. S. Department of Justice, 1970.

BARD, M., ZACKER, J., AND RUTTER, E. Police family crisis intervention and conflict management: An action research analysis. Mimeographed report submitted to the U.S. Department of Justice, 1972.

BENJAMIN, C. Consultee receptivity to consultation as a function of crisis. Unpublished doctoral dissertation. University of Texas, Austin, 1967.

BERGER, I. Bereavement and the acceptance of professional service. *Community Mental Health Journal*, 1969, *5*, 487–495.

BERK, M. Effects of mental health consultation on teacher-child interaction. Unpublished doctoral dissertation, University of Texas, Austin, 1971.

BINDMAN, A. J. The clinical psychologist as a mental health consultant. In L. E. Abt and B. F. Riess (Eds.), *Progress in Clinical Psychology.* New York: Grune & Stratton, 1966, 78–106.

BLOOM, B. The "medical model," miasma theory, and community mental health. *Community Mental Health Journal*, 1965, *1*, 333–338.

BLOOM, B. The evaluation of primary prevention programs. In L. M. Roberts, N. S. Greenfield, and M. H. Miller (Eds.), *Comprehensive Mental Health: The Challenge of Evaluation.* Madison: University of Wisconsin Press, 1968.

CAMPBELL, D. T. Reforms as experiments. *American Psychologist*, 1969, *24*, 409–429.

CAPLAN, G. The role of the social worker in preventive psychiatry. *Medical Social Work*, 1955, *4*.

CAPLAN, G. Mental health consultation in preventive psychiatry. *Boletin do Institute Antonio Ametio da Costa Ferreira*, 1958, *17*, 480.

CAPLAN, G. *Concepts of Mental Health and Consultation.* Washington, D.C.: U.S. Children's Bureau, 1959.

CAPLAN, G. Types of mental health consultation. *American Journal of Orthopsychiatry*, 1963, *33*, 470–481.

CAPLAN, G. *Principles of Preventive Psychiatry.* New York: Basic Books, 1964.

CAPLAN, G. *The Theory and Practice of Mental Health Consultation.* New York: Basic Books, 1970.

CAPLAN, G. *Support Systems and Mental Health.* New York: Basic Books, 1974.

CUTLER, R. L., AND MCNEIL, E. B. Mental health consultation in schools: A research analysis. Department of Psychology, University of Michigan, 1966.

DOHRENWEND, B., AND DOHRENWEND, B. *Social Status and Psychological Disorder.* New York: Wiley, 1969.

DOHRENWEND, B., AND DOHRENWEND, B., Psychiatric epidemiology: An analysis of "true prevalence" studies. In S. Golann and C. Eisdorfer (Eds.), *Handbook of Community Mental Health.* New York: Appleton-Century-Crofts, 1972, 283–302.

DUBOIS, R. J. *An Outsider's View of Action for Mental Health.* National Association for Mental Health, Miami, 1961.

EISENBERG, L., AND GRUENBERG, E. M. The current status of secondary prevention in child psychiatry. *American Journal of Orthopsychiatry,* 1961, *31,* 355–367.

ELINSON, J., PADILLA, E., AND PERKINS, M. *Public Image of Mental Health Services.* New York: Mental Health Materials Center, 1967.

ERIKSON, E. Growth and crisis of the healthy personality. In C. Kluckhohn, H. A. Murray, and D. M. Schneider (Eds.), *Personality in Nature, Society, and Culture.* 2nd ed. New York: Knopf, 1953.

FARIS, R. E. L., AND DUNHAM, H. W. *Mental Disorders in Urban Areas.* Chicago: University of Chicago Press, 1939.

GLASSCOTE, R. M., SUSSEX, J. N., CUMMING, E., AND SMITH, L. H. *The Community Mental Health Center: An Interim Appraisal.* Washington, D.C.: Joint Information Service, 1969.

GLIDEWELL, J. Research problems in community psychology. In A. J. Bindman and A. D. Spiegel (Eds.), *Perspectives in Community Mental Health.* Chicago: Aldine, 1969, 669–682.

GURIN, G., VEROFF, J., AND FELD, S. *Americans View Their Mental Health.* New York: Basic Books, 1960.

HALPERN, H. Crisis theory: A definitional study. *Community Mental Health Journal,* 1973, *9,* 342–349.

HOBBS, N. Mental health's third revolution. *American Journal of Orthopsychiatry,* 1964, *34,* 822–833.

HOLLINGSHEAD, A. B., AND REDLICH, F. C. *Social Class and Mental Illness.* New York: Wiley, 1958.

JACOBSON, G. F., WILNER, D. M., MORLEY, W. E., SCHNEIDER, S., STRICKLER, M., AND SOMMER, G. J. The scope and practice of an early access brief treatment psychiatric center. *American Journal of Psychiatry,* 1965, *121,* 1176–1182.

JAHODA, M. *Current Concepts of Positive Mental Health.* New York: Basic Books, 1958.

JOINT COMMISSION ON MENTAL ILLNESS AND HEALTH. *Action for Mental Health.* New York: Basic Books, 1961.

JOINT COMMISSION ON MENTAL HEALTH OF CHILDREN. *Crisis in Child Mental Health.* New York: Harper & Row, 1969, p. 398.

KARDINER, A., AND SPIEGEL, H. *War Stress and Neurotic Illness.* New York: Hoeber, 1947.

LANGSLEY, D. G., AND KAPLAN, D. M. *The Treatment of Families in Crisis.* New York: Grune & Stratton, 1968.

LEWIS, W. W. Continuity and intervention in emotional disturbance: A review. *Exceptional Children*, 1965, *31*, 445–465.

LIBERMAN, R. Police as a community mental health resource. *Community Mental Health Journal*, 1969, *5*, 111–120.

LINDEMANN, E. Symptomatology and management of acute grief. *American Journal of Psychiatry*, 1944, *101*, 141–148.

LIPSET, S. M. Why cops hate liberals—and vice versa. *Atlantic Monthly*, 1969, *233*, no. 3., 76–83.

MANN, P. A. *Psychological Consultation with a Police Department: A Demonstration of Cooperative Training in Mental Health.* Springfield, Ill.: Charles C. Thomas, 1973.

MANN, P. A. Student consultants: Evaluations by consultees. *American Journal of Community Psychology*, 1973, *1*, 182–193.

MCGEE, T. F. Some basic considerations in crisis intervention. *Community Mental Health Journal*, 1968, *4*, 319–325.

MICHAEL, C. M., MORRIS, D. P., AND SOROKER, E. Follow-up studies of shy, withdrawn children: II. Relative incidence of schizophrenia. *American Journal of Orthopsychiatry*, 1957, *27*, 331–337.

MILLER, K., AND ISCOE, I. The concept of crisis: Current status and mental health implications. *Human Organization*, 1963, *22*, 195–201.

NEWBROUGH, J. R. Community mental health: A movement in search of a theory. In *Community Mental Health: Individual Adjustment or Social Planning.* Bethesda, Md.: National Institute of Mental Health, 1964.

O'NEAL, P., AND ROBINS, L. N. The relation of childhood behavior problems to adult psychiatric status: A thirty year follow-up of 150 subjects. *American Journal of Psychiatry*, 1958, *114*, 961–969.

PHILLIPS, E. L. Parent-child psychotherapy: A follow-up study comparing two techniques. *Journal of Psychology*, 1960, *49*, 195–202.

PHILLIPS, E. L., AND JOHNSON, M. Theoretical and practical aspects of short-term parent-child psychotherapy. *Psychiatry*, 1954, *17*, 267–275.

PHILLIPS, L. The competence criterion for mental health programs. *Community Mental Health Journal*, 1967, *3*, 73–76.

PIERCE-JONES, J., ISCOE, I., AND CUNNINGHAM, G. Child behavior consultation in elementary schools: A demonstration and research program. University of Texas, Austin, 1968.

PLOG, S. C. Urbanization, psychological disorders, and the heritage of social psychiatry. In S. C. Plog and R. B. Edgerton (Eds.), *Changing Perspectives in Mental Illness.* New York: Holt, Rinehart & Winston, 1969, 288–312.

RAPOPORT, L. The state of crisis: Some theoretical considerations. *The Social Service Review*, 1962, *36*, 211–217.

RAUSH, H. L., AND RAUSH, C. L. *The Half-way House Movement: A Search for Sanity.* New York: Appleton-Century-Crofts, 1968.

RICHMAN, B. A test of the theme interference hypothesis. Unpublished doctoral dissertation, University of Texas, Austin, 1970.

RHODES, W. C. Training in community mental health consultation in the schools. Chicago: American Psychological Association, 1960.

ROMAN, M., AND SCHMAIS, A. Consumer participation and control: A conceptual overview. In H. H. Barten and L. Bellak (Eds.), *Progress in Community Mental Health*, vol. 2. New York: Grune & Stratton, 1972, 63–84.

ROSSI, P. H. Practice, method, and theory in evaluating social-action programs. In P. Cook (Ed.), *Community Psychology and Community Mental Health.* San Francisco: Holden-Day, 1970, 213–227.

SANFORD, N. The findings of the commission on psychology. *Annals of the New York Academy of Science*, 1955, *63*, 341–364.

SANFORD, N. Is the concept of prevention necessary or useful? In S. E. Golann and C. Eisdorfer (Eds.), *Handbook of Community Mental Health.* New York: Appleton-Century-Crofts, 1972, 461–471.

SARBIN, T. R. Notes on the transformation of social identity. In L. M. Roberts, N. S. Greenfield, and M. H. Miller (Eds.), *Comprehensive Mental Health: The Challenge of Evaluation.* Madison: University of Wisconsin Press, 1968, 97–116.

SARBIN, T. R. The scientific status of the mental illness metaphor. In S. C. Plog and R. B. Edgerton (Eds.), *Changing Perspectives in Mental Illness.* New York: Holt, Rinehart & Winston, 1969, 9–31.

SCHIFF, S. K. Free inquiry and the enduring commitment: The Woodlawn Mental Health Center 1963–1970. In S. E. Golann and C. Eisdorfer (Eds.), *Handbook of Community Mental Health.* New York: Appleton-Century-Crofts, 1972, 755–778.

SINDBERG, R. M. A fifteen-year follow-up study of community guidance clinic clients. *Community Mental Health Journal*, 1970, *6*, 319–324.

SMITH, M. B. Optima of mental health. *Psychiatry*, 1950, *13*, 503–510.

SMITH M. B. Research strategies toward a conception of positive mental health. *American Psychologist*, 1959, *14*, 673–681.

SMITH, M. B. Mental health reconsidered: A special case of the problem of values in psychology. *American Psychologist*, 1961, *16*, 299–306.

SROLE, L. LANGNER, T., MICHAEL, S., OPLER, M., AND RENNIE, T. *Mental Health in Metropolis: The Midtown Manhattan Study*. New York: McGraw-Hill, 1962.

SZASZ, T. *The Myth of Mental Illness*. New York: Hoeber-Harper, 1961.

TRIONE, V. The school psychologist, teacher change, and fourth grade reading achievement. *California Journal of Educational Research*, 1967, *18*, 194–200.

WHITE, R. W. *Lives in Progress*. New York: Dryden, 1952.

5. The Organizational Model

The study of the group and the relationship of individuals to groups has been the focus of much of social psychology. In 1946 a group of psychologists and educators met at New Britain Teachers College in Connecticut to plan a program of group discussion as a means of educating people about community and social relations. The leaders of this group were Kurt Lewin, Ronald Lippitt, Kenneth Benne, and Leland Bradford.

Lewin was a native German who was prominent in the field of Gestalt psychology.* He was especially interested in the application of this form of psychology to problems of personality and social issues, rather than its application to problems of perception, as were most Gestalt psychologists. He had conducted major and significant research on personality and on social problems while at the Child Welfare Research Station at the University of Iowa. He had founded and was head of the Research Center for Group Dynamics at the Massachusetts Institute of Technology.

Lippitt had been a student of Lewin at Iowa, and together with Ralph White they conducted a major social experiment on the effects of leadership styles on social climates in groups. In what was to become a well-known study, they demonstrated that democratic leadership produced greater participation and satisfaction among groups of boys than did either a *laissez faire* or an autocratic form of leadership (Lewin, Lippitt, and White, 1939).

*An interesting and detailed biography of Lewin is presented in Alfred F. Marrow's *The Practical Theorist* (New York: Basic Books, 1969).

Benne was an academician interested in philosophy of education, and especially in the pragmatic philosophy of John Dewey. Bradford, an educator, was concerned with problems of adult education and had extensive experience during World War II in mobilizing such programs for large numbers of people employed in various government agencies.

These men had in common several things that were important in influencing the work they would do. They had a strong belief in democracy as a human process and ideology. They were committed to a study of the group and group processes. And they believed in the possibilities of change and the importance of experience and learning in the change process. Moreover, they believed that a psychological study of these factors in combination was an important contribution for society and for the survival of mankind. It should be remembered that this meeting took place virtually in the shadow of World War II and the atomic bomb. One can only imagine the sense of urgency and importance that characterized their work. Yet they were also committed to the patient and careful analysis of experimental approaches to the problem of the scientist.

A chance event during these meetings led to what was to become a major part of the technique that evolved out of these initial sessions. The original format of the group sessions was to be the conduct of group discussions during the daytime, and a review and analysis of the processes in the groups by the staff each evening. Some of the participants asked to sit in on one of these review sessions, which provided them with an opportunity to confront feedback about themselves and to clarify the observers' inferences with descriptions of their own feelings and intentions (Back, 1972). Thereafter, this episode was made a part of the process, providing a comparison of intention with observation, of feeling with behavior.

The total process of learning was originally referred to as basic skills training (BST), of which what was to become known as the "T-group" was one part. It provided participants with an opportunity to learn about the impressions they created on others in a group setting, as opposed to the impressions they thought they were creating, as well as to learn about the psychological processes of group functioning (Bradford, Gibb, and Benne, 1964).

Central to this learning process is the concept that group members are "defensive" about the revelation of their true feelings to others in the group, and, as a consequence, the process of communicating real meanings to each other becomes distorted.

Starting in 1947, the laboratory training sessions were held each year in Bethel, Maine. Out of these experiences emerged the National Training Laboratory, based primarily on the principle of experiential learning through the T-group method. Originally, these sessions were conceived as a joint work effort of a trainer and a research team that made observations of group process. During the 1950s the group method became more consolidated and the research participants gradually moved toward more academic and theoretical pursuits, while the National Training Laboratories maintained the applied orientation.

One of many factors that led to this division of research and practice was the fact that the T-group was coming to have a life of its own, and participants came as often to learn the method or to achieve some therapeutic result (a goal not endorsed by the NTL leaders) as to learn about group process. No longer concerned with community and social problems as such, the T-group, sometimes called "sensitivity training," became a marketable commodity that was sought out increasingly by business organizations, church groups, and individuals.

The emphasis on the "here-and-now" experience in the group came to be shared by a number of new and sometimes esoteric forms of sensitivity, encounter, and personal development groups that were concerned with individual, rather than group, results. Back (1972) reviewed the evolution of these developments into what became a form of social movement, in which the "here-and-now" became an end in itself. Back feels that the extreme forms of this movement are largely an anti-intellectual movement in which feeling is valued more than thinking, and which promotes preoccupation with self and diminished concern with social problems. That these developments are not what the originators of the National Training Laboratory process had in mind is quite clear, not only from the standpoint of goals, but also from the standpoint of methods. As Harold Leavitt (1971), who was at MIT during the beginnings of the National Training Laboratory, said: "The original idea was that people should understand their feelings so that they would be able to think better, not that feeling is more important than thinking. To assume the latter implies that the natural state of man is infancy."

A problem that was recognized early with the laboratory training method was the carry-over of the training to the "back home" situation. Some attempts were made to handle this problem by including several persons from the same organization in groups, which were known as "family groups." However, the use of this training approach also became more frequently a part of the work of consultants attempting to solve organizational problems in what is now known as organizational development (O.D.).

At the same time as these developments were occurring, the Tavistock Institute in England was also developing a psychological approach to organizational problems. The Tavistock approach was strongly influenced by psychoanalytic thinking, viewing the entire organization as analogous to a "patient," with the corrective action termed therapy for the organization (Jacques, 1951). They also placed a heavy emphasis on the group, and the group-functioning theories of W. R. Bion (1961). Over the years there has been considerable exchange of views and personnel between Tavistock and NTL, and although the methods and assumptions vary in some important respects, the common focus has come to be on the organization or group as a whole.

During its developmental years, an important concern of the organizational approach was the humanization of the bureaucratic form of social organization that had come to predominate during the twentieth century. Throughout the writings of the leaders of this movement, one finds an emphasis on human values as opposed to the more formal and impersonal ones of the bureaucracy. As opposed to the directive- and efficiency-oriented school of management that had developed during the early part of the twentieth century, these organizational practitioners envisioned new organizational forms, in which social climate was more important than structure, with new values toward work and people, which they believed would improve the functioning of groups and organizations. It was this combination of human values with a specific methodology that was viewed with great favor during the 1960s by those concerned with institutional reform.

The prototype of those institutions in need of reform to make them more responsive to the people were the institutions serving the poor, especially the welfare bureaucracy. With the establishment of the Office of Economic Opportunity there was increasing emphasis on promoting the responsiveness and humaneness of those social institutions that served the poor. Similarly, momentum was growing to promote the organized attack on racial discrimination that marked much of the social activities of the 1960s.

As demands met with resistance, and confrontation led to conflict, there was a feeling of urgency for some means of achieving institutional reform. The report of the Kerner Commission (1968) on civil disorders of the 1960s came down heavily on white racism as a major focus of the problem. Rather than overt bigotry, this problem was defined as one of a latent lack of sensitivity and awareness among the majority citizens of the United States. At nearly every level of society a sense of pain and urgency had developed.

In addition to the Office of Economic Opportunity and its subsidiary programs—including Head Start, the Neighborhood Youth Corps, and the Job Corps—there were also such programs as the development of Community Mental Health Centers, which were to provide vastly increased services to segments of the population previously untouched by such services, and Volunteers in Service to America (VISTA), which was to employ large numbers of United States citizens in working with groups with which they had previously had little contact or understanding.

These programs had in common a need to recruit large numbers of persons to perform tasks that were new to them with a client population with which they were largely unfamiliar. These developments posed enormous management problems, but they also posed larger issues in the form of the problem of trying to incorporate the newly emerging ideology about human sensitivity into the administration of large-scale programs. While elements of the organizational approach, particularly sensitivity training, were applied to problems of many of these programs, more often this approach has been pressed into use in the face of mounting tensions, such as the racial and, later, student protest disturbances. As we shall see, the motivation for this latter employment of the model was more often an attempt to cool off the immediate situation than to effect any significant organizational change.

Assumptions

Many of the assumptions of the organizational model are influenced by a point of view advanced by Douglas McGregor (1960) that he called "Theory X" and "Theory Y." Theory X is the conventional management view of organization and, while phrased in the context of a business organization, is also applicable to other types of organizations. According to McGregor, Theory X consists of the following assumptions:

1. Management is responsible for organizing the elements of productive enterprise—money, materials, equipment, people —in the interest of economic ends.
2. With respect to people, this is a process of directing their efforts, motivating them, controlling their actions, modifying their behavior to fit the needs of the organization.
3. Without this active intervention by management, people would be passive—even resistant—to organizational needs. They must, therefore, be persuaded, rewarded, punished, controlled—their activities must be directed. This is management's task—in managing subordinate managers or workers. We often sum it up by saying that management consists of getting things done through other people. Behind this conventional theory are several additional beliefs—less explicit, but widespread:
4. The average man is by nature indolent—he works as little as possible.
5. He lacks ambition, dislikes responsibility, prefers to be led.
6. He is inherently self-centered, indifferent to organizational needs.
7. He is by nature resistant to change.
8. He is gullible, not very bright, the ready dupe of the charlatan and the demogogue.

McGregor's Theory Y consists of the following assumptions:

1. Management is responsible for organizing the elements of productive enterprise—money, materials, equipment, people—in the interest of economic ends.
2. People are not by nature passive or resistant to organizational needs. They have become so as a result of experience in organizations.
3. The motivation, the potential for development, the capacity for assuming responsibility, the readiness to direct behavior toward organizational goals are all present in people. Management does not put them there. It is the responsibility of management to make it possible for people to recognize and develop these human characteristics for themselves.
4. The essential task of management is to arrange organizational conditions and methods of operation so that people can achieve their own goals best by directing their own efforts towards organizational objectives.

The sorts of personal and psychological difficulties that this approach addresses have been documented amply in such writings as Whyte's (1956) *The Organization Man* and Riesman's (1953) *The Lonely Crowd.* While this antibureaucratic sentiment was popularly experienced as a reaction against personal conformity, during the 1950s and 1960s enlightened business management began to embrace the Theory Y orientation and sought help increasingly from organizational consultants employing this model.

The organizational approach clearly makes assumptions about a particular ideology concerning group work. These include the definition of organizational problems as human problems, rather than engineering problems, which require human solutions, as opposed to bureaucratic or structural solutions. This ideology contains specific values that favor participation over the concentration of power and indeed aims toward the redistribution of power within organizations. There is an emphasis on personal growth as a means of achieving cooperation within organizations, and an emphasis on openness about one's feelings and the promotion of trust in others as a means of improving communication.

An important difference in this approach from the bureaucratic approach is that the latter emphasizes a relatively static structure that attempts to minimize and resist change, while the organizational approach takes an orientation to ongoing change as a continuing process. It also provides a technology for change, based on experiential learning as opposed to the management development approach that provides for the manager to learn new ideas and instruct others to carry them out.

The distinction between management development and organizational development is an important one to understanding the organizational model. Burke and Schmidt (1971) have detailed several of these distinctions. The differences turn to a great extent on the degree to which one subscribes to a "key man" theory of group functioning as opposed to a social system perspective on the organization. For example, typical management development goals are to improve the functioning and skills of the manager. Consequently, change strategies in management development usually involve taking the manager out of the organization for specialized training. The time perspective in management development is short-range and tends to focus on the immediate problem. Resistance to management development is likely to come from the manager feeling threatened when someone suggests the need for his self-improvement.

In contrast, organizational development goals seek to improve the capacity of the organization to solve problems through greater commitment to organizational goals and more flexibility in the use of appropriate competence, rather than a reliance on structural roles in assigning responsibility for solving problems. The change strategy in organizational development emphasizes training on the job, and the time perspective is long-term, dealing with the anticipation of change and the problems resulting from it. Accordingly, resistance to organizational development stems from a greater degree of risk involved in the changing of role structures and power distributions, as well as the open-ended time commitment.

The distinctions between these two approaches fit with the differences that organizational theorists see between bureaucratic solutions to problems and the new conditions of life that the bureaucratic approach does not accommodate. Bennis (1966) delineates a number of these distinctions. He feels that the bureaucracy makes no accommodation to the need to integrate the individual and the organization. The reliance on legal-rational power and its implied correlate, coercive power, through a hierarchical structure with routinized procedures, all tend to insulate the bureaucratic structure against an adaptive response to changing conditions. He feels that new knowledge concerning human needs, rising aspirations, and human values make an integration of individual and organizational needs imperative. Such an integration is also required to solve conflicts arising from competing claims and to accommodate the increasing specialization and interdependence within organizations. Bennis feels that the increased communication, cooperation, and sharing of mutual goals that are necessary to solve these problems are all reduced in the bureaucratic form.

It is important to note that the implementation of this approach to solving organizational problems is based on a knowledge of social psychology, which also recognizes that many of the patterns of organizational practice are strongly internalized within the individual who has been socialized in such organizations. This internalization, as discussed in Chapter 3, has strong psychological roots, as well as strong psychological and social implications. For example, Parsons (1952) has described the superego, regarded in psychoanalytic theory as a strong and unyielding source of standards and prohibitions within the personality of the individual, as a reflection of the social organization of the individual's cultural milieu. But it should also be observed that this internalization of organizational patterns receives strong support in the social environment and is even propagated through social institutions. Illustrating this point, a study by Miller and Swanson (1958) found that the effects of parental child-rearing practices on children were mediated by the type of organizational structure in which the chief bread-winning parent was employed. They found that the same practices of "entrepreneurial" and "bureaucratic" parents had different effects on their children.

It is the recognition of the link between social institutions and processes of internalization on which the organizational model as a model of community psychology rests. The model assumes that the community is a collection of organizations of groups in which the important transactions of the community are conducted. More than just the collective action of individuals, the key organizations of a community set the norms and values that predominate in the community and by which individual behavior is regulated.

On the one hand, group processes are seen to affect individual behavior; on the other, the internalization of the effects of these processes means that changes in the patterns of behavior do not occur from mere intellectual awareness or discussion. Argyris (1969) documents this assertion with a number of experiences with different types of organizations. Despite McGregor's assumptions about the nature of man in Theory Y, he also points out that those currently socialized in organizations have resistances to change that arise from these internalized patterns, and methods of changing them must deal with the emotional force of this resistance.

While much of the discussion up to this point has relied on references to business organizations, we will turn now to some typical interventions that have been addressed to social and community problems, as a means of illustrating the community implications of this model.

Typical Interventions

The organizational model has evolved gradually into a collection of specific interventions that complement and reinforce each other. The integration of these interventions for an approach to specific organizations is the process referred to as organizational development (O.D.). This process of organizational change is ordinarily carried out by a consultant or team of consultants who are invited in by an organization to work with it for an extended period of time.

The O.D. approach has been employed primarily with business organizations, and it is extremely rare that the entire O.D. approach is applied to a community organization. Examples of community interventions using the organizational model are more likely to employ a single, limited intervention, for reasons that will be explored later. The following interventions, then, are selected as typical examples of the organizational approach in community settings.

SENSITIVITY TRAINING

Many of the general characteristics of the T-group method have been discussed already. Looking more closely, we find that the T-group is an attempt to create an environment, or, perhaps better, an experience, in which the individual and group become integrated harmoniously. That individuals are not automatically prepared for this experience provides for some of the powerful effects of the initial stages of the T-group experience.

The initial stage of the T-group is a deliberately unstructured one in which the individual's internalized patterns of group functioning do not fit. Thus, the members of the group must struggle with their expectations of the leader (trainer) to provide some structure, which the trainer declines to do. The resultant discomfort over dependency eventually turns to a counterdependent attitude, in which an attempt to deny the dependency feelings is acted out in rebellious behavior, followed by the formation of subgroups and the emergence of conflict. There follows a phase of identification among the members in which group forces exist that move toward the removal of individual identities. Resistance to these forces eventually results in a resolution of this conflict through increasingly authentic interpersonal communication. If this phase of development of the group is reached, a deliberate effort is made to reinforce this good group spirit in the final sessions of the group (Bennis and Shepard, 1956).

This procedure is based on Lewin's theory of attitudes and attitude change. He assumes that an individual's attitudes are firmly anchored to the norms of an individual's reference groups—those with which he identifies. In order to change these attitudes, it is necessary first to "unfreeze" the attitudes, to use Lewin's term, by a process of disconfirmation of the expectations concerning group behavior that are based on these attitudes. Once the attitudes are unfrozen, they are amenable to change. It is then necessary to refreeze them in the context of the group experience (Lewin, 1951).

In the initial NTL groups, a deliberate effort was made to diminish the familiarity of cues and increase the probability of "unfreezing" by assembling group members who were strangers to each other. However, this creates a paradox in that the new attitudes achieved in such groups are not then anchored in the old groups back home and should not be expected to last, according to the theory. The attempt to work with members of groups who are already in some organizational relationship to each other is an effort to solve the carry-over problem. It should be expected, however, that such groups would have more difficulty overcoming the initial inhibitions in the "unfreezing" stage. Let us examine some typical group interventions with this in mind.

Hassol (1970) was invited to develop a T-group format for a leadership training program for adolescents in a two-week summer camp format. The program had been in existence for some years and consisted of structured adult-adolescent discussions about leadership. The staff of the program, sponsored by a religious group, were ministers and their wives who were experienced in youth work.

As a consultant to the staff, Hassol provided training in T-group theory and technique and led a T-group experience for the staff members prior to the opening of the camp. Once the camp began, the staff members conducted T-group sessions each day with the adolescents, then had a session of their own each evening for supervision and review. The procedure is quite reminiscent of the original format described in the introduction to this chapter.

Hassol focuses on three events that occurred during the camp session that caused some concern among the adult staff, and how these issues were handled among the participants through the T-group experience. While each of the issues—the formation of cliques, the sexually deviant stereotyping of one of the campers, and the violation of smoking rules—was resolved positively through these sessions, Hassol finds that the important side effect of the resolution of these issues was increased trust and understanding that resulted between the adults and the adolescents through these experiences in mutual learning.

While he presents no statistical data on the effects of these groups, his anecdotal evidence is quite convincing on the effects of these groups' experiences in the camp setting. This is clearly significant in itself, since the issues he discusses are ones that adults and adolescents frequently find difficult to discuss, let alone resolve. He also does not present any data on the carry-over of these changes beyond the camp setting.

However, Hassol is clearly interested in the implications of this experience as a model for improving the democratic atmosphere in the more general school situation. Besides improving the interest and involvement of students, Hassol feels that experiences of this type that involve young people in the process of taking responsibility for making decisions affecting the group's welfare are important learning experiences in themselves, both for the adolescents and the adults.

Hassol notes that the adolescents seemed to move through the initial stages of the T-group experience somewhat faster than did the adults, which may suggest that their usual group attitudes were not as firmly anchored, or perhaps were not as strong because of the shorter life span during which they could become internalized. The question of what happens to these group attitudes when the adolescents return to a conventional group situation is not answered by this experience, however.

That there is a contrast between the conventional and "human relations"-oriented environments should be self-evident, and the conflict that has occurred in many communities over the use of participatory, experience-based educational strategies further emphasizes this point. One clear requirement for the successful implementation of such an atmosphere in a major social institution, the school, is its acceptance by the school staff.

Keutzer, Fosmire, Diller, and Smith (1971) demonstrated the effects of such an approach. Taking advantage of the event of the opening of two new, comparably sized high schools, they implemented a series of T-groups for the entire staff of one of the schools, which they termed Experimental High School (EHS), but not the other, which served as Control High School (CHS). The effects of the training on the social climate of EHS were measured by changes in students' perceptions from the beginning to the end of the first year. At EHS, students reported an increase in preferred events and a decrease in nonpreferred events, whereas at CHS the opposite tended to occur. Moreover, at the end of the year twenty four teachers requested transfers into EHS, while only two requested transfers away from it. The authors of this study supplement these data with several observations of increased purposive activity among students, and more frequent and relaxed student-teacher interaction as support for the perceived changes. They also caution that there were some students who seemed to have difficulty adapting to the requirements for self-discipline and control, but they felt the benefits outweighed these exceptional cases.

Boller and Boller (1973) and Hartzell, Anthony, and Wain (1973) also report positive changes in teachers' attitudes following sensitivity training. The latter study adds some interesting observations on the carry-over effect. Subjects in the Hartzell *et al.* study were student teachers. One group (Before) received training prior to their student-teacher experience; a second group (Concurrent) received the training along with their student teaching, and a third (Control) received none. While significant changes in human relations skills were found in both Before and Concurrent groups, the changes in the Before group were somewhat reduced following their student-teaching experience. The authors suggest a modeling effect based on low human relations skills scores obtained by the student-teachers' supervisors, but the study more likely demonstrates the advisability of integrating the T-group experience with the ongoing experience of the natural group.

Sensitivity training approaches have been conducted with another major community institution—the police department. The most publicized and by far the most ambitious of these programs was the Houston Police–Community Relations Project (Sikes and Cleveland, 1968). This project was developed by a group comprised of the mayor of Houston and several businessmen, who raised funds for a program to improve mutual understanding between policemen and community members during a time of intense racial unrest. Each human relations training laboratory met for three hours once a week for six weeks. A total of fourteen hundred police officers and a corresponding number of community members participated in these workshops.

Policemen attended the sessions in uniform, during off-duty hours, but were paid their regular salaries for attending. The sessions were held in community centers, most of which were located in poverty areas. Community members participated voluntarily and were not paid.

The results of these sessions indicated that the attitudes of community members changed more than did those of the police, a result that is probably understandable from a number of standpoints. The policemen were participating under less than voluntary conditions and were clearly on the defensive, given the social climate of the times. Furthermore, the police attendance in uniform and as paid, official representatives of the police department undoubtedly activated constraining social norms within the police organization against change, while the community members as a group were not so constrained by organizational visibility, although some of them may also have felt the pressure of reference groups (Mann, 1968). The authors make no claims for far-reaching changes, but they do point to some significant and dramatic changes in a few individual police officers in their attitudes and behavior, and to an overall educational impact in providing a sample of the reality of community attitudes toward the police.

Numerous other programs of this kind have been conducted, with mixed results. Frequently the evaluative data are either limited or ambiguous. For example, Lipsitt and Steinbrunner (1969) used small groups of policemen and citizens in a pilot project that found positive changes in group interaction over the course of the training, but mixed positive and negative attitudinal changes. Pfister (1975) and Sata (1975) report positive results, with mixtures of personality-scale and anecdotal data. More impressive is their use of the observations of others of the policemen's behavior. Sata reports favorable reactions by others to the behavior of laboratory-trained policemen during a riot situation, and Pfister used an ingenious device of soliciting questionnaire responses from citizens who had contacted the police for minor incidents. Comparing laboratory-trained with control policemen, whose group membership could not have been known to the citizens, the trained group were seen as more understanding, considerate, and cooperative than the controls.

On the other hand, Sacon (1971) found that sensitivity training tends to produce short-term attitude improvement, but that the changes do not persist on later follow-up, and in some cases may worsen. Teahan (1975) reports some worsening of interracial attitudes after an eighteen-month period of experience as policemen. Thus, the findings must be tempered with the repeated observation that such changes in attitudes as may be produced by T-group experience require a supportive organizational environment in order to continue, and a commitment on the part of the organization to maintain that support (Argyris, 1962). Accordingly, partial application of the organizational model through sensitivity training alone is unlikely to produce the extent of organizational change that is needed to sustain a human relations climate within the organization.

SURVEY FEEDBACK

The survey feedback technique was pioneered by Floyd Mann of the Survey Research Center at the University of Michigan (Mann, 1957). While many organizations utilize some sorts of surveys, suggestion systems, or other sources of information that could provide organizational feedback, too often this information is not integrated into organizational practices. Mann's survey feedback approach is designed to promote not just utilization of survey information, but internalization of the solutions derived from it, as well (Katz and Kahn, 1966).

Briefly, Mann's approach involves surveying an entire organization by an outside research team. The results of the survey are discussed with organizational "families," composed of a supervisor at any level and those reporting directly to that supervisor, starting with top management. This procedure provides for a linking between families, as the supervisors at one level will be involved, for example, in a "family" of supervisors at the next level. The researchers prepare results for each family that are directly relevant to that group, as well as summaries of the entire organization for comparison.

These results are "fed back" to the organizational families through group discussions in which the results are analyzed, questions raised, new surveys taken if required, and solutions proposed. An important aspect of this approach is the involvement of employees in the formulation of questions to be surveyed, as well as discussions on the results and their implications. It is this series of small group discussions that distinguishes survey feedback from the mere conduct of surveys. Besides the objective presentation of feedback information, it also promotes participation and involvement throughout the organization.

The goals of survey feedback are to provide more objective information about organizational functioning to its members, and to improve interpersonal relations and communication within organizational families. Katz and Kahn (1966) describe three conditions that are necessary for survey feedback to achieve these goals. First, there must be a factual, task-oriented atmosphere, which is facilitated by the use of organizational families. Second, there must be freedom at each family level to arrive at its own conclusions and implications for practice in order for the group process to develop. Third, results of group discussions must be fed back to higher-level families, as well as proceeding down the line to those lower in the organizational structure.

Mann's approach recognizes the realities of the hierarchical nature of organizations and provides a procedure that fits well with that structure. While there is a force created to promote increased participation and involvement at each level, relationships between families in this approach have to be carried out through those individuals who have cross-linking family memberships—the supervisors. Moreover, this approach does nothing to promote a change in organizational structure. While such a change could conceivably result from group discussion at the top levels of the organization, the survey feedback approach takes organizational structure as a given and makes no prior assumptions about the value of more horizontal organizational arrangements.

Studies of survey feedback by Beckhard (1959) and Mann (1957) in large organizations indicate that two phases are involved to achieve meaningful changes. First, the organization must learn to use the feedback process. Initial contacts between the research teams and organizations accomplished little more than this. Second, the organization can then proceed to solve problems and make changes. In both of these studies, organizations that had initially used survey feedback procedures were found to change during a second contact with the survey feedback team.

Miles, Hornstein, Callahan, Calder, and Schiavo (1969) report on a survey feedback intervention for a school system. They first fed back survey data to the top admininstrative group, then each school-building principal and staff received feedback and discussion. Following this, a cross-building task force model was used to discuss problems identified in the feedback process. This latter step is a departure from the process outlined by Mann, inasmuch as the "problems" were not continuously discussed in the groups in which they were identified. This group of task forces then made proposals for action that were fed back to the administration. While the research team noted significantly increased interaction and involvement in process analysis by the participants, and the participants reported significant increases in satisfaction with the group's decisions, they were unable to find any significant changes in a large number of measures of change that they employed. These measures had to do with power equalization, communication, and norms.

The Miles *et al.* study used an innovation in its evaluative procedures in that some of the survey data was withheld from feedback. The team used these measures for evaluation purposes, reasoning that their use in feedback sessions would contaminate them as assessment devices because the participants could become "testwise" through their discussions. However, they also commented that they felt these measures were relatively insensitive to change.

Interviews with administrative personnel indicated changes in communication and interpersonal relationships, but not in power equalization, and the recommendations of the task forces had not been acted upon at the end of the school year. The researchers concluded that no lasting changes had occurred as a result of the survey feedback process. However, it should be noted that there is nothing inherent in the survey feedback model that would predict changes in power relationships, and that the previous studies cited required a period of growth with the new communication patterns before active problem solving was undertaken through a second relationship with the survey intervention team. Perhaps the conclusions were premature.

Selltiz (1971) reports on a community campaign against racial discrimination in restaurants in New York City in the early 1950s in which action surveys were conducted by having designated white and black couples seek service in various restaurants and recording the results of equal or discriminatory treatment. The results of the survey were then discussed with the owners or managers of the discriminating establishments as well as with associations of restaurant owners and unions of restaurant employees.

Each of the individuals or groups was asked to sign a pledge making a commitment not to discriminate. Reports of the survey were also published in newspapers. A resurvey was conducted two years later. It was found that 42 percent of the restaurants in the first survey discriminated through poorer seating, poorer service or rudeness, or both, for the black couple. In the second survey, only 16 percent discriminated, a significant reduction.

While this survey was different from the survey and feedback through group discussion model, it illustrates an important precondition for the effectiveness of survey feedback and other interventions in organizations. The survey disconfirmed what some of the people believed they were doing as indicated by the surprised and disbelieving initial reaction of some of the restaurant personnel. The willingness of these persons and their organizations to sign pledges not to discriminate indicates that the prevailing social norm was against discrimination. When the survey indicated that practices were not in conformance with the norm, the former could be changed to align with the latter. Thus, when survey results differ from beliefs about practices, but not from the normative structure, then changes can be achieved.

A contrasting example is provided by Lester Maddox, a Georgia restaurant owner who was later to be elected governor of that state. When it was pointed out to Maddox that he was violating the law in discriminating against black customers in his restaurant, Maddox protested vigorously and received national attention. He refused to yield, and closed his restaurant instead and went into politics. It is a reasonable assumption that Maddox believed that normative support was with him, regardless of the law, and his subsequent election to statewide public office seems to support that assumption.

As a general principle, then, organizational intervention using the feedback process in its many forms would seem to depend upon normative support for the changes that are contemplated, either in the minds of the change agents or those of organizational members. Changes in normative structure itself are more likely to be linked to changing events in the external environment of the organization that are fed back to the organization, according to Katz and Kahn (1966). This point creates a significant difference between business organizations and public organizations.

The primary feedback linkage from the business organization to its external environment is productivity and profit. Decreases in organizational efficiency result in lowered productivity or profit, or both, and can be easily measured. While the efficiency of a public institution is also related to its product, no profit as such is readily measurable. Since business organizations today tend to rely heavily on mass-produced, standardized products, the potential consumer can easily depend on obtaining a product that is nearly identical to any other product that that organization may produce. However, since public institutions deal in human outcomes, standardization of product is impossible and even undesirable in a society that values individual liberties. Contrast, for example, public expectations toward police and schools with those toward public utilities, where the product is visible and standardized.

Thus, environmental feedback to public organizations is more likely to be in terms of questioning the inputs and their internal utilization, such as salaries for teachers or policemen, then it is to question the product that is produced. When the latter is done at all, it tends to take the form of criticism of the "raw material" or input. Ryan (1971) has called this process "blaming the victim." A humorous variation of this theme is attributed to a rather unreflective prison warden who is reputed to have said it would be impossible to have any successful rehabilitation in his prison until he started getting a better class of prisoners.

Rhodes (1972) has developed an elaborate conception of the interdependence among the majority culture bearers, institutions for controlling deviance, and deviant behavior. On a psychological level, Rhodes maintains that deviant behavior only arouses public response when it creates a sense of threat among the majority culture-bearer group. Public institutions for controlling deviance then need only to respond in a way analogous to the way defense mechanisms of individuals respond to anxiety, that is, to create the illusion of diminished threat. As long as this is done, according to Rhodes, the sense of threat is diminished and the deviance-controlling mechanisms will be maintained. In terms of the analysis presented here, this means they will continue to receive favorable feedback (inputs) from the external environment.

Within this framework, it is also worth noting another distinction, having to do with differences in operational freedoms that the two types of organizations enjoy. The general public has little or no concern with the manner in which business organizations go about doing their business as long as they do it in a way that produces a desired outcome. Besides the freedom of business organizations to engage in organizational development or not, relatively independent of public opinion, consider the difficulties encountered in attempting to change racially discriminating practices of some government contractors or the environmentally polluting practices of some manufacturing firms. Jobs for the employees and productivity are nearly always given greater weight. With public organizations, however, where people are not informed, or do not agree, on what the product should be, there is no way to control output through product feedback, so public opinion is concentrated almost entirely on process—how the organization conducts its affairs—and untested hypotheses about how that process affects outcomes.

The schools and the police are excellent examples of this distinction. Recently, the Kansas City, Missouri, police department conducted an elaborate, well-designed research study of the effects of motorized patrol on crime prevention (Kelling, Pate, Dieckman, and Brown, 1974). This study consisted of certain precincts assigned to routine patrol, others to intensified patrol, and still others to no patrol. The results showed that the type of patrol made no significant difference in the amount of crime reported or arrests made in these precincts, a finding that contradicts a long and widely held belief among policemen about the effects of patrol. When these results were announced, they were met largely with criticism and attempts to discredit them by police chiefs across the country, despite the fact that the police chief in Kansas City at the time of the study, Clarence Kelly, was later to become the director of the Federal Bureau of Investigation. This event vividly demonstrates the strength of normative structures in the face of contradictory information when there is no clear-cut feedback from the external environment. Were public opinion to mount to a significant level concerning the results of these studies and their implications, then almost certainly these normative beliefs, and the practices tied to them, would change. A more informed, interested, and concerned public would be required, however, for this to happen. In the face of presently mounting rates of crime in nearly every city in the country, the fact that such a public movement is not forthcoming tends to strengthen Rhodes's argument concerning the defensive nature of the relationship between the community and its deviance-controlling organizations. Perhaps this analysis sheds some light on the limited changes obtained in some of the schools and police departments referred to earlier in this chapter.

Typical Research

The number and variety of research methods used in the field of organizational psychology and related research on group dynamics is considerably larger than can be reasonably covered in this discussion. Accordingly, consideration of the research employed with the organizational model will be limited to a few examples of generic types of research methods most frequently employed in the processes discussed under interventions. These include a variety of *rating scales* for the assessment of self- and other-related attitudes and for assessing perceptions of organizational characteristics; systems for the *analysis of interaction processes*; and measures having to do with *organizational outcomes* or products.

Gibb (1970) has reviewed the results of sensitivity training research, which covers a broad range of topics and issues. He identifies six goals of sensitivity training and examines the evidence for the achievement of each of these objectives. The research has employed each of the three types mentioned above, and tends to find generally positive results, although this conclusion must be qualified with recognition of several methodological problems. The six goals are (1) increased sensitivity, (2) better management of feelings, (3) better management of motivations, (4) improved functional attitudes toward the self, (5) improved functional attitudes toward others, and (6) increased interdependent behavior.

Although a variety of research techniques are employed, typical research on the sensitivity dimension has involved the completion of rating scales either to predict how other persons will respond to the scale for themselves, or how they will rate the subject. While management of feelings and management of motivations are sometimes assessed through the use of personality inventories or projective tests (neither of which appear to be very sensitive to the effects of these types of training experiences), the better results seem to be obtained from the observations of others. However, the results on these two goals are the least impressive, in part because of ambiguities in operational definitions of appropriate outcomes. For example, a person who has gone through a T-group experience may quite reasonably be expected to be more expressive of feelings, but may also be rated by a supervisor as not managing feelings or motivations well.

The typical measurement of attitudes toward the self involves asking the subject to rate his perceived actual and ideal positions on some dimension of personality. Several studies report finding increased congruence between these two estimates, indicative of increased self-esteem. Gibb suggests that such changes are a necessary precursor to behavioral changes in groups. Attitudes toward others tend to be assessed using generalized attitude or personality scales, such as authoritarian, democratic, or humanistic values. These studies produce as many "no change" as positive results, and tend to follow the general pattern of less significant findings on generalized personality tests. Studies of interdependent behavior rely less on self-ratings and more on observational methods. These studies tend to find both positive and "no difference" results, for reasons perhaps similar to those mentioned above concerning the management of feelings and motivations.

The difficulties of conducting research in the T-group setting have led to a number of methodological weaknesses in these studies, the most frequent of which is the absence of a control group. In addition, the use of before-and-after measurements is especially subject to response bias and the knowledge on the part of the subject as to what is a "correct" response. Some observational studies, even where control groups are used, are biased by the observer's knowing the previous training experience of the subjects. All of these things, of course, render the results of such research ambiguous.

These methodological shortcomings are, however, a trivial limitation in assessing the outcomes of T-group experiences, since the overall concern is greater organizational effectiveness, which is not assessed by these methods. Many of the studies referred to above have been useful in generating hypotheses about group functioning and process that can lead to modifications of both practice and research. Following Lewin's tradition, research in the organizational model is action research.

An important step in the diagnosis of organizational problems is the assessment of interactions patterns (Bradford, Stock, and Horwitz, 1970). Bales (1950) developed a scheme for coding interactions, which can be used by an independent observer to record who communicated to whom and the content of the communication. There are twelve content categories that reflect positive and negative socioemotional messages and task-oriented messages. The twelve categories are:

1. Shows solidarity, raises other's status, gives help, reward.
2. Shows tension release, jokes, laughs, shows satisfaction.
3. Agrees, shows passive acceptance, understands, concurs, complies.
4. Gives suggestion, direction, implying autonomy for other.
5. Gives opinion, evaluation, analysis, expresses feeling, wish.
6. Gives orientation, information, repeats, clarifies, confirms.
7. Asks for orientation, information, repetition, confirmation.
8. Asks for opinion, evaluation, analysis, expression of feeling.
9. Asks for suggestion, direction, possible ways of action.
10. Disagrees, shows passive rejection, formality, withholds help.
11. Shows tension, asks for help, withdraws out of field.
12. Shows antagonism, deflates other's status, defends or asserts self.

The first three categories are in the positive socioemotional area, the next six cover instrumental or task-oriented, and emotionally neutral, areas, and the last three are in the negative socio-emotional area. An observer using a grid containing these categories can code interactions between group members over time and the observations can then be summed to determine both communication patterns and role taking within the group.

Argyris (1965) has constructed a somewhat different scheme to attempt to characterize the level of interpersonal communications in groups, which is related to his theory of organizational effectiveness. His scheme includes six categories of individual and six of interpersonal behavior on one level, and six categories on the group norm level. Each category is further divided into two subcategories: ideas (i) and feelings (f). His theoretical scheme leads Argyris to conceive of these categories as those that facilitate or impede interpersonal relationships. They are presented in tabular form below.

Categories of Behavior

LEVEL I				LEVEL II	
Individual		*Interpersonal*		*Norms*	
Experimenting	i	Help others to	i	Trust	i
	f	experiment	f		f
Openness	i	Help others to	i	Concern	i
	f	be open	f		f
Owning	i	Help others to	i	Individuality	i
	f	own	f		f
		Zero line			
Not owning	i	Not help others	i	Conformity	i
	f	to own	f		f
Not open	i	Not help others	i	Antagonism	i
	f	to be open	f		f
Rejecting	i	Not help others	i	Mistrust	i
experimenting	f	to experiment	f		f

SOURCE: Reproduced from C. Argyris, The incompleteness of social psychological theory, *American Psychologist*, 1969, *24*, 893–908. Copyright 1969 by the American Psychological Association. Reprinted by permission of the APA and the author.

Use of this scheme in observing 163 different meetings produced a predominance of ratings in only six categories. The categories "own i," "concern i," and "conform i" made up 75 percent of the observations, while "open i," "individuality i," and "antagonism i" were observed 20 percent of the time. The remaining categories together added up to 5 percent of the observations. Argyris observes that expression of feelings was rarely observed, and interpersonal helping or group norms of trust were seldom seen. He refers to this pattern as Pattern A. Groups in which feelings are expressed, which are characterized by interpersonal helping and norms of trust and individuality, are called Pattern B. Argyris notes that the typical T-group begins with Pattern A and, if successful, moves to Pattern B.

A final type of research involves the assessment of organizational impact in its transactions with the environment. Here a consideration of Katz and Kahn's (1966) conception of organizational effectiveness provides a useful theoretical framework. They first distinguish organizational efficiency as a component of effectiveness. Efficiency has to do with the internal workings of an organization, as has much of the research discussed to this point. It is defined as the ratio of input to output in the organization. Any organization requires input in the form of personnel, funds, and resources, and produces some output through the use of input. No organization is perfectly efficient, for some of the input is used up in the maintenance of the organization. From this standpoint, effectiveness, then, is the return to the organization of additional inputs from the environment. Increased efficiency may or may not result in increased effectiveness. Assessment of organizational effectiveness is moderated by one's frame of reference regarding the organization. For a business organization, effectiveness may be assessed by return to investors, employees, or improvements to productive capacity. Public organizations, on the other hand, are effective in the contributions they make to the overall community, in the form of transactions with citizens or other organizations.

Changes in public organizations such as schools may be assessed by a variety of educational and behavioral outcomes, including an increase in desirable outcomes, such as ratio of students graduated, admission of graduates to other appropriate institutions such as further education or employment, and similar criteria. Changes in police departments may be assessed by changes in arrest behavior, such as a decline in discretionary minor arrests and an increase in arrests that lead to prosecution (Shellow, 1975); increased cooperative inputs to other organizations such as referrals for mental health or other social services (Mann, 1973); or a decline in undesirable outcomes, such as public disturbances resulting from arrest behavior, supportable citizen complaints, and injuries to policemen and citizens (Bard, 1970; Bard, Zacker, and Rutter, 1972).

While many of these indicators of organizational effectiveness have the virtue of being relatively free of response and observer bias, they are also more difficult to relate precisely to any specific intervention. The use of such measures requires careful and sophisticated research design to reduce the sources of invalidity in their interpretation.

Typical Settings

The practitioner of organizational change is typically an outsider to the organization in which he intervenes, which means that while he brings a presumably noninvolved, objective point of view to that organization, he requires some base of operations to support his own work. The typical arrangement between an organization and a consultant is a fee-for-service agreement. However, the consultant may require rather elaborate resources for research and analysis of organizational problems aside from the client organization. In the field of organizational change today, three major institutes stand out: the National Training Laboratory, the Tavistock Institute, and the Institute for Social Research at the University of Michigan. Each of these is self-supporting through its work and relatively independent, the latter despite its university affiliation.

More numerous bases for organizational consultants are a few university schools of business and private consulting firms, where the consultation is also performed on a fee-for-service basis. Clearly, the large institutes and university-based groups have access to relatively abundant research facilities, and in the case of the university-affiliated consultant, the research may also contribute instrumentally to the consultant's standing and tenure in the university.

Because of the realities of financial support needs, it is unlikely that any of the existing large institutes can provide the sort of long-term consulting relationships in significant numbers that would be required to work with a sufficient array of community organizations to make a difference in overall community functioning. On the other hand, there is no local community agency or institutional base that could support such an effort at the local level, such as the community mental health center could conceivably do for the mental health model. As a consequence, most community organizations tend to rely on the importation of consultative help from outside the community for highly specialized and time-limited tasks, if they seek such help at all. As NTL discovered in its early years, there is not likely to be sufficient demand from the public sector to support locally informed private consulting organizations in very many communities without their having eventually to rely on private business organizations for the majority of their fee support, with the result that such firms have difficulty developing expertise in the special problems of community organizations.

Thus, the most viable setting for the organizational model is likely to remain the university-affiliated or the freestanding institute, in relatively small numbers, and the entrepreneurial consulting firm in predominantly large cities. As a result, the systematic application of the organizational model to community problems is unlikely to take place in any significant degree.

Assessment of the Model

Using the criteria generated previously (Chapter 3), the organizational model conceptualizes the community as a set of organizations that function according to the principles derived from the study of social groups. While social norms are an important regulating principle concerning the behavior of individuals, a heavy emphasis is placed on face-to-face relationships in both the diagnosis and solution of problems. More than just collections of interpersonal relationships, however, the organizational model is concerned with regularized interpersonal relationships directed to some end over and above that of the interacting parties. There are no assumptions about geographical areas, nor is there any set of assumptions concerning the superset of organizations that would constitute the community itself.

The value assumptions of the model are quite explicit in placing positive values on participation, the sharing of power within organizations, and the assumptions that individuals are self-motivating, given the appropriate organizational climate. These values, besides having considerable backing in a variety of organizational research studies, are based on conceptions of the individual personality as self-actualizing (Maslow, 1954) and on a psychology of humanism that supports the democratic ideology.

Change processes are conceptualized generally as the creation of a special group atmosphere in which the usual expectations of the group are disconfirmed (the Lewinian concept of "unfreezing");

support is generated for exploring new expectations, attitudes, and feelings; and a belief in the capacity of the group to come to a new formulation by which the group's capacity to resolve problems is improved. Particular attention is given to the emotions generated in this process, and while the organizational change process is conceptualized as a new growth process among normal individuals, it can be easily confused with a psychotherapeutic change method by those who are not conversant with the assumptions of the model. An aspect of the change process that is not fully conceptualized in the model, because it is not fully understood, is the process of the maintenance of change. It is assumed that the interventions of the organizational model lead to a new organizational climate in which sufficient openness is generated that a continual orientation to change is maintained. While some evidence to support this assumption is presented by Seashore and Bowers (1970), the process of change maintenance remains little understood.

Inasmuch as these change processes are conceived as internal to the organization, there is nothing in the model that deals with change at the community level, except, presumably, as a summation of changes in separate organizations. However, just as we recognize that changes in one part of a social system tend to create changes or resistances to change in other parts, it would be expected that some forces similar to these would operate across organizations. Problems at the social system level of the community, and interorganizational problems, cannot be conceptualized adequately within the organizational model itself. Indeed, if the problems with public organizations discussed earlier can be taken as an example, it may be that such groups are less free to implement organizational changes of the kinds described here *because* of their relationships with other organizations, public and private, in the community. Where, then, does one begin the organizational change process? Nothing in the model itself can answer this question.

It is conceivable at least that improvement of the intraorganizational climate may facilitate the internal workings of community organizations without necessarily influencing the organization's transactions with the external environment. The question of how intraorganizational improvements in human relations translate into improvements in the extraorganizational community environment is a deficiency in the model that requires more elaboration in transposing the organizational model from the business organization to the community organization.

The organizational model values participation, and in fact utilizes participation as a vehicle for change, as well as a state to be achieved. On the other hand, it is clear that the organizational model as conceived is largely accountable to top administration, and the level of accountability would only change if the intervention would lead to a radically more horizontal form of organization, a state that is unlikely to be completely attained. It is this aspect of the model that leads some critics, particularly those in labor and trade unions, to suspect that the model serves primarily the interests of management to avoid improvements in wages and benefits while achieving a boost in productivity. In some instances this conflict of values can be a significant problem if unresolved.

The organizational model is conceived as a relatively long-term enterprise, and thus survival value is a significant question. However, the eventual aim of the intervention is to produce an organization that is capable of self-sustaining change. One of the intermediate goals of this objective is the development of intraorganizational change agents, or groups of change agents, who can take over the functions of the external consultant. The number of consultants to organizations who report continuing contacts over a period of several years, although not as intensive as the original contacts, leads to the impression that the relationship between consultant and organization is relatively open-ended. Moreover, Gibb (1970) suggests the need for periodic follow-ups of human relations training sessions to promote the carry-over effect. With T-groups, and with organizational change in general, the model is simply not old enough that it is possible to answer this question with any degree of precision.

In summary, the organizational model is high on values of participation, openness to change, and humanism; is clear in its assumptions about values, the locus and process of change within organizations; but is limited in its conception of overall community systems, the relationships between organizations, and the change process related to this level of community functioning. Because the model has limited settings that can support its application to community work, the factors noted earlier are likely to lead to its partial and less effective implementation on a tactical, rather than a strategic, basis. Real organizational development for the community has not really been attempted and will require solution of the problem of the setting and interorganizational transactions in order to be implemented. In Katz and Kahn's (1966) conception of organizational effectiveness, these latter problems are seen as political, rather than organizational, challenges.

References

ARGYRIS, C. *Interpersonal Competence and Organizational Effectiveness*. Homewood, Ill.: Dorsey, 1962.

ARGYRIS, C. *Organizations and Innovation*. Homewood, Ill.: Irwin, 1965.

ARGYRIS, C. The incompleteness of social psychological theory. *American Psychologist*, 1969, *24*, 893–908.

BACK, K. *Beyond Words*. New York: Russell Sage, 1972.

BALES, R. F. *Interaction Process Analysis*. Cambridge, Mass.: Addison-Wesley, 1950.

BARD, M. *Training Police as Specialists in Family Crisis Intervention*. Washington, D.C.: U.S. Department of Justice, 1970.

BARD, M., ZACKER, J., AND RUTTER, E. Police family conflict management: An action research analysis. Report prepared for the Department of Justice, Law Enforcement Assistance Administration, April 1972.

BECKHARD, R. Helping a group with planned change: A case study. *Journal of Social Issues*, 1959, *15*, 13–19.

BENNIS, W., AND SHEPHARD, H. A theory of group development. *Human Relations*, 1956, *9*, 415–437.

BENNIS, W. G. Changing organizations. *Journal of Applied Behavioral Science*, 1966, *2*, 247–263.

BION, W. *Experiences in Groups*. New York: Basic Books, 1961.

BOLLER, J. D., AND BOLLER, I. D. Sensitivity training and the school teacher. *Journal of Educational Research*, 1973, *66*, 309–312.

BRADFORD, L., GIBB, J., AND BENNE, K. (Eds.). *T-group Theory and Laboratory Method*. New York: Wiley, 1964.

BRADFORD, L., STOCK, D., AND HORWITZ, M. How to diagnose group problems. In P. Golembiewski and A. Blumberg (Eds.), *Sensitivity Training and the Laboratory Approach*. Itasca, Ill.: Peacock, 1970. 141–156.

BURKE, W. W., AND SCHMIDT, W. H. Primary target for change: The manager or the organization? In H. A. Hornstein, B. B. Bunker, W. W. Burke, M. Gindes, and R. J. Lewicki (Eds.), *Social Intervention*. New York: Free Press, 1971.

GIBB, J. The effects of human relations training. In A. E. Bergin and S. L. Garfield (Eds.), *Handbook of Psychotherapy and Behavior Change.* New York: Wiley, 1970. 2114–2176.

HARTZELL, R. E., ANTHONY, W. A., AND WAIN, H. J. Comparative effectiveness of human relations training for elementary student teachers. *Journal of Educational Research*, 1973, *66*, 457–461.

HASSOL, L. Adults and adolescents: An experiment in mutual education. In D. Adelson and B. Kalis (Eds.), *Community Psychology and Mental Health.* Scranton, Pa.: Chandler, 1970. 220–237.

JAQUES, E. *The Changing Culture of a Factory.* London: Tavistock Publications, 1951.

KATZ, D., AND KAHN, R. *The Social Psychology of Organizations.* New York: Wiley, 1964.

KEUTZER, C. S., FOSMIRE, F. R., DILLER, R., AND SMITH, M. D. Laboratory training in a new social system: Evaluation of a consulting relationship with a high school faculty. *Journal of Applied Behavioral Science*, 1971, *4*, 493–501.

LEAVITT, H. Address at the School of Business, University of Texas, Austin, 1971.

LEWIN, K., *Field Theory in Social Science.* New York: Harper & Row, 1951.

LEWIN, K., LIPPITT, R., AND WHITE, R. Patterns of aggressive behavior in experimentally created "social climates." *Journal of Social Psychology*, 1939, *10*, 271–299.

LIPSITT, P. D., AND STEINBRUNER, M. An experiment in police-community relations: A small group approach. *Community Mental Health Journal*, 1969, 5, 172–179.

MANN, F. C., Studying and creating change: A means to understanding social organization. *Research in Industrial Human Relations*, Industrial Relations Research Association, no. 17, 146–167.

MANN, P. A. Discussion of the Houston police-community relations project. Part of a symposium at the Texas Psychological Association Meeting, Houston, December 1968.

MANN, P. A. *Psychological Consultation with a Police Department.* Springfield, Ill.: Charles C. Thomas, 1973.

MASLOW, A. H. *Motivation and Personality.* New York: Harper, 1954.

MCGREGOR, D. M. *The Human Side of Enterprise.* New York: McGraw-Hill, 1960.

MILES, M. B., HORNSTEIN, H. A., CALLAHAN, D. M., CALDER, P. H., AND SCHIAVO, R. S. The consequence of survey feedback: Theory and evaluation. In W. G. Bennis, K. D. Benne, and R. Chin (Eds.), *The Planning of Change.* New York: Holt, Rinehart & Winston, 1969. 457–467.

MILLER, D., AND SWANSON, G. *The Changing American Parent.* New York: Wiley, 1958.

PARSONS, T. The super-ego and the theory of social systems. *Psychiatry*, 1952, *15*, 15–26.

PFISTER, G. Outcomes of laboratory training for police officers, *Journal of Social Issues.* 1975, *31*, 115–122.

RHODES, W. *Behavioral Threat and Community Response.* New York: Behavioral Publications, 1972.

RIESMAN, D. *The Lonely Crowd.* New Haven: Yale University Press, 1950.

RYAN, W. *Blaming the Victim.* New York: Pantheon, 1971.

SACON, S. *An Intensive Training Program for a Police Department.* Washington, D.C.: American Psychological Association, September 1971.

SATA, L. S. Laboratory training for police officers. *Journal of Social Issues*, 1975, *31*, 107–114.

SEASHORE, S., AND BOWERS, D. Durability of organizational change, *American Psychologist*, 1970, *25*, 227–233.

SELLTIZ, C. The use of survey methods in a citizens campaign against discrimination. *Human Organization*, 1955, *14*, 19–25.

SHELLOW, R. Evaluating an evaluation. *Journal of Social Issues*, 1975, *31*, 87–94.

SIKES, M., AND CLEVELAND, J. Human relations training for police and community. *American Psychologist*, 1968, *23*, 766–769.

TEAHAN, J. E. A longitudinal study of attitude shifts among black and white police officers. *Journal of Social Issues*, 1975, *31*, 47–56.

WHYTE, W. H., JR. *The Organization Man*, New York: Simon & Schuster, 1956.

6. The Social Action Model

The war on poverty, conceived during the administration of President John F. Kennedy and enacted under the administration of President Lyndon B. Johnson, arose in a time of unprecedented affluence in the United States and was aimed at eliminating poverty. That such a program could command as much of the attention of a society that was, relatively speaking, as well off economically as United States society was at that time provides an important clue to the problem that the war on poverty addressed. Despite rising levels of the standard of living, the distribution of income within society was becoming increasingly skewed, with the poorest segments of society receiving a declining share of the economic pie (Levitan, 1969). The strategy of the war on poverty was to equalize opportunity for upward social mobility on the one hand, and to make available increased social resources on the other. While seeking to improve the condition of the poor, the programs of this strategy sought also to change the social and psychological characteristics of the poor so that they could participate more fully in society.

By the early 1960s it had become apparent that the huge expenditures of the many social welfare programs that were begun in the 1930s were not affecting the most serious problems. Roman and Schmais have summarized the primary assumptions behind the recognition that new and different approaches were needed during the 1960s:

> 1. The need for comprehensive efforts to deal with deep-rooted and interrelated social problems.

2. The recognition that the sources of these problems lay in the social structure.

3. The awareness that existing services and facilities were both unresponsive and inadequate in dealing with widespread need.

4. The development of community action competence, through the organization and involvement of residents, would be an important factor in devising effective solutions. (1972, p. 65)

In one of the major analyses of the war on poverty, Levitan (1969) delineates four purposes of these programs: mobilization and coordination of community resources, involvement of the poor, provision of jobs and improvement of employability through training, and stimulation of self-employment and the development of small businesses through loan programs. The center of these efforts was the Community Action Program, an innovative and controversial attempt to stimulate local responsibility and participation in programs dealing with social problems. We have discussed already the complications associated with the concept of "maximum feasible participation," but it should also be noted that the creation of the Office of Economic Opportunity at the federal level put this new office in potential conflict with federal bureaucracies that conducted existing programs, most notably the Department of Labor and the Department of Health, Education, and Welfare (Levitan, 1969; Moynihan, 1969); at the local level the Community Action Programs were in potential conflict with welfare departments and school districts, as well as with local government officials (Marris and Rein, 1967).

On a political level, Davidson (1969) observes that the planners of the war on poverty in the Johnson administration were wary of the ability of states to administer the new programs effectively because they represented an intermediate level of social structure, and because they feared that certain governors might try to obstruct the programs. Having before them the model of the Peace Corps working directly with citizens of foreign countries, the framers of these programs decided on a strategy of "the New Federalism" that would allocate funds directly to community groups and bypass the state and local governments that were judged to have been unresponsive to the needs of the poor in the conduct of the ineffective programs of the past. The Economic Opportunity Act of 1964, and its amendments of 1965, did not develop this concept in pure form, since provisions were made for governors to veto selected programs in their states, such as VISTA, but the OEO Director was authorized to reverse the vetoes after a thirty-day period.

It has been suggested that one of the motivating forces behind this program was the increasing concern in the Democratic party that the proportion of support that the party received from poor and black voters was declining, in part due to the newly gained enfranchisement of black voters in the South who had previously been unregistered because of state poll taxes or similar requirements, and because of the increased migration of southern blacks to northern urban areas, who were politically unsocialized (Roman and Schmais, 1972). Indeed, of thirty governors' vetoes of OEO programs during the first three years, at least some seem to have been for political effect:

> Governors Wallace of Alabama (both George and Lurleen) and Ronald Reagan of California were the champion vetoers, accounting for three of every five vetoes. While Governon Reagan's actions received considerable attention, the ten vetoes he exercised during his first year of office accounted for less than one percent of the total funds allocated by OEO to California; and some of the vetoed projects became effective after expiration of the thirty-day waiting period. (Davidson, 1969, p. 3)

A more explicit perception of the political challenge surfaced in Syracuse, New York, where the Republican mayor accused an OEO-funded political action training program of registering discontented poor, mostly Democratic, voters. Ultimately, the Syracuse grant was terminated, and the OEO extended the veto power to city and county officials as well. The Green amendment to the CAP legislation made it possible for local government officials to assume control of these programs, but 96 percent of the CAPs funded in 1968, prior to the Green amendment, were nongovernmental organizations, while government-sponsored CAPs were found in the larger cities (Davidson, 1969).

To dismiss this approach as mere national politics would be shortsighted. To be sure, any effective program will no doubt benefit the administration in office, but such programs might take several forms and certainly in this case could have taken less politically controversial ones. For example, another of the problems linked to poverty, and to these particular solutions, was that of manpower and employment. During the 1950s there had been increasing concern with the displacement of workers through automation and the inability of manufacturing segments of the economy to provide sufficient employment opportunities. From 1929 to 1963 there had been a 255 percent increase in output in the manufacturing sector, with only a 4 percent increase in the work force. During the same period a three-fold increase in the output of the service sector of the economy had required nearly a doubling of the manpower force in that area (Arnhoff, 1972). Furthermore, manpower shortages in the service area, particularly in health care and social services, were forecast (Albee, 1959).

If the continuous, although gradual, gains made in civil rights since the 1954 Supreme Court decision against school segregation were to have any meaning, additional job opportunities would have to be generated. While the early years of the Kennedy administration saw increased numbers of blacks employed by the federal government (Pettigrew, 1964), and although the Department of Labor argued forcefully for a jobs program (Levitan, 1969) as the main thrust of the poverty program, this is not the route that was chosen. While a jobs program could have been clearly effective in promoting votes, the planners of the war on poverty had their attention on other factors. One of these was the widely assumed apathy of the poor; another was the assumption that unemployability was as large a problem as unemployment, that is, that lack of relevant skills was tied in with lack of opportunity; and, finally, that many areas inhabited by the poor lacked community organization and structure. These considerations, along with a history of concern with community development that was coming to particular historical salience at that time, combined to form a programmatic thrust that not only was concerned with economic improvement, but saw economic problems closely associated with social and psychological conditions.

While the concept of community organization is traced by a number of writers to the development of community organizations in Chicago in the 1930s to combat delinquency (Clark, 1964; Rubin, 1969), in fact, the origins of this movement can be traced to the latter part of the nineteenth century in the form of the settlement houses, such as Jane Addams's Hull House in Chicago, which were established to provide a means of integration into society for numerous European immigrants (Levine and Levine, 1970). Indeed, many of the social problems, solutions, and political obstacles seen during the 1960s were strikingly similar to those described by the Levines in their insightful book. They attribute the social problems of that era to the difficulties encountered by newly arrived immigrants in assimilating into the social structure of the United States, and they draw a convincing analogy to the problems of blacks attempting to "immigrate" into largely northern American society in the 1960s, and to the similarity of the programs developed to deal with them.

The events that shaped the particular form of the antipoverty program were more recent, however. During the 1950s, concern over the increasing population in central cities, which strained available urban resources, had stimulated the Ford Foundation's "gray areas programs," which attempted to mobilize community resources to recognize and solve these problems (Marris and Rein, 1967). Kenneth Clark (1968) traces the origins of the community participation aspects of the antipoverty programs through four stages. Beginning with the concern with providing increased services to deal with the problem of juvenile delinquency, which had proven ineffective, he cites the next phase as the programs initiated under the President's Committee on Juvenile Delinquency and Youth Crime in 1961. Based in part on a modernized version of the sociologist Durkheim's views of the effects of anomie (Cloward, 1959), in which it was reasoned that youth turned to illegitimate means for achieving goals when the access to legitimate means was blocked, and in part on Leonard Cottrell's concepts of individual and community competence (Cottrell, 1964), these programs sought to use youth and community involvement as a preventive approach to delinquency. Among the sixteen programs funded under this act, Harlem Youth Opportunities Unlimited (HARYOU) is perhaps the best known. The strategy of community involvement led to the participation of youths and adults in the Harlem area in self-help programs, including membership on the governing boards. The program evolved into a series of economic and civil rights actions, which quickly put it in conflict with the city's political establishment.

In the third phase, the concept of community participation developed in these earlier programs was carried over into the broadened conception of social intervention in the OEO programs, which, rather than focusing on community organization as such, provided for the participation of the poor, or their representatives, in the planning of the programs. The role of participation, however, was never well defined, as has been discussed in Chapter 3. Probably more than any other factor, the resistance of local establishments to the threat of change in the social structure posed by these programs led to a coalescence between community action programs and the increasing civil rights militancy of the day, with its emphasis on black separatism. Thus, the fourth phase identified by Clark was the emphasis on community control of the programs, as a response to the perceived resistance.

The loose alliance between federal planners and community activists bypassed local officials not only in an administrative sense, but also in the important sense that in at least a few communities such programs had been a reservoir for dispensable political favors in the past. If CAP activities were to provide increased employment opportunities in public jobs for poor people, there were suddenly increased potential opportunities for local politicians to reward constituents with employment. In short, as these programs affected the political and social structure of the community, the elements of that structure began to resist and react. Moreover, during the late 1960s riots broke out in many urban areas, particularly in Detroit and Newark, which had been the recipients of large amounts of federal funds for such programs. The riots provided an engaging stimulus for diverting blame onto the antipoverty programs, despite the fact that this was not the finding of the Kerner Commission, which investigated the causes of the riots. Despite claims that the war on poverty was "stirring up the poor," poor persons in many target cities actually received a minority of the funds. Of the OEO money provided, poor persons received 30 percent of the Detroit funds, 44 percent of the Newark funds, and 42 percent of the New Haven, Connecticut, funds (National Advisory Commission on Civil Disorders, 1968, p. 80). Following these events there was a steady erosion of funding, and debate and political machination continued over the future of OEO. Any of those who were working with such programs during this time observed the markedly reduced effectiveness that ensued as job insecurity became a fact of life and plans could not be made realistically beyond the end of the next year's funding expiration.

The participation of social scientists in these programs was evident from the planning stages to the implementation of programs, involving workers from virtually every discipline in almost every conceivable sort of role. Psychologists, sociologists, and social workers were employed in government and nongovernment roles as researchers, evaluators, implementers, and advocates. The simultaneous development of increased service programs, such as community mental health centers and community organization programs, often involved professionals in conflicting roles of service providers and community participants. During this same time the role of the community psychologist began to emerge, with the same conflicts and confusions that characterized much of the activity of that time. We will attempt to construct here a somewhat organized view of the activities of community psychologists in what constituted the social action model.

Assumptions

The basic assumptions underlying the social action model have been articulated best, and most often, by Robert Reiff. A former laborer and labor organizer, Reiff obtained his Ph.D. in clinical psychology at the University of Kansas, where he was also exposed to the ecological psychology of Roger Barker. Many of the assumptions were presented in Reiff's address as the first president of the Division of Community Psychology of the American Psychological Association, in 1967.

The first assumption is that traditional psychological views of human behavior are excessively intrapsychic, influenced heavily as they are by psychoanalytic theory, and give insufficient attention to social factors. When social factors are included, they are generally in the form of interpersonal concepts. As Reiff puts it, "Such tangible social conditions as housing and transportation, or even such nontangible social conditions as literacy and free speech, play little or no role in the clinician's conceptualizations of individual behavior" (Reiff, 1968, p. 525). While asserting that the fact of mental illness cannot be denied, Reiff feels that the psychiatric model of illness is an inadequate base for a psychology of social problems inasmuch as it defines normality by concepts derived from the behavior of the mentally ill and equates abnormality with mental illness, that is, with individual defects or deficiency. More than just on a theoretical level, these assumptions are deeply embedded in the policies and practices of many social agencies dealing with social problems, but are simply inadequate for an understanding of individual behavior at the social level, or for understanding the behavior of large groups of people by extrapolation. This limitation poses a significant obstacle for addressing the problem of services for poor people who are alienated both from such concepts and from the social institutions that embody them.

Further, Reiff feels that the traditional psychological assumptions obscure an understanding of the real problems faced by society. Thus, the second assumption is that the level of understanding that is required is a perspective in which the primary object is an aggregate of people and factors that affect their normal—that is, usual—behavior. Thus, there is a need for a body of knowledge about how social systems effect psychological reactions, as well as a knowledge of the operation and modification of social systems themselves. Perhaps nowhere is this better illustrated than in the outbreak of violence that followed the gains in civil rights and economic opportunity. Just as a social system appeared about to be doing something about conditions that had been tolerated for years, these conditions became suddenly intolerable. Thus, the concept of relative deprivation and the dynamic social power of hope are seen as more powerful psychological forces than the past histories of individual deprivation and whatever presumed deficits or personal conflicts these might have engendered.

Just as many of the concepts of traditional clinical psychology are focused on internal processes, so are they largely derived from and related to concepts that are relevant for a middle-class way of life. Reiff feels that a psychology of self-actualization is unrealistic for the poor and that the emphasis should be on self-determination. While many of the problems that face poor people are very real manifestations of their social position, the psychological impact of their relationship to the social structure is a sense of powerlessness. Thus, a second assumption is that interventions should have self-determination as their goal. However, Reiff does not believe that this goal can be approached from a focus on the autonomy of the individual; rather, he believes that there must be a concentration on the concept of freedom in society (Reiff, 1975). This point of view ties these first two assumptions together.

A third assumption has to do with a further questioning of the usual perspectives on the relationship between man and society. Reiff quotes Plato as saying that society is man writ large, and points to the Freudian view of man's inherent biosocial conflicts as consistent with the traditional American view of individualism. He also quotes Marx as saying that man is society writ small, but he asserts that both the Freudian and Marxist views are wrong in that they assume an isomorphic relationship between man and society that Reiff does not believe exists in that simple form, whichever point of view one takes. Examination of the true nature of the relationship between man and society may lead to a more viable approach to social problems and their psychological counterparts, Reiff believes. What is suggested is a quest for new knowledge about social structures and individuals, with an emphasis on social, rather than individual, values. Rather than presenting a systematized theory, this model makes assumptions about the nature of the theory that is required, and, admitting that an adequate theory is not at hand, suggests a pursuit of knowledge about the concepts that are relevant to this level of concern through participation in and analysis of elements of social policy. Strong emphasis is placed on how the definition of problems effects subsequent interventions, and on the applicability of "participant-conceptualization" to generating the required knowledge.

Like the organizational model, the social action model values participation. However, it takes a more explicit stance toward the question of redistribution of power. One might say that while the organizational model works from the top down to encourage power sharing, the social action model works from the bottom up to assist those in the underprivileged class to press for their share of power. It is instructive to note that the assumptions of the organizational model imply that it is in the best interests of the organization to share power in this way. Where the organizational model is successful, this assumption is shared by management. It is difficult to find an example of a total community where this attitude toward the sharing of power—i.e., that it is in the best interests of the community—exists. While the conditions addressed by these two models have some similarities, there are also some important differences. The management of an organization would seem to have less difficulty seeing the workers in the organization as part of the same social system they inhabit than the "managers" of a community seem to have in seeing the poor and minority groups as part of the same social system, particularly where this view of "includedness" is contrary to social norms, cultural traditions, or institutional beliefs. Accordingly, the social action model assumes that the "power structure" of a community tends to be unaware of the needs and desires of the poor and the alienated, and does not necessarily share the assumption that it is in the community's interest to share power.

Typical Interventions

Two major interventions were suggested by the form of the legislation enacted during the 1960s, which can be seen as instrumental, in theory at least, to meeting the multidimensional goals of those programs. One of these was the development of members of the target population as service workers in the new programs. The other was the organization of consumers of services to control the activities of the programs.

THE INDIGENOUS NONPROFESSIONAL

Despite the unfortunate connotations of this term, a more accurately descriptive euphemism has not yet been developed. The strategy behind the training of residents of program target areas as case aides, outreach workers, or facilitators, was designed to serve a number of goals. First, inasmuch as it was known that the intended recipients of these services were not inclined to utilize such services, it was assumed that these new employees could provide a liaison function with the community that the community members would be more likely to trust, and thus encourage use of services. Second, since it was known that the professionals providing many of the services were unfamiliar with the felt needs of the recipients, the nonprofessional worker could provide important input into planning of programs that would be more relevant to the needs of potential recipients. Third, the increased employment opportunities thus created would provide "new careers" for the poor, which were needed both by the employees and by the service sector of the economy, particularly in the health services (Pearl and Riessman, 1965; Reiff and Riessman, 1965; Riessman and Scribner, 1965).

Finestone and Sobey (1969) surveyed 185 projects that used a total of 10,417 nonprofessional workers, primarily in hospital settings. There were thirteen different job titles employed, ranging from "tutor-teacher aides" to nursing and ward personnel. The majority of the projects employed more nonprofessional than professional personnel. Over half the workers were females, with males occupying fewer job categories, mainly case aides. The majority of the workers had high school educations or more, leading to the conclusion that those with less than high school education were underselected. About 40 percent of the workers could be considered "indigenous," that is, with problems similar to those in the target populations.

The researchers found that the nonprofessional staff were highly valued by their employers, more than anything else for their ability to provide informal support and communication with the clientele of the projects. They also found that the use of nonprofessionals created some interpersonal and role problems within the projects, which caused the agencies to examine themselves more critically, and sometimes painfully.

A survey of nonprofessionals employed in mental health facilities (NIMH, 1970) as of January 1968 showed over 138,000 persons employed as attendants and aides or mental health workers. Of these, 14,596 were in the latter category. These positions had the lowest vacancy rates of all positions, professional and nonprofessional, listed. The largest percentage of these, however, were employed in state and county mental hospitals, while the smallest number were employed in outpatient psychiatric clinics. Of 221 such workers listed as employed in outpatient facilities, 128 were in New York State, while the largest state in use of nonprofessional mental health workers in state and county mental hospitals was North Carolina, with a total of 1,012. While there is obviously a difference between states in the number of these different types of facilities available, these figures do indicate quite different usage of nonprofessionals in different localities.

The Lincoln Hospital Community Mental Health Center, serving an urban ghetto in the South Bronx in New York City, had a program for utilization of nonprofessional mental health workers that was widely cited as a model for the employment of the nonprofessional strategy. Nonprofessional workers were utilized in three functional roles: direct service, community organizer or neighborhood worker, and facilitator or expediter who served to link clients with appropriate services (Kaplan, Boyajian, and Meltzer, 1970). In the Lincoln program, one important function of the indigenous nonprofessional was to function literally as a translator, since 60 percent of the target population were Puerto Rican, and many did not speak English. But there are many cultural and social factors that create barriers between the professional services offered and the orientation of the residents of the service area, barriers that could only be overcome by the nonprofessional worker.

A detailed plan for the selection and training of the ten applicants for every position in the Lincoln program is described by Jacobson, Roman, and Kaplan (1970). It is clear from their account that they realized the sensitive nature of the relationships between the institution and the community, of which they and the nonprofessional were the respective representatives. Trainees were given a core of training in the mental health field, followed by on-the-job training through supervision.

However, in 1969, the Lincoln Hospital program was wracked by what has variously been termed a "strike," a "work stoppage," or a "confrontation" (Shaw and Eagle, 1971), centering on the issue of community control of the program. This event really has two separate but interwoven implications for our discussion here. While we will consider the issue of community control later, there are aspects of the role of the nonprofessional worker that relate to this problem, also, although they have larger implications for the occupational role itself.

A serious limitation in the nonprofessional worker strategy is the question of a career ladder. It was known before these programs were undertaken that the majority of positions that those eligible for nonprofessional roles could enter initially were low-paying, dead-end jobs, with no career ladder for advancement without considerable further training. This, of course, accounted for the large unfilled need at this level. Arnhoff (1972) notes the difficulties in recruiting workers for these positions, even with increased funds available, because the positions are largely in the health and welfare fields that traditionally are seen as women's jobs. Indeed, the majority of workers recruited to these positions have been women, and the turnover rate has remained high.

An inherent issue in such positions is the relationship of the nonprofessional to the professional, with questions bound to arise over the functions that nonprofessionals would be allowed to perform versus the prerogatives of the professionals to claim certain types of tasks as their own. Often these nonprofessional positions were characterized by unclear job specifications, as is understandable in a time of innovation, but the functional ambiguity of job domain has also contributed to the problems. Underlying this problem is the question of continued low status for such workers, who are at the same time told they are indispensable for the success of the program. Thus, the limitations of the absence of a career ladder and role ambiguity tend to reinforce each other in creating intraagency tension.

Added to these difficulties is the further problem of role-strain. The nonprofessional worker is often placed in the conflicting position of being an employee of an institution and being expected to represent an alienated segment of the population in its demands for change from that institution. To expect persons placed in such a situation of divided loyalties to be effective agents of social change while occupying the lowest status positions in the organizations they are expected to change, and to keep their jobs at the same time, is totally unrealistic. The worker thus conflicted has open only the alternatives of quitting the job or agitating for community control. Faced with power struggles between their own position and others within the institution, and power struggles between the institution and the community, it is indeed surprising that the Lincoln Hospital incident was not repeated more often.

The nonprofessional worker continues to be of importance in the service-delivery system. In mental health programs, social services, and educational settings nonprofessional workers continue to be used, despite the fact that the "New Careers" program has been eliminated. Karlsruher (1974) has reviewed the literature on the use of nonprofessionals as psychotherapeutic agents and finds that they are clearly effective in working with adult psychotic inpatients, probably effective in working with adult outpatients, but that the research to demonstrate their effectiveness with other groups, or in comparison with professionals, has not yet been conducted. Cowen and his associates (Cowen, Dorr, Izzo, Madonia, and Trost, 1971; Dorr and Cowen, 1973; Dorr, Cowen, and Kraus, 1973) have found the nonprofessional workers to be effective in a program of secondary prevention with school children in an economically disadvantaged area. Sandler, Duricko, and Grande (1975) replicated these results in an area that was similarly economically deprived, and which included a large percentage of children of Mexican-American descent.

The nonprofessional worker is clearly a valuable addition in the field of human services for the unique contribution that that worker can make to delivering services. The use of the nonprofessional has not been a successful strategy, however, in changing the distribution of social power. The question of power is a central one in the social action model. We will turn now to consideration of another type of intervention, the quest for community control.

COMMUNITY CONTROL

Traditionally, the participation of citizens in health and social service functions has been a middle- or upper-class domain, characterized by serving on agency boards or funding organizations. Typically, there has been no conflict between citizens and program administration, as there has been agreement on the values and goals of such programs between the participants and the administration (Roman and Schmais, 1972).

This sharing of values and goals did not exist between the same administrators and the intended recipients of programs designed to serve the poor. The confusion generated by the concept of consumer participation has been noted already in Chapter 3 and earlier in this chapter. This confusion was not one-sided, however, and the conflicts that have arisen over community control seem to have resulted more than anything else from resistance at the administrative level to meaningful participation by the poor as the poor defined it, which coalesced with the development of racial militancy and the community organization emphasis of many of the programs.

Reiff, Levin, and their co-workers in the Lincoln Hospital programs (Levin, 1970) were concerned from the beginning with the question of community organization and self-determination referred to earlier. Their strategy was to increase the competence of the residents of the target population to solve their own problems. Requests for new programs or services were handled by involving the residents in the preparation of grant requests, collecting relevant data, and meeting with the appropriate governmental bodies to request such services. While the psychologists served as consultants to the residents, the emphasis was on the organization and participation of the residents as a means of increasing both their skills and their sense of efficacy.

This approach is, of course, consistent with both the spirit of the antipoverty legislation and the recent history of a number of social programs in New York, referred to earlier. As Roman and Schmais put it:

> The central ideological contribution of the major government-initiated efforts has been the recognition, *as reflected in public policy*, that specific social problems (juvenile delinquency, youth employment, inadequate health care, mental illness) can only be understood and affected in terms of broader pathologies such as poverty, institutional elitism, economic disenfranchisement, and racial discrimination. (1972, p. 70. Italics in original.)

In the midst of the political and poverty implications of these programs, it should not be overlooked that the community organization strategy has important implications in its own right concerning the prevention of social problems. A wealth of literature suggests that highly cohesive groups have higher morale and productivity (Shaw, 1971), and that mental health problems are lower in both cohesive combat units (Kardiner and Spiegel, 1947) and in well-organized communities (Leighton *et al.*, 1963). Typically, poverty areas are characterized by social disorganization and powerlessness, relative to more affluent areas.

Traditionally, American ideology holds that the individual is responsible for his or her economic fate; thus, it would follow from this ideology that the poor are poor because they are deficient in some way and therefore unable to organize themselves or to participate in organizations. The goal of organization following this ideology would be to teach social skills through the process of organization. However, if one assumes that the poor are poor because they have been systematically excluded from opportunities to participate in community institutions, and that this exclusion puts them in a position of powerlessness, then different consequences for organizational strategies follow. Organization would be planned for the purpose of seeking greater power. It should be noted that the term power as used here does not necessarily connote influence over others, but rather the power of self-determination, which implies freedom from being controlled by others and freedom to participate in planning and policymaking that affects them directly.

In either case, the task of community organization is a formidable one. Traditionally, social programs have been provided to the poor in the name of individual improvement; the poor have tended to be apathetic toward these programs. The same degree of apathy exists toward community organization, however. Roman and Schmais have noted some of the factors contributing to this kind of apathy: "(1) hostility and cynicism toward political involvement; (2) deep-rooted distrust based on unkept promises of the past; (3) exposure to indignities and insult at neighborhood agencies in the present; (4) a lack of skills necessary to sustain organizational momentum; and (5) the soft and, sometimes, intangible nature of health and mental health problems which may not be immediately apparent" (1972, p. 76).

While much has been written about the dependency of the poor, it should be made clear that this term refers to economic dependency, not to personality characteristics usually connoted by the term dependency. Similarly, the concept of disorganization must be seen relative to the larger economic and social system; it does not imply that there is not a degree of social organization within the urban ghetto. It is perhaps ironic that the major organizational linkages with the larger society are crime (Clark, 1970) and politics. In addition to the economic dependencies of the ghetto population, the traditional attitude of service providers that the consumers are dependent on services whose plans and policies are made by others creates a political dependency that reinforces the sense of powerlessness. As conceptualized in the social action model, the community control strategy is designed to address what is seen as a central element in the maintenance of these dependency-generating structures: social power.

Within this perspective, it is possible to view the Lincoln Hospital event as both a success and a failure. While conflicting accounts of the event have been given, it is clear that the central conflict was one of power. Some accounts tend to blame the radicalizing and inflaming of the nonprofessionals by ideologues on the staff as being responsible for the conflict, while others fault the lack of faith on the part of the hospital in what they saw as a commitment to community control (Shaw and Eagle, 1971). The precipitating event seems to have been the successful application for a community mental health center staffing grant, obtained in 1968. More than anything else, this grant seems to have signaled a decrease in perceived community control, the relative deprivation of which Reiff has spoken.

The fact that the grant would be so perceived demonstrates that the residents of the area had developed some feeling of participation and at least the expectation of power sharing. The employment of nonprofessionals from the area can thus be seen as a central part of that strategy, providing a linkage to the existing social organization of the population. The strike itself is testimony to overcoming apathy. On the side of administration, however, the event indicates a lack of education as to how the program was perceived by the residents of the community, or a lack of commitment to sharing of power, or both. Thus, while apathy may have been overcome, economic and political dependency were not, as indicated by the precipitating issue—an event that raised the question of control of funds and, subsequently, programs.

There is some evidence that community participation increases the utilization of services by the poor (Roman and Schmais, 1972), increases the effectiveness of educational programs (Sandler, Duricko, and Grande, 1975; Schiff, 1972), and is viewed as beneficial in mental health programs where it has been implemented (Windle, Bass, and Taube, 1974). At the same time, it is clear that participation by service recipients has not been widely employed. In their review of community mental health programs, Windle, Bass, and Taube (1974) found that few centers have accomplished meaningful involvement of consumers in planning and policymaking, and that this deficiency is cited more than any other in evaluations of mental health center programs.

In a study of the effectiveness of seventeen Community Action Programs in creating change in educational programs, Babarick (1975) hypothesized five social change strategies employed by these programs. These were: creating an alliance with those who had resources or influence, such as a university, church, or industry; integrating cognitive processes with emotional and socializing functions that were appropriate for the group served; maintenance and utilization of a cadre of professionals who could confront professionals in established positions on an equal level of status and expertise; moving resources into "community no-man's land," where services or programs did not exist; and maintaining a change-agent posture outside the traditional local community system. He then tested these hypotheses by determining whether or not these tactics were used by four agencies that were judged effective and six agencies that were judged ineffective in achieving community development goals. The agencies were selected so that they were geographically dispersed, although all but one of them represented urban areas. The results indicated that the successful agencies could be distinguished from the unsuccessful ones by their use of the first four hypothesized tactics, while the fifth tactic, maintaining a change-agent posture outside the system did not consistently discriminate successful and unsuccessful programs. However, one of the ineffective programs, the only one located in a rural area, employed three of the five hypothesized tactics. Since the rural program contributes the largest source of inconsistency in the data, it may be that the results should be considered to apply mainly to urban, but not necessarily to rural, programs.

It is clear that the conflicts and excesses generated in these programs have commanded more than their share of attention, making the programs vulnerable to their political detractors. People are more likely to read headlines than research reports. The conflicts that occurred can be viewed from a social-psychological perspective as a reverse form of relative deprivation. That is, when the powerless demanded to share in social power, this was perceived by those who had power as a potential illegitimate loss, even though they probably would have retained the greater amount of power. Rather than seeing community control efforts as directed at self-determination, they appear to have seen them as a win-or-lose proposition in which losing would mean being controlled.

This perception of the situation is referred to as a "zero-sum game" by game theorists, one in which whatever one party wins, the other loses (Thibaut and Kelley, 1959). This perception results in turn from the participants' seeing themselves in competition for control of a single community subsystem. Had either participant defined the situation differently, the zero-sum condition would not have existed. Advances in community development and reduction of community conflict could have resulted from the authorities' seeing that it is in the interest of the community social system to allow meaningful participation, but they evidently did not see it that way and there is no evidence that it was ever presented to them in that fashion by those seeking control.

"Changing the social structure" is a different-sounding battle cry than "sharing in the determination of policy," yet the difference in what these phrases mean to various audiences is a subtle and elusive one. Overall, the scene is testimony to the difficulties of blending federally conceived programs with the political and social realities of the local community. The community action programs, and others like them, contained the possibilities of meaningful community participation, but the federal plans failed to spell out and deal with the issues of social structure and vested interest. Instead, they attempted to bypass them. When the federal programs failed to back up the autonomy of the local programs, the poor and their local allies were left to fight a political battle without reinforcements. As one community action program director said of the war on poverty, "The sword is too short." The poor fought a battle, and they lost. The war continues, but with greatly reduced resources. The successor strategy to these programs, federal revenue sharing, has played directly to the existing political structures, and, consequently, an incomparably smaller amount of funding has been devoted to programs for human services at the local level, the money going instead largely to sewer and road construction.

As Reiff has noted, the residual impact of these programs has been to demonstrate that the poor can become involved in efforts on their own behalf, and to make society more aware of the nature of the problems to be faced. The issues of freedom and consumer participation have been broadened to the population in general (Roman and Schmais, 1972). The programs have not, however, alleviated either poverty or the manpower questions (Mangum, 1969). Perhaps more than any other contribution, they have demonstrated that these problems are not problems of personal deficiencies, but problems of social structure.

These efforts at community organization have created opportunities for leadership that were not previously available. They undoubtedly contributed to the development of competence and skill on the part of many individuals and some community areas, opening up an opportunity structure for at least some individual members of those communities. However, these same reasons were the ones the author heard once from a southern school administrator in justifying segregated schools; that is, that minorities would have fewer opportunities for leadership in integrated schools. They have not contributed materially to social integration, and whether the gains made outweigh the disappointment and disillusionment that followed remains to be seen.

Typical Research

The 1960s must have been one of the most heavily socially researched decades in history. Particularly following the urban ghetto riots, the residents of the areas in which these disturbances took place were interviewed by social psychologists and sociologists seeking attitudinal bases for the riots; to the point that it became a common joke that the next riot would be a reaction against social scientists. The broad-scale social programs implemented during this time called for massive evaluative research efforts. As with the programs themselves, however, the research process became strongly politicized.

Research at this level presents numerous difficulties; selection of appropriate definitions of criteria, use of appropriate control groups, and the control of numerous coacting factors such as economic and political trends, maturation effects of samples (particularly young persons), and changes in programs. For example, suppose one develops an alternative educational program designed to reduce the number of school dropouts. Over a three-year period it may develop that employment opportunities for those with less than a high school education may increase in that locality, increasing the incentive to drop out; or the opposite may occur; with a decline in job opportunities, more students may elect to remain in school. Neither of these effects could be attributable to the educational program. Similarly, a major factor with the antipoverty programs was that any gains made were more than wiped out by inflation in the economy.

One of the major problems with research of this type is the problem of "weak effects" (Rossi, 1970). This is particularly a problem in a highly affluent, highly educated society. In times of economic depression, when large numbers of people are out of work, it is relatively easy to demonstrate gains in employment or earnings with virtually any intervention that results in improvement. However, in an economy that has a high employment level, additional gains are going to be only marginal because of "ceiling effects" and will be hard to demonstrate. A similar limitation affects educational interventions. Where the rate of literacy is low, any educational program may show a large increase in literacy; where it is already high, gains in educational attainment that are greater than the errors of measurement in the assessment devices are difficult to show. Such gains as are made are likely to be sufficiently undramatic that their interpretation may be ambiguous and subject to disagreement and debate. Thus, the two major factors of multiply determined problems and weak effects of intervention make research interpretation in this area extremely difficult.

It is not surprising, then, that the findings of national studies, such as those of the Kerner Commission (National Advisory Commission on Civil Disorders, 1968) and the evaluation of Project Head Start (Westinghouse Learning Corporation–Ohio University, 1969) would be subject to dispute and political manipulation (Lipsky, 1971; Williams and Evans, 1969). In Lipsky's account of the riot commission study, there was considerable controversy between the social scientists conducting the research and the commission lawyers who were to put the report together over what was to be included and how the interpretations were to be worded. In the Head Start evaluation, primary emphasis was given to evaluating gains in intellectual development, despite the fact that Head Start also made important contributions in health care, nutrition, and parent involvement. Seldom taken into account in evaluating these programs is the fact that the majority of Head Start children did not have such services available to them except at costs they could not afford. This is a question of coverage, rather than impact, and research would only need to demonstrate that services were being delivered sufficiently to those in need. The question of impact, on health as well as intellectual development, is another question. The proof of the popularity of Head Start is perhaps best exemplified by the fact that the program is still continuing and is one of the few to maintain a meaningful role for parental involvement, despite the spirited controversy over intellectual gains that the program sparked in academic circles in the well-known "Jensen debate" (Jensen, 1969; Cronbach, 1969; Jencks, 1969; Silberman, 1970).

Accordingly, not only are research findings likely to be subject to the political process, but the implementation and maintenance of programs themselves are, as well. In a study particularly germane to this topic, Aiken (1969) conducted a survey of different communities to determine the factors that influenced their decision to adopt innovative programs requiring mobilization of community forces. He was particularly interested in the relationship between the adoption of programs and the type of power structure that characterized that community.

He used measures of the degree to which thirty one communities participated in four federal programs: public housing, Urban Renewal, Model Cities, and the war on poverty. These measures were correlated with an index of diffusion of community power that located the communities as one of four types of power structure: pyramidal, factional, coalitional, or amorphous; from most centralized to most diffused. His results supported the hypothesis that the implementation of these programs was associated with more diffuse power structures. However, the effects were weak, and it was impossible to separate the diffuseness of power variables from the fact that the communities with more diffuse power were also more diverse in their demographic structure, including such factors as racial and socioeconomic composition of the population. He concluded that the effectiveness of particular organizations around particular issues would be a more appropriate level of analysis than would be the community as a whole.

Aiken's results concerning the power structure are thus confounded with the nature of the issues, having to do with concerns that are heavily weighted with racial and poverty implications. Subsequent studies concerning other issues, not so laden with these latter concerns, might shed more light on the relationship between power and innovation. Thus, an approach akin to that recommended by Campbell and Fiske (1959) concerning the assessment of personality characteristics would seem to be applicable here, that is, the use of multiple methods to assess multiple manifestations of both program and power structure variables.

Guttentag (1972) presented data on the effects of a community-controlled school district in Harlem on a number of educational, personal, and social variables. She found improvements in the social climate of the school, participation of parents, children's achievement and sense of personal identity in the community-controlled school district, compared to a neighboring centrally controlled district. While these results appear to support the concept of community control for educational purposes, it is impossible to determine the effect of history in this particular district's becoming community controlled; that is, it could be that there was something about the parents of these particular children that led them to become more militant in seeking community control of the educational institution. Neither do we know what the long-term effects of such an intervention will be. These are not meant as criticisms of the research itself; rather they are factors that are typically not considered in the planning and implementation of such social experiments. From what we know about socialization practices, for example, it is reasonable to assume that the important long-term effects of any of these social policy innovations will be the extent to which they influence social norms that can provide a cultural context for sustaining whatever gains may be made in the short run, whether with racial or economic problems. It is unlikely that such effects can be meaningfully assessed in less than a two-generation time span.

The multiple-time-period, multiple-criteria approach is necessary not only to assess the long-term experimental impact of such programs, but also to assess the occurrence of unintended consequences. Papers written about the success of the Lincoln Hospital nonprofessional program, for example, apparently did not anticipate the disruptive events that were to occur before some of the papers appeared in print. On a longer-term basis, the movement for community control in the middle sixties could not have anticipated the large-scale social reactions to the Vietnam war, the change in student culture that accompanied that reaction, and the spread of consumer concern to the economy at large. It is clear that this generalized concern with community control does not have the same implications for changes in the social structure as those who developed the concept in working with poorer segments of the population had envisioned.

Probably the most significant aspect of research in the social action model, however, is a change in the purpose of research and the perspective from which it is done. In part because of reactions from those who were the subjects of such intense research activity during the 1960s, and in part because of the strategy of the social action model, social research has taken on a different character.

For years, social scientists had conducted research studies using subjects who were never informed as to what the researcher learned from the study. If there was anything of direct relevance for them in the research, seldom if ever were these results fed back to the participants. It must be admitted that the conduct of such research sometimes appeared to be quite cavalier to the subjects. Partly in reaction to this attitude, partly because there was a dawning realization that social scientists were building their own careers through the subjects who did not see any benefit for them in the research, and partly because the subject groups disagreed with some of the interpretations that were made from the research, such subjects became increasingly resistant, even hostile, toward research participation. While some of this reaction was interpreted as an "experimenter bias" effect, owing to the racial or social-class differences between researcher and subject, and attempts were made to correct for this bias by employing racially or ethnically matched researchers and subjects, it is clear that a major thrust of this reaction was that the poor and minority subjects of these studies were demanding a piece of the research action, too. The often dramatic contrast of the white, middle-class researcher with research subjects was an all-too-obvious indication of the researcher's status as a representative of the "establishment."

As a consequence, organized groups that emerged during this time began to demand a voice in the research that was conducted, and to obtain knowledge of the results. The study conducted by Guttentag mentioned earlier was specifically requested by the parents in the community-controlled school district, *who outlined the questions that they wanted answered.* This tendency has since spread to become policy in many, if not all, school systems and other community institutions. The author conducted a research study in a police department that had established a policy that the design of the study was to be reviewed by the police department prior to the collection of data, and any publication of the results was subject to the approval of the department. Thus, again, a policy that began in the response of disadvantaged groups spread to become adopted by other community institutions.

Involvement of subjects in research was a key principle of the social action model itself, however, as part of the strategy of improving the self-help skills of the population being served. At the annual meeting of the American Psychological Association in 1969, which was devoted to the theme "Psychology and the Problems of Society," George Miller, then president of the association, urged psychologists to "give psychology away to the people" (Miller, 1969). Those psychologists who followed the social action model had been doing just that some years prior to this exhortation.

Teaching the residents of poverty areas to conduct their own research as part of the process of helping them gain skills in grant applications, and thus improving their ability to gain control over funds, has been one of the important aspects of this strategy. Arthur Pearl (1970) tells an amusing but all too poignant story of a group of adolescents whom he had trained in some of the basic principles of research design confronting a sociologist with some of the flaws in the design of a study that he was about to conduct on them.

To subsume these changes under the rubric of "relevance" hardly does justice to the significance of this rather new direction in research, particularly in view of the triteness that has come to be associated with that term. The concept that research conducted with and for disadvantaged groups should be useful and meaningful for them is certainly consistent with the use of research in many other fields. Because of this fact, the degree of rhetoric and rationalization that has been expended to justify this type of research is some testimony to the irrationality of the objections sometimes raised to its legitimacy. It does not follow that all research should or must meet the same criteria of "relevance." This is, after all, a debate that is more germane to concern with academic careers, having to do with the setting of the university rather than the setting of the community.

In the university setting, emphasis tends to be placed on two defining qualities of research: elegance of research design and the development of a "research program" by the individual researcher, which indicates a progression of research on the same type of problem in such a way that it promises to lead to some greater ultimate contribution to knowledge. Both of these requirements are obviously met much more easily in laboratory research than in field research. It is also true, however, that there is an inherent tendency for the well-designed, relatively quickly accomplished laboratory studies to be confined to problems of such limited scope that their generalization to the real world is limited, while those questions that are of more immediate relevance to the real world are more difficult to study through the use of elegant research design. In part, the fault lies in assuming, falsely, that the model of physical science research should be the criterion for judging social research. But the problem is also compounded by the fact that adequate research studies of this nature require large quantities of resources, usually in the form of government grants, to sustain them. Unfortunately, the priorities for funding research change as the political policies and concerns of government change, making it difficult to sustain such research over the time periods required. In the 1960s many universities established "urban affairs institutes," utilizing, and providing a funnel for, research funds that were available from the government. As priorities changed from, say, studying the causes of riots during the 1960s to studying how to control social unrest in the 1970s, funds were suddenly unavailable, and either the focus of these research institutes changed or they went out of business.

While these factors contribute to the instability of university-based programs for the study of social problems, the implications of these policies for the poor are clearly more devastating. Besides communicating a lack of commitment from the larger society, and a sense that their importance to that society is dependent on what happens to be fashionable at the moment, this policy leaves open the equally serious question of who will serve to demonstrate the needs of the poor to the rest of society through research. Thus, that aspect of the social action model that involves the poor in conducting research on their own problems assumes more importance.

Typical Settings

Many of the adherents of the social action model have been persons who work in university or community mental health settings, or both. While either of these settings may provide a somewhat appropriate setting for this model, depending upon its commitment to community participation, the fact that social policy concerns must compete with other priorities in such settings is a very real limitation. The ideal setting for this model is the Community Action Program, or those agencies of community organization that perform functions similar to such programs (Reiff, 1966). By their very nature, they are likely both to employ members of the community and to be open to community participation or control.

Levin (1970) describes her work as that of an employee of the community that ran the multiservice center. It was mentioned previously that Guttentag's research was done in response to questions to which the community members wanted answers. The theme here is accountability of the professional to the community, and it is a central part of the social action model. While much has been written, said, and formulated about "accountability" in both social legislation and politics, this self-concept of the professional as community employee captures the spirit of what is intended by the term better than much of what has been forthcoming in either legislation or political debate.

During the 1970s, the programs of the community action agencies have been drastically reduced, and whether the community action agency or some similar counterpart will endure as a meaningful community agency is problematic. No similar community structure is presently visible that could provide the basis for community control and participation within a specifically targeted set of programs, as did the concept of the community action program. At the same time, however, many of the principles of citizen participation, accountability, and employment of indigenous workers that marked these programs have at least gained normative legitimacy, if not reality, in community institutions. For example, legislation enacted in the 1970s, providing federal funding of state social service programs, has mandated that the planning of such programs receive citizen input and review. Despite the fact that much of the visibility and the "social action" over community action programs has diminished, these principles are an important legacy of those programs.

Perhaps the setting for the social action model is not the appropriate level of concern. The point of view of consumer planning and control is one that is applicable to professional work in a number of settings. The model serves well as a "consciousness-raising" mechanism for professional and community as well—again, another important contribution. However, these generalized principles do nothing in particular to resolve those social problems to which these programs were addressed originally. Indeed, the evidence of the middle 1970s is that the problems are probably worse than ever.

Thus, the establishment of these principles notwithstanding, the gains for society have been small indeed. For society, and certainly for those who are alienated and denied full participation in it, principles are of little value unless they lead to something relatively concrete and, if not immediate, at least foreseeable. Some sort of tangible community organization that is immediately accessible to its constituents provides at least the hope of self-help. Raising hopes beyond the power or the intent of the community to deliver can, as it has been demonstrated, produce disastrous results. But it should be remembered that the social upheavals that occurred during the 1960s *did not occur* in the majority of communities that had community action programs, and the linking of the programs themselves to civil disturbances is illogical. Community action programs did not invent social unrest.

However, changing trends in funding patterns, the key element in both the development of settings and in community control, make the development of viable community settings for the social action model quite difficult. The concept of federal revenue sharing, developed in the 1970s, moved funding away from even semiautonomous groups and into the funneling process of governmental structures. Increasingly, funding of social and health services began moving in the direction of "private enterprise" models of service delivery, which are funded through purchase-of-service contracts with government funding sources (Demone and Schulberg, 1975). The net effect of these changes is to continue the service elements of the social programs of the 1960s, but at reduced levels and under more direct governmental control. The community organization aspects of the programs were effectively eliminated. It is unreasonable to expect that a setting as compatible with the social action model as was the community action program will develop in the near future. As a program of service delivery without a component of community organization, it seems unlikely that these programs can do anything to alleviate the economic and political dependencies of the poor; indeed, it is conceivable that they will strengthen those dependencies.

Assessment of the Model

The concept of community in the social action model is defined by a particular constituency within the community as that term is ordinarily used. Thus, community action programs refer to a particular part of the community, not to the community as a social system. The primary focus of the social action model is on the conflict between the structural organization of society and the human needs of the poor. Community processes are conceptualized in terms of conflicting interests between groups. If one group appears to control power in the community, the task of redistributing that power consists of organizing an appropriate constituency to confront what is seen as an illegitimate holding of power by the dominant group. The organizational process involves creating increased consciousness of common concerns among the potential constituency so as to coalesce that group into a cohesive, functional organization. The task of organization is seen as a means of creating increased pressure on the dominant group to recognize what are generally seen as *legitimate* claims in a democratic society. The view of the community that emerges from this approach is a political and economic one. The conceptions of community processes and the strategies involved are quite analogous to labor union organization and union-management confrontations.

As has been mentioned, the social policy model values freedom and participation in social programs. Human needs are given precedence over economic and political ones. It is assumed that these values are best met in a context of self-determination. Yet the model sees the limitations on achieving these values as stemming from economic and political structures, leading to the conclusion that economic and political equity are precursors to the satisfaction of these needs. Thus, the model values political action as instrumental to the achievement of higher value goals. The values made explicit in the model are consistent with basic societal ideology, if not with its frequent practices.

In conceiving of the process of social change as one of mobilization of power, the social action model is taking a revolutionary, rather than an evolutionary, position. Despite its consistency with the central social ideology, there are a number of social and psychological considerations that led to the revolutionary character of the model's posture toward social change. This revolutionary position is furthered by the juxtaposition, and at times, fusion, of the model with civil rights causes and the youth protest that began with the Vietnam war. These three movements had many similar interests and overlapping constituencies. Indeed, the latter may have been a consideration in furthering the fusion of these causes so as to create a larger constituency. However, the social-psychological consequences of this fusion go far beyond the question of constituency and require careful analysis.

Pettigrew (1968) reviewed the progress of racial integration in the context of intergroup relations. He concluded that the consequences of racial separatism were more separatism, and, while gaining a measure of autonomy, the thrust for community control of a separatist social organization would not lead to integration. He pointed out that community control without control of the tax base was no control at all, and he faulted the comparison of contemporary blacks with former immigrant groups on the grounds that their history was significantly different. Pettigrew advocated direct integration into the mainstream of the social system as the only viable route. The community control strategy goes contrary to this advice.

Studies of social conflict underscore Pettigrew's contention and point to a paradox in the community organization strategy. A number of studies have indicated that high in-group cohesiveness tends to be maintained by conflict with out-groups (Coser, 1956), and conflict is thus seen as an important step in creating community organization (Alinsky, 1946). This same cohesiveness, however, tends to increase the likelihood of conflict with other groups. Williams (1972) has developed a theory of conflict in which he hypothesized that conflict is more likely to occur between groups that are interdependent, unequal, and that decrease interaction with each other. Friedman and Jacka (1969) have shown that group cohesiveness impairs intergroup negotiations. All of these considerations point to increased intergroup conflict as a result of community organization that seeks either to change or to circumvent the social structure. A concentration on a strategy of community organization that seeks participation in community institutions through the use of its power also generates reactions within the bureaucratic structure of the total society, which may set up a circular process of repression, organization, separatism, conflict, repression, and so on.

A brilliant analysis of the functions of the bureaucratic nature of the American social system presented by Katz (1966) illustrates these mechanisms. He points out that participation and concensus are only possible at the lowest levels of a bureaucracy, after which the system operates on a process of compromise and accommodation in which the majority rules. The higher in the system the process goes, the more it becomes a majority of power rather than numbers. Any bureaucratic system contains in it the remnants of the old order, which has maintained its stability in the past, even while it is changing, and these elements will resist change. The bureaucratic system is well established to absorb conflict and dampen dissent if it threatens to reduce the effective functioning of the system. Katz refers to these mechanisms as "defenses in depth." He notes that the civil rights movement had made as much progress as it had, largely in the legal and political realms, because the movement's ideology was basically consistent with that of the system. Separatism, however, was not. Moreover, the antiwar protests and the youth movement went directly against this ideology. Accordingly, the process of the community action movement was caught up in a larger social process that heightened its revolutionary character and probably contributed to the strengthening and quickening of social reactions against its thrust. Still, as with any revolutionary force, a period of reaction is to be expected, as noted in Chapter 2. In the early 1970s the evidence of antithetical reaction was quite prevalent. Yet there remain the gains noted previously, and how these will be integrated into a synthesis of an evolutionary social change remains to be seen.

The social action model values participation of a limited constituency and emphasizes accountability to it, but it tends to ignore participation and accountability to the larger social system because of its narrow definition of the "community." Accordingly, this revolutionary aspect of the model limits its survival value severely as part of the ongoing community process. This is a central paradox that the model does not solve, in that it could undoubtedly survive better within the normative structure of the community, but it would then be placed in conflict with some of its own constituency who would see such a move as a sign of accommodation with an out-group.

Unlike the organizational model, the social action model does provide a framework for intergroup relationships within the community. social system, but it defines these relationships in conflict terms, rather than from the perspective of a social system. Its limitation of the definition of community to a particular subsystem similarly limits its ability to account for the operation of the economic, political, and social aspects of the system on an overall, rather than an adversarial, basis. However, consistent with Lewin's dictum that if you want to understand how a system works, try to change it, the model has contributed to a better realization of how the contemporary social system operates.

References

AIKEN, M. Community power and community mobilization. *Annals of the American Academy of Political and Social Science*, September 1969, *385*, 76–88.

ALBEE, G. W. *Mental Health Manpower Trends.* New York: Basic Books, 1959.

ALINSKY, S. *Reveille for Radicals.* Chicago: University of Chicago Press, 1946.

ARNHOFF, F. N. Manpower needs, resources, and innovations. In H. H. Barten and L. Bellak (Eds.), *Progress in Community Mental Health*, vol. 2. New York: Grune & Stratton, 1972, 35–64.

BABARICK, P. Field-force intervention strategies: Changing the educational status quo in a community. *American Journal of Community Psychology*, 1975, *3*, 47–58.

CAMPBELL, D. T. AND FISKE, D. W. Convergent and discriminant validation by the multitrait-multimethod matrix. *Psychological Bulletin*, 1959, *56*, 81–105.

CLARK, K. (Ed.). *A Relevant War Against Poverty*. New York: Metropolitan Applied Research Center, 1968.

CLARK, K. *Dark Ghetto*. New York: Harper & Row, 1965.

CLARK, R. *Crime in America*. New York: Simon & Schuster, 1970.

CLOWARD, R. A. Illegitimate means, anomie, and deviant behavior. *American Sociological Review*, April 1959, 164–176.

COSER, L. A. *The Functions of Social Conflict*. New York: Free Press, 1956.

COTTRELL, L. S., JR. Social planning, the competent community, and mental health. In L. J. Duhl (Ed.), *Urban America and the Planning of Mental Health Services*. New York: Group for the Advancement of Psychiatry, 1964, 391–402.

COWEN, E. L., DORR, D., IZZO, L. D., MADONIA, A., AND TROST, M. A. The primary mental health project: A new way of conceptualizing and delivering school mental health services. *Psychology in the Schools*, 1971, *8*, 216–225.

CRONBACH, L. J. Heredity, environment, and educational policy. *Harvard Educational Review*, 1969, *39*, no. 2.

DAVIDSON, R. H. The war on poverty: Experiment in federalism. *Annals of the American Academy of Political and Social Science*, September 1969, *385*, 1–13.

DEMONE, H. W., JR., AND SCHULBERG, H. C. Human services trends in the mid-1970's. *Social Casework*, 1975, *56*, 268–279.

DORR, D., AND COWEN, E. L. Nonprofessional mental health workers' judgements of change in children. *Journal of Community Psychology*, 1973, *1*, 23–26.

DORR, D., COWEN, E. L., AND KRAUS, R. Mental health professionals view nonprofessional mental health workers. *American Journal of Community Psychology*, 1973, *1*, 258–265.

FINESTONE, S., AND SOBEY, F. *Non-professional Personnel in Mental Health Programs*. Washington, D.C.: National Clearinghouse for Mental Health Information, 1969.

FRIEDMAN, M., AND JACKA, M. E. The negative effect of group cohesiveness on intergroup negotiations. *Journal of Social Issues*, 1969, *25*, 181–194.

GUTTENTAG, M. Children in Harlem's community controlled schools. *Journal of Social Issues*, 1972, *28*, 1–20.

JACOBSON, S. L., ROMAN, M., AND KAPLAN, S. R. Training nonprofessional workers. In H. Grunebaum (Ed.), *The Practice of Community Mental Health*. Boston: Little, Brown, 1970, 625–643.

JENCKS, C. Intelligence and race. *The New Republic*, September 13, 1969.

JENSEN, A. R. How much can we boost IQ and scholastic achievement? *Harvard Educational Review*, 1969, *39*, no. 1.

KAPLAN, S. R., BOYAJIAN, L. Z., AND MELTZER, B. The role of the nonprofessional worker. In H. Grunebaum (Ed.), *The Practice of Community Mental Health*. Boston: Little, Brown, 1970, 591–624.

KARDINER, A., AND SPIEGEL, H. *War Stress and Neurotic Illness*. New York: Hoeber, 1947.

KARLSRUHER, A. E. The nonprofessional as a psychotherapeutic agent. *American Journal of Community Psychology*, 1974, *2*, 61–78.

KATZ, D. Group process and social integration: A systems analysis of two movements of social protest. *Journal of Social Issues*, 1967, *23*, 3–22.

LEIGHTON, D., HARDING, J., MACKLIN, D., MACMILLAN, A., AND LEIGHTON, A. *The Character of Danger*. New York: Basic Books, 1963.

LEVIN, H. Psychologist to the powerless. In F. Korten, S. Cook, and J. Lacey (Eds.), *Psychology and the Problems of Society*. Washington, D.C.: American Psychological Association, 1970, 121–127.

LEVINE, M., AND LEVINE, A. *A Social History of Helping Services*. New York: Appleton-Century-Crofts, 1970.

LEVITAN, S. A. *The Great Society's Poor Law*. Baltimore: Johns Hopkins Press, 1969.

LIPSKY, M. Social scientists and the riot commission. *Annals of the American Academy of Political and Social Science*, March 1971, *394*, 72–83.

MANGUM, G. L. The why, how, and whence of manpower programs. *Annals of the American Academy of Political and Social Science*, September 1969, *385*, 50–62.

MARRIS, P., AND REIN, M. *Dilemmas of Social Reform*. Chicago: Atherton, 1967.

MILLER, G. A. Psychology as a means of promoting human welfare. In F. Korten, S. Cook, and J. Lacey (Eds.), *Psychology and the Problems of Society*. Washington, D.C.: American Psychological Association, 1970, 5–21.

MOYNIHAN, D. P. *Maximum Feasible Misunderstanding*. New York: Free Press, 1969.

NATIONAL INSTITUTE OF MENTAL HEALTH. *Staffing Patterns in Mental Health Facilities 1968*. U.S. Public Health Service, publication no. 5034. Washington, D.C.: U.S. Government Printing Office, 1970.

PEARL, A. The poverty of psychology: An indictment. In V. L. Allen (Ed.), *Psychological Factors in Poverty*. Chicago: Markham, 1970, 348–365.

PEARL, A. AND REISSMAN, F. *New Careers for the Poor*. New York: Free Press, 1965.

PETTIGREW, T. F. *A Profile of the Negro American*. Princeton, N. J.: Van Nostrand, 1964.

PETTIGREW, T. F. Racially separate or together? *Journal of Social Issues*, 1969, *25*, 43–69.

REIFF, R. Mental health manpower and institutional change. *American Psychologist*, 1966, *21*, 540–548.

REIFF, R. Social intervention and the problem of psychological analysis. *American Psychologist*, 1968, *23*, 524–531.

REIFF, R. Of cabbages and kings. *American Journal of Community Psychology*, 1975, *3*, 187–196.

REIFF, R., AND REISSMAN, F. The indigenous non-professional. *Community Mental Health Journal*, monograph series, no. 1, 1965.

Report of the National Advisory Commission on Civil Disorders. New York: Bantam Books, 1968

REISSMAN, F. AND SCRIBNER, S. The under-utilization of mental health services by workers and low income groups: Causes and cures. *American Journal of Psychiatry*, 1965, *121*, 798–801.

ROMAN, M. AND SCHMAIS, A. Consumer participation and control: A conceptual overview. In H. H. Barten and L. Bellak (Eds.), *Progress in Community Mental Health*, vol. 2. New York: Grune & Stratton, 1972, 63–84.

ROSSI, P. H. Practice, method and theory in evaluating social-action programs. In P. E. Cook (Ed.), *Community Psychology and Community Mental Health*. San Francisco: Holden-Day, 1970, 213–227.

RUBIN, L. B. Maximum feasible participation: The origins, implications, and present status. *Annals of the American Academy of Political and Social Science*, September 1969, *385*, 14–29.

SANDLER, I. N., PURICKO, A., AND GRANDE, L. Effectiveness of an early secondary prevention program in an inner-city elementary school. *American Journal of Community Psychology*, 1975, *3*, 23–32.

SCHIFF, S. K. Free inquiry and the enduring commitment: The Woodlawn Mental Health Center 1963–1970. In S. E. Golann and C. Eisdorfer (Eds.), *Handbook of Community Mental Health*. New York: Appleton-Century-Crofts, 1972, 755–777.

SHAW, M. E. *Group Dynamics: The Psychology of Small Group Behavior*, New York: McGraw-Hill, 1971.

SHAW, R., AND EAGLE, C. J. Programmed failure: The Lincoln Hospital story. *Community Mental Health Journal*, 1971, *7*, 255–263.

SILBERMAN, C. E. *Crisis in the Classroom*. New York: Random House, 1970.

THIBAUT, J. W. AND KELLEY, H. H. *The Social Psychology of Groups*. New York: Wiley, 1959.

WESTINGHOUSE LEARNING CORPORATION–OHIO UNIVERSITY. *The Impact of Head Start: An Evaluation of the Effects of Head Start on Children's Cognitive and Affective Development*, Yellow Springs, Ohio, 1969.

WILLIAMS, R. Conflict and social order: A research strategy for complex propositions. *Journal of Social Issues*, 1972, *28*, 11–26.

WILLIAMS, W., AND EVANS, J. W. The politics of evaluation: The case of Head Start. *Annals of the American Academy of Political and Social Science*, September 1969, *385*, 118–132.

WINDLE, C., BASS, R. D., AND TAUBE, C. A. PR aside: Initial results from NIMH's service program evaluation studies. *American Journal of Community Psychology*, 1974, *2*, 311–328.

7. The Ecological Model

In his formulation B = f(P,E), Lewin (1951) emphasized the interdependence of the person and the environment in determining behavior. As early as 1943, Lewin had suggested that an analysis of "psychological ecology" should proceed by first examining nonpsychological factors before proceeding to the examination of psychological ones. Yet nonpsychological environmental characteristics have been largely ignored by the majority of psychologists, who have been more concerned with theories that emphasize the determining qualities of intrapersonal factors. Whether influenced by the intrapsychic supremacy inherent in Freudian theory, or the interest in response variability to restricted and controlled stimulus conditions of the behaviorists, few psychologists have been inclined toward either the naturalistic observation or the examination of environmental characteristics that are suggested by Lewin's formulation.

Lewin's concept of the life space has been a more attractive version of the "environment" for many psychologists than has his original emphasis on the nonpsychological environment. The life space includes "all facts that have existence and excludes those that do not have existence for the individual or group under study" (Cartwright, 1951, p. xi). While often taken to mean the phenomenological field at the moment for an individual or group, the life space can also include factors of which the individual or group is not consciously aware, but which may still influence behavior. However, this orientation toward the phenomenological field has been more compelling for many psychologists using Lewinian theory than has the nonpsychological environment. It is not, however, the ecological environment.

One psychologist who has taken seriously the concern with the nonpsychological environment is Roger Barker. Barker and Herbert Wright established the Midwest Psychological Field Station at Oskaloosa, Kansas, in 1947, and began a series of studies to describe and conceptualize the environment of that small community. In 1954, a companion station in Leyburn, Yorkshire, England, was established for comparative studies. These communities are referred to as "Midwest" and "Yoredale," respectively, in the several publications that Barker and his associates have produced since then.

Among the first tasks in the study of the environment is that of defining and clarifying the terms of the study. Barker (1968) cautions that if one is to examine the interrelationship of behavior and environment, these two factors must be studied independently in order to avoid a tautological situation. For example, in pointing out the interdependence of person and environment in determining behavior, Lewin (1951) notes that one can say that the person is a function of the environment, and that the environment is a function of the person. To distinguish among the behavior of the individual, the individual's perception of the environment (life space), and the ecological environment, it is helpful to keep in mind that these are events that exist on different levels and are comprehended by different means. Consider, for example, viewing a football game through the medium of television. If one is naive about the rules and procedures for the game, one cannot understand the behavior of the players from viewing the field alone (the physical environment) prior to the arrival of any of the contestants; it is necessary to view the game in progress in order to understand the interrelationships between the players' actions and the hash marks, yard markers, and goal lines that make up the environment. One can acquire some insight into a part of the game by watching the performance of a wide receiver or a running back on an isolated replay view of a single play, which is analogous to studying the behavior of individuals, but one cannot from this alone comprehend the behavior of the game. Similarly, one can gain further knowledge by listening to a postgame interview of one of the players giving the reasons why he acted in a particular way in a particular situation, which would be analogous to examining the individual's life space, but, again, this is not sufficient to understand the behavior of the total game. The game itself would consist of a collection of physical entities, including people and objects, that make up a *behavior setting* in Barker's terms, a concept he developed to describe the link between ecology and psychology. The playing of the game would be a behavior episode. As the defining properties of behavior settings are examined, these characteristics will become clearer.

Behavior settings are eco-behavioral units that contain behavioral episodes. Barker outlines seven defining characteristics of behavior settings. These are (1) standing patterns of behavior; (2) standing patterns of behavior-and-milieu; (3) the milieu is circumjacent (enclosing, encompassing) to the behavior; (4) the milieu is synormorphic (similar in structure) to the behavior; (5) the behavior-milieu parts are synormorphs (both physical and behavioral attributes). Structurally, a behavior setting is a set of synomorphs; (6) synomorphs have a specified degree of interdependence; (7) synomorphs have a greater degree of interdependence among themselves than with parts of other behavior settings.

The behavior setting has a locus in both time and space, is clearly discriminated from entities outside the setting, has its own internal structure, and exists independently of any particular observer. As such, a behavior setting has all of the desired properties of an objective eco-behavioral unit, and can be reliably identified by trained observers working independently (Barker, 1963).

Barker suggests three tests to determine if part of a community is a behavior setting. One is a *structural* test. A part of a community qualifies on this test as a behavior setting if it is a behavior-milieu synomorph. Another is an *internal dynamic* test. A part qualifies as a behavior setting on this test if it shows a specified degree of interdependence among synomorphs that are structurally within that part. A third is an *external dynamic* test. A part qualifies as a behavior setting if it shows a specified degree of *in*dependence from synomorphs that are external to that part. Using these three tests, Barker has shown that a number of synomorphs, or structurally similar behavior-milieu parts, can be assessed to determine whether they constitute behavior settings. These behavior settings are the eco-behavioral units that make up a community. In Midwest, a community of 830 persons, Barker identified 884 settings during a one-year period. Thirty-five percent of these settings occurred only one day during the year, while 2.8 percent of them occurred nearly every day of the year. In addition to variability in occurrence, Barker has outlined a number of other variable properties of behavior settings, that is, ways in which behavior settings differ from each other. Yet it is the stability of particular behavior settings over time that makes the concept important for ecological analysis. As Barker has noted:

> One of the striking features of communities is how, year after year, they incorporate new people, despite the idiosyncratic behavior and personality traits of these people, into the characteristic patterns of their stable behavior settings: of Rotary Club meetings, of doctors' offices, of garages, of bridge clubs. Obviously, whatever it is that impresses the characteristic array and flow of behavior settings upon their interior entities and events is largely independent of the persons who participate in them. (1963, p. 20)

For Barker, the stability of behavior settings results from a quasistationary equilibrium of forces, a concept that is familiar from Chapter 3. The inhabitants of the setting maintain this quasistationary equilibrium by carrying out its essential functions; the inhabitants are at once the source and the recipients of many of these forces. Thus, the population manning of settings is an important variable in Barker's theory.

Barker assumed that the number of forces within a behavior setting is a constant. Therefore, with optimal manning or overmanning these forces are distributed among more people than is true when the setting is undermanned. In the optimally manned setting, each individual would experience less force, and in the undermanned setting each would experience more force. In the undermanned setting, individuals would experience more range of directions of the forces acting in the setting than would be true in an optimally manned setting. Accordingly, Barker predicted that the inhabitants of undermanned settings, compared to those in optimally or overmanned settings, would be more active within the setting in a greater variety of actions. These predictions have been confirmed in numerous studies (Barker, 1968). The predictions hold true, of course, within a limited range of undermanning, since a population too small to carry out the essential functions of the setting would change the setting to a different behavior setting. In the example that Barker used, a game of baseball might be transformed into a game of workup.

Aside from being an objectifiable attribute of the environment, the importance of the concept of behavior setting is that it allows predictions directly from the environment to behavior, rather than statistical or probabilistic statements, and these predictions have been verified and replicated several times. Studies by Rausch, Dittmann, and Taylor (1959, 1960) have shown as much variation in behavior across settings in the same individuals as across individuals in the same settings, clearly supporting the Lewinian view of the interaction between person and environment. The effects of population manning of the setting have also been found in a variety of settings (Barker and Gump, 1964; Barker, 1968). Thus, analyses on one level can be related to phenomena across boundaries to an entirely different level. Ecological principles refer to the environment and permit assessment of the environment independently of behavior; yet these principles can be used to extend knowledge of behavior by bridging the levels of persons and environments and increasing the understanding of their interdependence.

James Kelly (1968) has undertaken such an extension by formulating a set of principles derived from ecological theory that serve as a conceptual framework for examining settings and behavior: understanding maintenance and change processes in the setting, studying varieties of adaptive behavior, and devloping plans for interventions to enhance adaptation to changing conditions. These principles constitute the major assumptions of the ecological model of community psychology.

Assumptions

The assumptions of the ecological model can be thought of as comprising two categories. The first of these is a set of ecological principles that govern the assessment of settings for the purpose of identifying problems and generating a set of alternative interventions. The second is a set of principles that guide the change process derived from the study of the ecosystem under consideration. We will examine the assumptions in each of these categories in turn.

ECOLOGICAL PRINCIPLES

The ecological model assumes that the community is an ecosystem that can be characterized and understood through the concepts governing ecosystems. At present, many of these concepts must be applied as analogies, since the necessary research to establish valid applications is limited. Nevertheless, such analogies provide a useful conceptual framework for community processes. Kelly (1968) has proposed four principles to guide the ecological analysis of community settings.

1. The principle of interdependence. This principle is based on the ecosystem principle in biological ecology. It asserts that the units within an ecosystem are interdependent. Three types of interdependence are recognized: between living and nonliving parts of the environment; among living elements; and between structure and function of parts of the ecosystem. The principle of interdependence means that any change in a componenet of an ecosystem effects changes in the relationships between other components of the system as well. Not all relationships are changed to the same degree, and some are only detectable over longer time periods than others. Deevey (1963) provides a useful example of this interdependence by suggesting an analogy to a heating system in a house. Consider a bedroom that is some distance away from the thermostat located in another part of the house. As temperature drops in the bedroom, air currents eventually carry the temperature change to the thermostat, which activates the furnace sending heat to the bedroom. In the process, heat is sent to other rooms in the house as well, even though their temperatures may not be dropping as much. Of course, these other rooms also contribute air temperature information to the thermostat, so that the temperature at the thermostat is never the same as in the distant bedroom or in any other particular room of the house. Yet the heat supply to any room can be affected by the temperature in any of several other rooms.

Along with interdependence, Kelly introduces the concept of limiting factors, which points up the fact that while ecosystems contain many complicated functions, some are more critical than others. Generally, the most important functions are those that are in relatively short supply and high demand. This concept provides the ecologist with a point of entry into the complex functions in an ecosystem.

In a human ecosystem, the principle of interdependence is important for understanding the social structure of a community: how are persons linked to roles, and roles to each other? This structure is important for understanding the form and extensity of mutual need satisfaction or frustration, and the generation of cooperation and conflict within a community ecosystem. The way in which contrasting environments affect interdependence also has implications for understanding the consequences of alternative interventions on the interdependence of functions, and thus on the form of the functions themselves, within an ecosystem. For example, we mentioned in Chapter 1 how the increased enrollment of those eligible for welfare benefits placed increased pressure on the institution of public welfare for new solutions to the welfare problem because of public alarm at the increasing numbers. The community mental health movement has created a similar problem through its move to discharge state hospital patients into communities without adequate provision for their support or for integration into new roles. This problem exists at the level of the community social system, and the mental health model's focus on individual and dyadic levels does not provide a perspective for this problem.

2. The principle of cycling resources. This principle refers to both the utilization and the replacement of energy forms in an ecosystem. In natural environments this principle is illustrated by energy transformations and food chains. In the human environment this principle has to do with how the ecosystem creates, develops, and utilizes new resources for changing requirements.

Trickett, Kelly, and Todd (1972) emphasize the importance of assessing how the setting defines and utilizes its resources as a first step in any attempt to create a change program. The history of the identification and utilization of talent within an ecosystem is of particular significance for this analysis. In turn, this analysis is important to understanding how the setting shapes and influences adaptive styles of its inhabitants. A relatively unchanging environment, for example, tends to look for and employ persons with the same histories and abilities to occupy the same roles over time, while the relatively changing environment encourages and utilizes persons with a diverse range of talent.

3. The principle of adaptation. The principle that the environment shapes adaptation is central to the ecological thesis. Levins (1966) defines adaptive behavior as the relative diversity of environments in which a unit of evolution can survive and reproduce. He assumes that environmental uncertainty increases niche breadth, or the range of environment to which the organism can adapt, while environmental constancy leads to specialization of adaptive capacity. Thus, adaptation is relative to a particular environment, and behavior that is adaptive in one environment may not be so in others.

This principle has led Kelly (1971) to the study of the adaptive potential of different coping styles in contrasting environments. The primary environmental characteristic employed in these studies has been population exchange: the rate of turnover of population from one year to another. The setting in which these studies have been conducted is the high school, which provides for a range of environments in which individual selection of the environment is reduced as long as other variables, such as social class, are controlled. These studies have begun with naturalistic observation of the setting according to ecological principles, followed by examinations of social processes, and finally studies of individual behavior. Environments with high exchange rates provide a fluid environment, which varies systematically in its social structure, interaction patterns, norms, and opportunities from an environment with a low exchange rate, which is characterized by environmental constancy (Kelly, 1969). Studies by Kelly and his co-workers have confirmed that these environments tend to support different patterns of social interaction and different individual coping styles (Kelly, 1971a).

4. The principle of succession. This principle points up the fact that natural communities are not stable, but are in a constant process of change, giving rise to changing demands for adaptive capacities in both social and individual behavior. A community exists in a dynamic equilibrium with its environment, and changes in the environment create forces for change in community structures.

The succession principle emphasizes the need for a long-range time perspective in assessing environments and planning interventions. Change processes need to be examined for both their short- and long-term effects. Succession means that as environmental conditions change, either as a result of natural conditions or as a consequence of intervention efforts, new adaptive behavior styles will be required. The principle underscores the need to predict and make accomodations for these changes. Here the concern is with the opportunities available for persons taking new roles under changing conditions, changing or creating new socialization processes, and making efficient use of resources.

Finally, the succession principle increases the visibility of the problem of the interaction between naturally occurring and deliberately planned changes. In this sense, the ecological model provides a view of the community as a changing entity rather than a static background of individual behavior.

INTERVENTION PRINCIPLES

When the development of community mental health centers was in its beginning stages, Kelly (1966) outlined several principles to guide the development of new services, based on ecological principles. In a later article, Trickett, Kelly, and Todd (1972) elaborated these principles in more specific detail. The following is a summary of those principles:

1. The intervention deals directly with local conditions. This principle recognizes the interdependence of change efforts and ongoing processes in the environment. It also emphasizes the need to tailor interventions to the particular requirements of a specific setting, rather than relying on assumptions about universally acceptable methods, which are more likely to have been successful in some other setting but are not necessarily valid for the setting in question. This principle also implies that accountability derives from effectiveness in a particular setting, not just from the application of a predetermined change program.

2. Interventions are based on longitudinal assessment of the local setting. Assessment is seen as an inherent part of the change process, building evaluation and accountability into the intervention. An important part of this assessment is to determine the likely response of the environment to the disruption caused by the intervention, and to use this knowledge to build in mechanisms for dealing with this anticipated reaction, thus increasing the chances of survival for the change process.

3. Effects of the intervention on inhabitants of the setting are anticipated, and efforts are made to reduce negative effects and enhance positive effects. Along with concern about accountability, future side effects of the intervention are anticipated by virtue of the interdependence and succession principles in ecological theory. Accordingly, an important goal of the change process is the development of a planning capacity in the setting to deal with expected future changes. Some care needs to be taken to specify the meaning of "expected" here. It means that the fact that changes will occur is assumed; it does not mean that the exact form of these changes can be predicted. The type of changes that are "expected" may be both predictable and unpredictable.

4. A wide variety of potential interventions are included. This principle implies that consideration of alternative interventions provides a basis for contemplating the various effects that can be anticipated and reduces the chances that stereotyped solutions will be implemented. It also recognizes the interdependence and adaptation principles of ecological theory, such that interventions that create one kind of change will very likely require other changes to deal with the effects of the first change. At a minimum, the devel-

opment of a planning capacity to deal with future changes would be required along with any other single or multiple change effort to enable the intervention to follow ecological principles.

The complexity of ecosystems and the interrelationships among these ecological principles may appear to represent an overwhelming problem. However, the ecological psychologist need not work with all of these complexities in order to employ the ecological model. In studying the high school, Kelly and his co-workers have focused on a particular ecosystem within the larger community ecosystem. They have found that the variable of population exchange accounts meaningfully for differences between contrasting environments. Unlike such variables as size or social class, which have been the subject of numerous studies, the use of population exchange rates provides a dynamic variable that can be expected to be related to changes in the environment over time in ways that other variables are not. A variable such as population exchange also provides a basis for understanding inputs and outputs in relation to the larger ecosystem of which the high school is a part. Similarly, the study of change processes in other limited ecosystems may proceed in the same way. The ecological model calls for working with a social system according to a set of concepts and principles derived from ecological theory. It does not define specifically the scope of the social system *a priori*. The importance of the ecological analogy is in the application of ecological principles from both a historical and a future perspective.

Typical Interventions

The relative newness of the ecological model is such that the model is in a transitional stage from theory and research to definitive interventions. Examples of actual interventions that have followed this model and have been evaluated for effectiveness are not available. It is possible, however, to consider some suggested interventions that would follow the model, and to use some actual interventions to illustrate the application of the model.

ORGANIZATIONAL REDEVELOPMENT OF HIGH SCHOOLS

Trickett, Kelly, and Todd (1972) have detailed the tasks of an intervention program for high school environments according to the four ecological principles discussed above. They derive different specific intervention activities according to each one of the four principles. These principles are considered as having implications for intervention in chronological order according to the following points:

> The principle of interdependence is salient for conceptualizing the entry process and the initial assessment of the client systems; the principle cycling of resources is useful in generating predictions about the potential of the organization's development; the adaptation principle is relevant for developing hypotheses about the social norms for effective and ineffective behavior emerging in the organization; while the principle of dynamic equilibrium and succession is valid for developing hypotheses regarding the long term development of the social setting. (1972, p. 392)

Entry into the ecosystem by the ecological psychologist is typically precipitated by some crisis in the setting: a chronically disruptive individual, a serious social upheaval resulting from student dissatisfaction, a systemic crisis brought on by court-ordered desegregation changes in the student body. While the psychologist may be brought in by a key administrative figure in the setting—the school principal or superintendent—the psychologist sees himself or herself as a part of a relationship between a change process and an ecosystem. Other parts of that relationship may include other outside professionals, key individuals within the social setting, and the setting itself. The goal is to develop this relationship as a long-term process that goes beyond the immediate presenting problem.

In the example described by Trickett, Kelly, and Todd (1972), disruptive behavior of an individual is taken as a hypothetical precipitating problem. Entry would begin by assessing the individual resources available for managing the problem. While the frequent solution for such behavior in the school setting is referral to an outside helping resource, such as a clinic, or exclusion from the setting, Trickett, Kelly, and Todd note that these solutions exclude both the teacher and the individual student from the definition of the problem as it occurs in the setting of the school. The school is limited in the number of times it can employ this solution. Clinics may become overcrowded; the individual most often will be reintroduced into the setting where the problem must still be managed; and such solutions are not solutions at all for large-scale disruptions. Exclusion solutions increasingly define the ecosystem as unable to adapt to problem conditions that arise in the setting. The combination of disruptive behavior and pressures for exclusion alert the ecological psychologist to look for disturbances in the interdependence within the system.

For Kelly (1964, 1970) this situation calls for an examination of naturally occurring help-giving roles in the setting. Where these seem blocked or limited, such as a definition of helping troubled or troubling students as being outside the teacher's role, an effort may be made to redefine the role in ways similar to the function of the consultant in the mental health model. The difference from that approach in the ecological model is in the consultant's focus on the interdependence of behavior in the setting and in the consultant's attention to factors in the ecosystem beyond that particular teacher-student relationship. Relevant questions concerning interdependence and help giving include the range of settings in which teacher and pupil interact, the nature of the settings in which interaction is effective and those in which interaction is ineffective, and the existence of other informal relationships, such as with peers, in which help might be available.

A second concern is the redefinition or development of supplementary helping roles, such as conferences with the principal, a tutorial relationship with a peer, or the development of a liaison relationship between school and family. These and other role resources are dependent in turn on the ecological makeup of the school setting. Kelly (1968) has hypothesized that in a school environment with low exchange rates and a resulting constant environment, student problems are more likely to involve difficulties with adherence to rules. Such settings more narrowly restrict the range of roles available to both faculty and students and also limit the opportunities for success. In such an environment, Kelly suggests that intervention programs will have to be tailored toward in-service training for teachers to enhance and support their help-giving efforts. In environments with high exchange rates and resulting fluid environments, students are expected to present more problems of alienation and diffusion of identity. In such environments, Kelly suggests a program of extracurricular activities to engage students in the setting as an appropriate intervention. It would be expected that the principle of interdependence would lead to greater need for and more support for the development of new helping roles in the fluid environment than in the constant environment. These roles might include recreational leaders, work-study coordinators, and persons whose functions would be to link the school setting with the surrounding community in a variety of functions.

The cycling-of-resources principle bears on such an intervention in terms of how the setting will define new roles for participation in help-giving activities. The setting's history of identifying and utilizing talent, the existing opportunities for student-teacher interaction in a variety of settings, and the communication patterns that define roles—who initiates such communications and who has opportunity to provide input into role definitions—are all important aspects of defining the pattern of resource utilization. Trickett, Kelly, and Todd suggest that the development of mechanisms for assessing goals for the setting is at once an important and a difficult aspect of actualizing this principle. As both external and internal conditions create new demands on the setting, mechanisms for reassessing goals are conceivably powerful, yet often neglected, sources of initiating adaptive change.

This process feeds into considerations relevant to the principle of adaptation. The school setting generates norms for the regulation of internal behavior. These patterns tend to generate styles of adaptive behavior that are rewarded within the setting. However, utilizing the principle that behavior that is adaptive in one setting may not be adaptive in another, the important question is how criteria for adaptive behavior within the setting generalize to the environment external to the setting.

Here the extent to which the high school environment approximates the community social system has important implications for the socialization of adaptive behavior. The functions of the environment of the school in identifying and meeting students' needs; providing relevant curricula for post-high school requirements, either vocationally or academically; providing opportunities for experiences in democratic processes and individual decision making; and developing channels for the expression and development of individual skills—all are important aspects of the adaptation-enhancing function of the high school environment. Kelly (1968) suggests that the high school environment with low exchange rates will provide more limited, standardized, and unchanging opportunities along these lines than will the high-exchange-rate, fluid environment. In the constant environment, adaptive help for students would consist of increasing ways for students to define as important for themselves adaptive directions that are at variance with the traditionally defined avenues; in the fluid environment, relevant help would consist of assistance in making choices from among a wider range of alternatives.

The principle of succession predicts that interventions cannot be expected to have useful effects for unlimited time periods. Starting with the assumption that crisis situations in human ecosystems often result from a failure of the setting to change with changing external conditions, ecologically based interventions must plan for subsequent changes in the relationship between the change program and the social system. For the inhabitants of the setting, these changes have to do with changes in the social structure of the setting. Three concerns having to do with these changes are criteria for membership, mechanisms for crossing status lines in social interaction, and changes in coping styles while a member of the setting (Trickett, Kelly, and Todd, 1972, pp. 398-399). For the setting, these changes are best evidenced by the development of a planning function within the setting that monitors change processes occurring in the exchange between the setting and the surrounding community. Most school systems, for example, maintain some sort of monitoring process to predict changes in enrollments, and building programs and staff recruitment are adjusted accordingly. Few if any of these processes, however, use this information to generate hypotheses about the effects of changing school size, exchange rates, and other accompaniments of enrollment fluctuation on behavior in the school setting; changing needs of students; and changing demands on the social structure of the school. The addition of this input to the school setting can be a unique contribution of the ecological analogy.

These proposals for a change program for the high school environment have focused on individual development in a key community institution established specifically for that purpose. The intervention deals with the larger community as a surrounding environment, but not as an ecosystem in itself. It is also possible, however, to apply the ecological model to the community system. In this sense, we will consider problems of community development from an ecological standpoint.

COMMUNITY DEVELOPMENT

A community is a naturally occurring form of social organization that is ubiquitous throughout plant and animal life. As such, a community is an *implicit* form, whereas human institutions, such as those addressed in Chapter 5 in the organizational model, and earlier in this chapter in the form of the high school, are *explicit* forms (Moe, 1959). As a collection of behavior settings, communities comprise both implicit and explicit forms. Barker views the behavior settings of a community as linked together by "authority systems," a view that is akin to the organizational, explicit form of the community. Indeed, such a view is also taken for granted in many of the community programs established by law that have been discussed previously. The ecological perspective permits an integrated view of both implicit and explicit aspects of community systems through the application of ecological principles that are independent of the organizational and social forms that may exist in a particular community. This dynamic, rather than structural, view allows for consideration of community processes as ongoing, naturally occurring changes, as well as deliberate planned changes.

While communities vary in a number of visibly obvious ways, such as size, economy, racial and ethnic integration, cultural and political traditions, they also vary in important dynamic ways that can be captured from an ecological perspective. While the ecological model deals with the question of community development from the standpoint of planned change to alleviate some problem, it also takes account of unplanned, naturally occurring changes. In this sense, the model emphasizes evolutionary development and change.

The history of the United States itself has been one of continual development in size and location of population. This development has been accompanied by a growth mentality that has only recently been questioned. Only occasionally in the past have concerns been aired about the form this development takes. Writers at least as early as Thomas Jefferson expressed concern about increasing urbanization, which they saw as a hazard to the quality of life compared to rural agrarian living. Yet industrialization has brought increasing urbanization and, with it, two conflicting themes. One of these is economic: a concern with luring further industrial growth to provide jobs and to increase the urban tax base to support services. The other is largely aesthetic: a concern with preserving some of the natural features of the environment, such as green spaces and parks.

Carried along by the growth mentality, the economic interest in community development has far outweighed the aesthetic interest. Only occasional conflicts over zoning laws and the granting of variances, and the development of a few "green belt" planned residential communities during the early part of this century (Weimer, 1962) have been exceptions to this trend. Rarely has the goal of community development been the promotion of adaptive human behavior, except indirectly.

As a result, many efforts at community redevelopment have repeated the errors of the past in new forms by ignoring the human behavior aspect of development in favor of a design based on economic and architectural structure considerations. Notable among the failures of this approach were the disruptions caused by forced relocation of persons living in urban renewal areas, and the social and psychological disasters embodied in the high-density, multifamily dwellings erected in these areas. In Boston's West End, Fried (1964) found serious increases in the incidence of depression among persons displaced from that area by an urban renewal plan that failed to take account of the strong cultural organization that existed there. In St. Louis, the Pruitt-Igoe high-rise housing development was deliberately destroyed by dynamite only a few years after its construction because of the skyrocketing rates of crime and social disorganization that occurred in buildings that were once thought to be a means of producing just the opposite effect.

In the 1970s, increasing awareness that man's developmental activities were making the environmnent less habitable, through air, noise, and water pollution, coupled with a developing psychology of scarcity, whether real or contrived, has caused a questioning of the growth mentality and provided some reflection on ecological questions. A coexisting economic problem, inflation combined with recession, with high unemployment, has increased the salience of economic concerns, however, and limited the psychological and political freedom to act on ecological concerns.

Part of the federal revenue-sharing program are funds marked for "community development." These programs require opportunities for citizen input into local decisions on spending the funds, but in many cities this process is a *pro forma* superficiality, having little impact on the actual use of the money. The actual use of these funds typically goes for such developments as sewers or parks.

Concern with an integrated conception of human and physical aspects of community development has not been an exclusive nor a very important province for psychologists. Some architects and city planners have a long-standing interest in such an integration. It was, for example, a major assumption in Frank Lloyd Wright's architectural designs that constructions should serve to unite man with nature rather than alienate him from it, as Wright assumed the majority of buildings did. Patrick Geddes's (1915) description of desired aspects of the study of cities is strikingly similar to many more recent suggestions for the role of the modern community psychologist:

> Still more must we take our share in the life and work of the community if we would make this estimate an active one; that is, if we would discern the possibilities of place, of work, of people, of actual groupings and institutions or of needed ones, and thus leave the place in some degree the better for our life in it; the richer, not the poorer, for our presence. Our activity may in some measure interrupt our observing and philosophising; indeed must often do so; yet with no small compensations in the long run. For here is that experimental social science which the theoretic political economists were wont to proclaim impossible; but which is none the less on parallel lines and of kindred experimental value to the practice which illuminates theory, criticising it or advancing it, in many simpler fields of action—say, engineering or medicine for choice. It is with civics and sociology as with these. The greatest historians, both ancient and modern, have been those who took their part in affairs. Indeed with all sciences, as with the most ideal quests, the sample principle holds good; we must live the life if we would know the doctrine. Scientific detachment is but one mood, though an often needed one; our quest cannot be attained without participation in the active life citizenship. (Geddes, 1915, p. 111)

The efforts of those architects and city planners who have been concerned with the human implications of community development have not found a useful body of knowledge in psychology concerning the environment, and as a consequence the integration of these concerns with physical building and human development has been impaired. The ecological model applied to community development has promise of contributing to such an integration.

Moe (1959) describes a typical community development process that employs groups of community members meeting together. Moe describes a number of important steps in the community development process, including the need for the community to set its own goals, the need to broaden membership of the original groups to make them representative of the community, the need to cast the consultant's expertise in an appropriate perspective so that it is not overvalued to the point that the community becomes dependent on the consultant, and the need to blend together appropriate amounts of planning and action. Notable in his description is the rejection by the community of preconceived or "packaged" programs of action in favor of programs developed by the community to fit their own particular needs.

These are elements that derive from the experience of consultants whose background training may range from psychology to agricultural extension work. While this process aspect of community development is important to the conduct of the intervention, it does not provide a framework for guiding the content of the intervention by which the appropriate questions concerning the development of the community may be asked.

The author has used the ecological framework in designing different intervention programs for two parts of a community that face very different problems, both currently and in the future. Although this program was developed while the author was working in a mental health setting, the use of the ecological model allows for a planning perspective that is quite different from the usual mental health intervention. While some of the activities are similar to those found in other models, they are cast in a different theoretical framework that alters their function within the intervention design.

One area was identified through an analysis of census data. Ten social indicators were selected for the analysis:

1. Percent unemployed, male.
2. Percent unemployed, female.
3. Percent school dropouts.
4. Number of families below poverty line.
5. Percent of families below poverty line.
6. Number of families receiving public assistance.
7. Percent of families receiving public assistance.
8. Percent of families with children under eighteen and a female head of household.
9. Percent black population.
10. Percent families in same residence last five years.

Of thirty-seven census tracts in the county, eight consistently appeared in the top ten tracts on these indices. Three were in the top ten on all ten variables, while one appeared five times. These eight census tracts comprise the central city of the community. In addition to the variables listed above, these tracts together have a population density that is double the median density for the county.

These indices have been shown to be highly related to the prevalence of both crime and mental disorders (Bloom, 1965; Lindorfer, 1972). Data on the prevalence of mental disorders as such for this area are not available. However, admissions for service at the county mental health center in 1974 indicate that 36.5 percent of the patients come from families with incomes below the official poverty guidelines; that admission rates for nonwhites are slightly higher than for whites, relative to their numbers in the population; and that low-income patients have consistently been the largest number, by income group, seen at the mental health center. In absolute numbers, patients from the low-income group have consistently increased from 1968 through 1974. In 1974, 559 patients from this income group were seen at the mental health center. A health survey conducted in 1973 included an incidental sampling of persons with "chronic nervous conditions" in the central city area and found the rate of persons with this condition to be 5 percent of the residents. Applying this rate to the central city population of 29,781, it can be estimated that 1,489 persons would be included in this category. This data on chronic nervous disorders clearly underestimates the total number of mental health problems that would be expected to exist in the area. Since the 559 patients from low-income families seen at the center do not all reside in the central city area, it is safe to assume that there are large numbers of untreated cases who do reside in the area, and additional numbers of persons who are at high risk of mental health problems.

From a psycho-social standpoint, this area is characterized by a relative lack of personal and social resources. The especially high percentage of families with children headed by females (three times the rate of the county as a whole), and the high percentage of females employed at relatively low incomes (over half of the female-headed families are below the poverty line in income) comprise a particularly high-risk group. Moreover, the 20 year forecast prepared by the planning commission predicts that this area will experience a decline in the number of employed residents and an increase in the number of children enrolled in school during the forecast period. This forecast is based on survival rates for five-year age group cohorts, and employment rates based on forecast employer demand, with no change in in- or out-migration rates (currently the highest in the county).

While blacks are not a majority in the area as a whole, or in any of the individual census tracts, three-fourths of the black citizens of the county live in this area. In the county, the median educational level is 12.1 years for whites, 10.6 years for blacks, and 10.9 years for Spanish-speaking residents. In the central city area, the average educational level is 10.9, but the range is from 9.1 in one tract to 12.0 in another. In general, median level of education is higher in tracts further from the downtown area and the river within this area. While the differences in educational level are not large, in a society that holds high school completion as a minimum entry credential for many occupations, these are differences that make a difference in economic terms.

Treating this central city area as an environmental entity, ecological principles can be applied to construct a description of key behavioral transactions within this ecosystem, and as an aid in planning appropriate interventions. Kelly's (1968) four principles of interdependence, cycling of resources, adaptation, and succession can be employed for this purpose.

ECOLOGICAL ANALYSIS

INTERDEPENDENCE

A structural analysis of the central city area identifies the existence of high concentrations of old, substandard, and overcrowded housing. The highest percentages of vacant dwelling units are found here, with a declining number of renter-occupied dwelling units, a trend that accompanies a gradual decline in total population in the area.

However, the black population increased significantly in this area from 1960 to 1970. These trends indicate a degree of "white flight" from the area, although perhaps as much due to the relative scarcity of adequate housing, upward economic mobility, and changes in the age structure of the population, as to racist attitudes, although the latter cannot be discounted. During the 10-year period cited above, there has been a slight decline in the percentage of children in the area, while a significant percentage of persons sixty-five and over remains (33 percent in one tract, an average of 14.5 percent for the area, compared to 9 percent for the county).

With these shifts, the area is characterized by a high rate of population exchange and retains the highest population density in the area. High exchange rates mark the area as a fluid environment with a number of associated characteristics: relatively changing and unclear social norms; a relatively high reliance on informal and unoffical social functions, in contrast to highly institutionalized social functions; and a diverse but poorly defined set of behaviors regarded as successful in the setting. High population density tends to increase the level of social stimulation in an environment (Calhoun, 1963; Desor, 1972). When added to the fluidity of the central city area, it can be expected that these environmental effects will be magnified relative to an environment with lower density.

For this particular environment, then, the combination of a high exchange rate, associated primarily with a large in-migration of blacks and out-migration of whites, high population density, and the persistence of a large percentage of senior citizens, would predict a high degree of conflict between new and old residents, and probably between perceived innovation and tradition.

Cycling of Resources

The cycling-of-resources principle identifies as relevant such questions as, how have resources in the environment been utilized in the past? How are helping roles defined in the environment and how are specific individuals identified and recruited to those roles? The cental city area contains the physical facilities of eight different child-serving social agencies and seven different adult-serving agencies. The cycling-of-resources principle can be addressed to the use of these agencies' services by residents of the area as a means of assessing how these resources can be better utilized within the area, including questions of overlap and duplication of services; relationship of services to needs defined from the ecological perspective; and how additional needed resources can be generated.

Adaptation

The relevance of this principle is to examine what behaviors are seen as adaptive in this environment, who participates in defining adaptive roles, how changes in adaptive requirements can be anticipated, and what socialization structures exist for shaping adaptive behavioral styles. Of particular importance for the central city area with its relatively high population exchange rate is the process of generating normative acceptance and support for a wide range of adaptive styles.

Succession

The principle of succession has relevance for both the socialization of newcomers to the area and the preparation of residents for anticipated changes in the community. If the predicted loss of employed residents and increase in school-enrolled children is realized, what changes in adaptive role requirements will be created? If these changes are viewed as undesirable, and not inevitable, what efforts are required to divert the evolutionary process in another direction?

ALTERNATIVE INTERVENTIONS

INTERDEPENDENCE

The central question concerning interdependence for this area is how to promote an increase in social organization and cooperation within the area. At present, the main visible forms of institutionalized organization are the social agencies, including three neighborhood centers. The problem is that these agencies have a history of independent, noncooperative activity. Planning of new programs tends to be preemptive and competitive. This tendency appears to be a carry-over of a cultural style of the community as a whole, and not just a characteristic of this particular area. The tradition is continued by virtue of the direction of social services coming primarily from board members of the various agencies who are not residents of the area. The noninstitutionalized, informal level of social organization within the area tends to clash periodically with the more traditional organizational structure, adding to the noncooperative atmosphere.

The task for intervention is to begin to build a degree of cooperation through the existing social agency structure on an informal, task-oriented basis. The mental health center has a history of case consultation with nearly all of these agencies on an individual basis, but it has not attempted previously to conduct a task-oriented group approach. Pooling of these relationships in a group consultation format (Altrocchi, Spielberger, and Eisdorfer, 1965) provides a means for approaching this task, with the ecological principles identified by Kelly (1968) as an agenda for planning the course of interventions.

The initial task focus will be on multiproblem cases that overlap agencies, and the interagency problems that exist, with the goal of defining new helping roles and identifying unutilized or underutilized resources. Anticipated developments in this process can be derived from Rhodes, Seeman, Spielberger, and Stepbach (1968) and Mann (1973). Mental health center staff will work on this project in two teams, one dealing primarily with child-serving agencies and one dealing mainly with adult-serving agencies.

CYCLING OF RESOURCES

The cycling-of-resources principle raises the question of how resources can be transformed to meet anticipated needs, and what the likely response to the intervention will be. Both these questions can be addressed by dealing with the history of noncooperation in the area, finding examples of cooperative behavior, and identifying superordinate goals that can promote cooperation. Assessment of needs and joint planning that involves both the formal and informal levels of social organization within the area, the social service agencies and the residents, can serve as a vehicle for mutual involvement and cooperation. The goal of community organization on this level is not the appropriation of political power from outside the area, but the development of internal resources and the creation of a means of providing recognition and support for the positive activities of residents. The definition of problems and needs would appropriately result from this process, but a number of these needs can be anticipated.

The relatively high proportion of working female heads of households, together with the projected increase in school-age children and decrease in employed residents in the area underscores the need for low-cost day- care facilities in the area to provide adequate child care and socialization resources. At the present time, the availability of such facilities is severely limited. Assuming that outside funding is either limited or unavailable, mechanisms for identifying and utilizing the skills of residents in the area in a cooperative day-care program would be an important example of resource transformation to meet ecologically defined needs. The staff of the mental health center can provide training and consultation support for such an enterprise, but the emphasis would be on the identification and utilization of local talent, similar to a program described by Rappoport and his co-workers (1975).

A second important need would be to examine how the resources of the schools in the area can be transformed into usable output for the residents. One existing example of such a resource transformation is the development by one social agency of a lighted-schools program, in which the otherwise unused facilities of the schools are available during evening hours for recreational programs. Other possibilities include the development of a child care curriculum at the junior high school level, which could feed into the need for such services as mentioned above, as well as to provide important educational and socialization experiences for the older students. Similarly, means for expanding the opportunities for work-study and vocational training could be explored with a view to providing consultative help to prospective employers and teachers in help-giving skills. Important aspects of this approach would be an assessment of the operation of informal help-giving roles in the peer culture at various age levels in the population, and the identification of mechanisms for redefining and creating needed new roles to provide help.

ADAPTATION

A high-priority task is to generate an understanding within the area, among social agency personnel and residents, that the characteristics of the environment at the present time will generate a wide range of adaptive behaviors. In part, this is an educative and consultative task, working with significant caregiver groups to develop an acceptable set of diverse norms for adaptive behavior, and recognizing the contributions that these behaviors make to the individual and to the social environment.

Given the old and dilapidated character of much of the housing in the area, it is important to anticipate that some sort of housing replacement program will be likely to develop, and input from the standpoint of human adaptation should be an important part of the process. Starting with the recognition that high-rise, high social stimulation housing is a benefit to the adaptation of many senior citizens, while low-rise, low-density housing patterns enhance adaptation among families with young children, input can be made to relevant planning and zoning bodies operating in the area.

A third task derived from this principle is the development of a monitoring capability within the resulting community organizational structure to assess changes in requirements for adaptive behavior over time as the fluidity or constancy of the area changes. Another aspect of the principle of adaptation is the assessment of mechanisms for welcoming and integrating newcomers to the area.

SUCCESSION

This principle calls attention to anticipated effects of the intervention on residents of the area, and on changes that can be expected in the relationship between the intervention and the community. Ordinarily, one might expect an initial increase in demand for services as the visibility of helping resources is increased, followed by a decline as some needs are met and expectations are clarified concerning the efficacy of the services. However, for this area this development is assumed to have occurred already, with the intervention program representing a change in, rather than an introduction of, services.

Accordingly, the initial focus is expected to be on the clarification of expectations and the anticipation of the effects of the intervention. Inasmuch as emphasis will be placed on the development of local resources and capabilities, the problem of excessive increase in expectations is not anticipated to be as much of a problem as is the maintenance of a moderately increased level of expected benefits tied to internal resource development. The maintenance of mutual goal definition among agencies and residents thus becomes a crucial ongoing task.

Along these lines, as additional local capabilities are developed, problems can be anticipated in developing changes in the definition of roles of various social agencies. As individual competencies increase, what mechanisms will be required for providing increased access of residents to policymaking positions, such as membership on agency boards of directors? How will such changes be viewed by those groups currently represented on the boards but not residing in the area? What provisions can be made for increasing interaction between residents of the area and groups in the surrounding community for facilitating this transition?

Criteria for assessing this intervention over time include a decrease in duplicated efforts and an increase in more responsive services; an increase in citizen participation in cooperative, mutual planning functions, and a decrease in preemptive, unilateral planning activities (Kelly, 1970).

Another area of the community is a predominantly rural area that is moving rapidly in the direction of suburbanization. The area is a collection of several small villages and rural areas that have combined to form a single school district. This district is composed of one entire census tract and parts of two other tracts that contrast with each other to some degree. While the school district compares favorably with the county averages on social indicators derived from census data, significant differences between the tracts are obscured by these averages.

The central tract, in which the district offices and the high school and junior high school are located is the most populous. It is characterized by average levels of education, income, unemployment, housing value, and the like. Most of the residents of this tract are employed outside the area, and the proportion of working wives and children enrolled in day-care and preschool programs is higher than the average for the county.

The two bordering tracts are characterized by lower levels of education, income, and employment. Women with young children in these tracts are less likely to be employed outside the home, with the result that fewer young children are enrolled in preschool and day-care programs. Thirty-eight percent of the workers in these tracts are employed in agriculture, more than double the percentage in the central tract. Similarly, the population exchange rate in these bordering tracts is significantly lower than in the central tract.

School counselors report a significant proportion of problems among junior and senior high school students in the district associated with families feeling alienated from and uninvolved with the school system, and the problem seems more pronounced among residents in the bordering tracts. Population projections for the school district forecast that it will be the fastest-growing area in the county in the next 20 years, with virtually all of the growth occurring in the central tract. The population in the central tract is expected to double in twenty years; the enrollment in the school system has already increased by 31 percent in the last five years.

Besides posing a significant problem for school growth, including construction costs and the resultant need for citizen support of bond issue referenda, these increases pose significant problems in changing requirements for adaptive behavior. The following is an application of principles of the ecological model to these problems.

ECOLOGICAL ANALYSIS

INTERDEPENDENCE

In this relatively low-density, dispersed environment, the school system provides the single unifying social structure. While the level of parental involvement in the schools is reported to be low, past experience with offering courses for parents in child-rearing techniques has produced a surprisingly good turnout. Social services are located both physically and psychologically at a distance from the area, and the schools provide a major source of organized social and recreational activities for adolescents in the area.

Cycling of Resources

Population growth will create growing demands for services that are already in short supply. It is unlikely that an increase in services to the area will come anywhere near matching the increase in population. Although an increase in large industries located in the area has occurred recently, and continued increases are likely, it is not known how these developments will effect increases in the tax base of the area to finance increases in human services. Existing resources in the schools, 4-H clubs, and the extension service of a major state university will likely experience changing demands for programs and services.

In the probable absence of an increase in institutionalized help-giving resources, the development of informal help-giving networks among the residents becomes important. While the existing resources can provide a vehicle for initiating these changes, it will also be necessary to redefine norms concerning help-giving roles during a transitional period of growth.

Adaptation

As these changes occur, it is anticipated that interdependent, cooperative behavioral norms outside of formal institutional structures will assume more importance in defining adaptive behavior. An increase in diversity of adaptive styles within the area will likely create some strain and conflict with existing norms concerning successful adaptation. These changes will require a redefinition of expected behavior in a variety of settings, most importantly in the school setting. The development of increased communication channels between schools and residents thus assumes heightened importance.

Succession

Prediction of alternative forms of the growth curve for the area has important implications for the development of functions in the community. Since the exact form of the growth curve cannot be predicted, alternative possibilities must be considered. Of the alternatives, a linear growth model seems the least likely to occur, with negatively accelerating, S-shaped, and positively accelerating curves comprising the remaining possibilities, stated in order of most to least likely, based on past and present trends. Within any of the latter three possibilities, a period of rapid transition will occur —the only remaining question being when this phase will occur.

Given these uncertainties, the development of two capabilities within this environment are critical: one is an increase in citizen participation in developing social organization within the area; another is the establishment of a planning capability concerning land use and zoning.

The significance of these functions can be illustrated by the possibility that large-scale construction of multiple-family housing in the area would rapidly increase both population and school enrollment without adding proportionately to the capability of providing increased human services. A second possibility would be the conversion of the area's prime agricultural land, its major resource, into housing developments, which would have the effect of creating an irretrievable resource loss for the area.

ALTERNATIVE INTERVENTIONS

INTERDEPENDENCE

Staff members of the mental health center have established a consulting relationship with staff members of the junior and senior high schools in the district. Using the school staff's positive past experiences in providing helping services to parents, it is planned to bring together a nucleus of representatives from a small number of services already operating in the district to meet with small groups of residents in their homes for informal discussions of problems and needs. Key residents will be identified in each of the areas served by the elementary schools in the district who will invite other residents to attend these discussions. These meetings will be used to promote familiarity between residents and school and other helping persons, and familiarity of potential help-givers with needs and resources. Results from these meetings will be fed back to appropriate school and government officials for further discussion and for the development of planning activities.

CYCLING OF RESOURCES

This project provides for a minimal introduction of new personnel and resources into the area initially, but a key task will be the linking of existing resources with needs and problems identified through the informal meetings, and the redefinition of roles to meet those needs. The mental health center staff and school staff representatives will meet frequently with other help-givers, including residents, to coordinate activities and define needed role functions.

In addition to this informal process of needs assessment, a more structured form of assessment of perceptions of community structure and function will be required both to assist in the definition of problems and to monitor effectiveness of the change processes.

Adaptation

Two necessary functions can be identified from the ecological perspective. One is the development of a mechanism for welcoming and integrating new members of the community, and for providing means by which new and old community members can become acquainted. Development of this function should be based on an analysis of the existing process by which new members are introduced. This function will assume increasing importance in the school setting as growth continues.

Another function is the development of communication and cooperation between planning and zoning organizations and the coordinating group that will be developed, so that the social and behavioral impact of planned new developments can be assessed along with the study of the physical environmental impact of such developments. While an overall planning capability exists for the county, there is no provision for organized community input into this process, nor is there any provision for assessment of the social and behavioral impact of new developments. The planned intervention can contribute to this process by helping the community to develop social and behavioral criteria for adaptation, which can be used in the planning process. In turn, participative definition of such criteria can have a powerful impact on realization of these goals, which cannot be achieved otherwise.

Succession

A community of five or six thousand widely dispersed persons, as this area was a few years ago, can possibly afford a minimum of readily available human services. However, a community of more than fifteen thousand persons, as the area is projected to become, with a significant increase in population density in the central tract, will require increasingly more accessible organized services. Although it is anticipated that such services will be undersupplied until a point of population stabilization is approached, the planned intervention described here should be thought of as a temporary forerunner to the establishment of more organized and stabilized services.

Moreover, the intervention proposed here may well serve to delay the development of a critical need for such services if it is successful. If the development of increased services were imminent, intervention of the type proposed here would be unwise; but since increased services are not readily available, it can serve an important transitional function. The plan must anticipate, however, that community needs will change, and that the planning function established through this project should help to develop its own transition to a more formalized organization that would assess the needs, desired locations, and suggested functions of more organized services as community stability is achieved.

These two interventions for contrasting environments are derived from a consideration of characteristics unique to the ecology of each setting. They are designed from the perspective of change agents entering the ecosystems from a mental health setting, and they rely necessarily on the preexisting relationship between the change agents' system and the ecosystems, and the contributions which the former can provide to the latter. It should be noted, however, that these interventions do not mark the mental health setting as the exclusive or necessary origin of such interventions.

Change agents coming into the ecosystems from other settings might design ecological interventions along different lines. For example, an ecologically designed intervention originating from a planning and zoning setting might focus the coordination and development of resources around land use and housing issues as they affect human adaptation; an intervention designed from a community action program setting might focus on employment and income issues. These approaches would have in common a concern with how the intervention into the community ecosystem affects adaptation over time and the development of a planning function to assess changing adaptational requirements.

Typical Research

The concept of the stimulus as an influence on behavior has a history in psychology as old as the field itself; yet the amount of research dealing with the effects of environmental stimulation on behavior is strikingly small within the body of psychological research. The research that has been done, such as in the field of mental retardation and early childhood development, has tended to focus on the minimal environmental conditions for minimally healthy development, leaving other behavioral factors to the study of individual differences.

No doubt this trend has also been influenced by the proclivity in American psychology for linear, quantitative, atomistic theory and research, which is more at home in a closely controlled laboratory setting than in the natural environment. Much of the descriptive, naturalistic observation of environmental characteristics has been conducted by sociologists, such as Herbert Gans's (1962) insightful study of Boston's West End. These naturalistic studies seldom deal with the impact of the physical environment itself. Some beginnings in this direction are represented in the studies of a newly developing field of environmental psychology (Proshansky, Ittleson, and Rivlin, 1970). However, all of these approaches stop short of providing a linkage between a conception of the environment as a dynamic, changing entity, and individual adaptation as an ongoing process.

Research within the ecological model is conducted in a number of different ways. The identification of a particular environment may make use of demographic or census data, such as that cited in the interventions described earlier. Such data consists of characteristics of the population and its distribution within specific geographical boundaries called census tracts. Once the environment for study is identified, a second type of research might involve the identification and characterization of behavior settings through naturalistic observation. This might be followed by assessment of inhabitants' perceptions of the environment through questionnaires or other surveys. Finally, some form of evaluation of planned intervention might follow such an activity, employing any of these above methods. Research within the ecological model is not highly developed. However, it is possible to review some typical patterns of research and suggest some of its possible uses.

BEHAVIOR SETTING RESEARCH

Naturalistic observation as a research method typically consists of either time sampling or episode sampling. Time sampling involves having an observer record all of the occurrences of a given behavior or set of behaviors during a specified interval of time. The group observational methods discussed in Chapter 5 are a type of time sampling in which the observer codes the occurrences of interpersonal behavior during the time the group is in session. More frequently, time sampling would select short intervals, such as one minute or five minutes, and record, for example, the occurrence of aggressive or helping behavior among a group of nursery school children. These sampling intervals would then be repeated several times over a longer period, such as a school day or several days. Episode sampling consists of an observer recording the occurrence of preselected events, such as the aggressive or helping behavior mentioned above, as often as they occur during a much longer time period. In time sampling one limits the interval of observation, while in episode sampling one limits the class of behavior to be observed.

Barker and his co-workers (Barker, 1968) discovered that behavior episodes constituted a meaningful unit of observation that had an identifiable beginning and ending point, but that numerous observations of behavior episodes showed more variability between settings than they did between children. This form of episode sampling led to the identification of the various behavior settings in which they occurred. In Midwest, Barker and his associates identified a total of 884 behavior settings during the year 1963–64. Some of these settings occurred only once, some occurred every day. In addition to recording the frequency of occurrence, the researchers recorded the duration of each setting. They found that these two attributes were highly positively correlated.

The number, occurrence, and duration of behavior settings can be expressed as percentages of the total in each attribute category for the entire community, and then averaged to yield an Ecological Resource Index (ERI). Barker points out that these attributes—number, duration, occurrence, and ERI—provide a measure of the extent of the availability of behavior settings to the residents of the community. He considers such an inventory analogous to a land survey: the number of behavior settings is comparable to the number of acres of land; the number of different genotypes of behavior settings is comparable to the variety of soil types contained in the acreage of land.

The Occupancy Time (OT) of a behavior setting is the sum of time spent by individuals in a behavior setting. Not entirely an attribute of the setting, it results from the interaction of the setting with individual decisions to enter or leave the setting. The OT is one index of the utilization of behavior settings by the residents. Following Barker's analogy, if number, duration, occurrence, and ERI are compared to a land survey, then OT can be considered analogous to a land-use survey.

Since residents follow a standing pattern of behavior while occupying a behavior setting, OT is also a measure of behavior output, and, expressed according to types of settings, it is an index of the output of particular classes of behavior. The residents of Midwest had a total OT of 1,125,134 hours in the various behavior settings during 1963–64, ranging from one hour in one setting to 87,376 hours in the setting Trafficways, which includes streets and sidewalks. OT and ERI are also highly positively correlated, but some behavioral settings *undergenerate* (rank lower in OT than in ERI) and other settings *overgenerate* (rank higher in OT than in ERI). The least productive in this sense are behavior settings where religion is the main action pattern; the most productive are settings where nutrition is prominent (public dining settings).

Price and Blashfield (1975) performed factor and cluster analyses on data collected by Barker in Midwest for 1968–69. They analyzed 43 variables pertaining to 455 behavior settings. The categories in which variables appeared were Class of Authority System (5 variables), Action Patterns (8 variables), Member Characteristics (9 variables), Performer Characteristics (9 variables), Target Characteristics (6 variables), Size of Behavior Setting (2 variables), Duration (3 variables), and Frequency of Occurrence (1 variable).

A principle components factor analysis produced thirteen factors that together accounted for only 62.2 percent of the total variance. These researchers concluded that this procedure did not produce a strong factor structure, since there was a large number of factors with no one factor accounting for more than 15 percent of the variance and most factors accounting for considerably smaller proportions of the variance. There were nine factors from this analysis that yielded interpretable results. These were: Adult members and targets; Religion vs. government; Young performers; Young members and targets; Female members and targets; Business; Duration; Adolescent members and targets; and Male members and targets. These results suggest that age, sex, and role grading of inhabitants, action patterns, and duration are important ways in which these settings vary, but the variability among settings is not easily or entirely reducible to these factors. The factorial dimensions appear to yield more information about the bases for segregating behavior settings than about the settings themselves.

As part of the same study, Price and Blashfield performed a cluster analysis on the same data, this time attempting to group together similar behavior settings. This analysis yielded twelve clusters: Youth performance; Religious; Women's organizational; Elementary school; High school; Adult; Men's organizational; Local business; Large membership; High school performance; Family oriented; and Government. This procedure yields a typology of behavior settings along dimensions quite similar to those in the factor analysis. The resulting factors or clusters are a significant reduction from the 138 genotypes that Barker found among the 455 behavior settings in the 1968–69 survey. The categorization of settings by genotype appears to be tied closely to clusters of behavioral episodes centered on key performers, while the categories produced by Price and Blashfield are more closely related to social structure and social interaction. These dimensions presumably tell us something important about this community insofar as the organization of its behavior patterns is meaningful. It would be interesting to know if factor or cluster analysis of other communities' behavior settings would line up the same way.

It would also be interesting to learn why there were more behavior settings in Midwest in the 1963–64 survey than in the 1968–69 survey. Whether this is due to a change in methodology or to a change in the community is unknown. If it were the latter, the reasons for this change and the processes by which it occurred would be an extremely meaningful contribution. Assuming that this change was a real one, it underscores again the importance of anticipating natural change in community structures, not just in the abstract or psychological environment, but in the concrete eco-behavioral system.

These classification studies are extremely important aspects of the study of the environment of human behavior. They are time-consuming and complex undertakings. It is, of course, not necessary to survey an entire community in this way, as Midwest is a rather small town and most communities are considerably larger. Such an undertaking would be nearly prohibitive in most communities. One can, however, survey smaller environments than an entire town in this way with quite useful results, provided the area selected is meaningful for the observer's purposes.

Kelly's (1969) studies of the high school environment, for example, began with naturalistic observations of selected behavior settings in high schools that differed in their rates of population exchange. In one school this rate of turnover was 42 percent, which was termed a fluid environment, and in another the rate was 10 percent, which was considered a constant environment. The settings selected for observation in the two schools were hallways, principal's office, and cafeteria. Observers of six hallways found that in the fluid environment there was varied dress among students, varied membership in conversation groups, and more body and gestural movements; in the constant environment dress was so similar as to be nearly uniform, there were few shifts in conversation groups, and conversations were conducted on a low level of noise. Observations of the principal's office showed that in the fluid environment there was a range of 30 to 110 entrances by students and faculty during a three-minute period, while in the constant environment the range during three-minute observation periods was 1 to 15. In the fluid environment, students and faculty entered in nearly equal numbers to talk with a variety of persons in the office; in the constant environment those entering were mainly faculty who held lengthy conferences with the principal.

Observations in the cafeteria presented a problem related to the environmental differences between the schools. In the fluid environment there was so much activity that it was difficult to code, while in the constant environment students were so conscious of being observed that it seemed to restrict their behavior even more. These problems were overcome by having several observers sample brief time periods in the fluid environment, and in the constant environment fewer observers made several repeated observations over a longer time. The cafeterias in the two schools revealed differences consistent with the other observations: more conversations between groups, more table hopping, and more conversations between tables in the fluid environment than in the constant environment.

These findings were consistent with Kelly's hypothesis that the fluid environment provided more public settings for personal expression, while in the constant environment personal expression would be limited to private settings. The study had also called for observations in lavatories, but when permission was refused to make such observations in the constant environment, Kelly reasoned that it may have been related to the greater need to maintain the privacy of such a setting in that environment. The results are generally consistent with Kelly's assumption that fluid environments provide generally more emphasis on personal development and reward diversity, while constant environments emphasize "fitting in" and reward conformity.

PERSON–ENVIRONMENT INTERACTION

Barker and Gump (1964) used school size as a critical environmental variable in investigating the effects of undermanning vs. overmanning* on the inhabitants of a behavior setting. They found that students in smaller high schools reported twice as many pressures to take part, participated in 2.5 times as many responsible positions, and reported more satisfactions on a number of dimensions of personal development and involvement with the setting than did students in larger high schools. Psychologically, the smaller school resulted in more emphasis on a person's functional importance to the setting (What can this person do?), while in the larger school, evaluations were more often made in terms of personality attributes (What kind of person is this?).

Kelly (1969) interviewed students in the fluid- and constant-environment schools described above. He found that in the constant environment newcomers were given the silent treatment until they declared themselves and then were either accepted or hazed depending upon the evaluation made of the newcomer. Adaptation of newcomers in this setting was facilitated if they had a visible competence that was in short supply in the setting and were willing to become absorbed in and dominated by the setting. Students in the fluid environment formed a welcoming committee to orient newcomers, point out the appropriate settings for various kinds of behavior, and to identify the newcomer's interests and needs.

Kelly found that students in the constant school were limited to a few well-defined positions of status, while a wider range of success opportunities were available to the fluid-environment students. Students in the constant environment were more concerned with their place in the school, and students in the fluid environment were concerned with their own personal progress. Based on scores

*The reader should note that the use of these terms antedates the concern with the implication of sex-role stereotyping associated with the use of the English language.

on a questionnaire designed to identify preferences for an exploratory coping style, defined as preference for novel experience, Kelly found that students with high exploration preferences were more likely to be identified as deviant by faculty in the constant-environment than in the fluid-environment school.

In another series of studies conducted in a different set of high schools that again differed in population exchange rates but were similar in other respects, Kelly and his co-workers found results that support the hypothesized differences between the settings. Newman (1971) surveyed students and faculty in two high schools, one with an exchange rate of 18.7 percent (fluid) and one with an exchange rate of 8 percent (constant). In line with the results above, he found that students reported more interactions with adults in the fluid school than in the constant school, and more interaction with peers in a variety of settings in the fluid school compared to the constant school. Newman felt that these differences in interaction patterns may have contributed to the fluid-environment students seeing themselves as more involved in the school, reporting a clearer perception of norms, and having greater identification with both social and work goals in the setting than did students in the constant environment. Of additional interest is Newman's finding that faculty in the constant-environment school reported poorer morale and less satisfaction with the school than faculty in the fluid-environment school.

In an ongoing longitudinal analysis of these school settings, Kelly and his associates (Kelly, 1971a, 1971b, in press) have found that the fluid environment continues to provide greater support for exploratory behavior and personal development than does the constant-environment school. That these socialization experiences have some carry-over effects on personal development is suggested by a study by Mann (1972). Reasoning that college students with a history of frequent geographical mobility would be more likely to have had experience in a diverse set of fluid environments than would those with little previous history of geographical mobility, Mann compared the responses of college students who differed in their mobility history to a set of personality and classroom preference questionnaires. High mobility was associated with personality differences only for male students and not for female students. High-mobility students, compared to low-mobility students, were more intellectually oriented, placed more value on autonomy and independence, and reported less anxiety in a stress situation. Geographical mobility did not contribute to differences in preferences for types of classrooms, but social mobility differences did, with upwardly socially mobile students expressing less preference for classroom structure than socially nonmobile students. It was assumed that the college environment is a relatively complex, fluid environment, and these high-mobility students would presumably adapt to it well. However, the same might not be true in a more constant environment.

Although these studies have been discussed at some length, research in the ecological model is still in its beginning stages. If one were to lay out a diagram of the possible studies that could be made even within the framework of the studies that have been discussed here, one would find several empty spaces in which studies have not been conducted. Inasmuch as the ecological model emphasizes the importance of research as an integral part of the process of planning and change, there is considerably more work to be done in this area. Not even mentioned here is the importance of evaluative studies of intervention programs, since such studies have not been conducted within this model as of the time of this writing.

Typical Settings

Ideally, the ecological model seeks to become an integral part of the community in which it is employed, and the emphasis on the community is an important consideration in the appropriate setting for the model. The problem is similar to that of the cultural anthropologist who seeks to learn about a particular group's life from day-to-day observation. However, an added dimension of considerable import for the model is its emphasis on change, which marks it as significantly different from many historical examples. Barker's pioneering development of a research field station comes somewhat closer to a desirable setting, but, again, such a setting is not identified with change processes, although presumably it could be. The desired combination of community embeddedness, involvement with change, and research capability is a demanding set of criteria for such a setting.

The interventions described in this chapter would originate from a university or community mental health center setting, but there are many constraints operating on such settings. While the university provides the research capability and the involvement with change, its relationship to the community, particularly concerning the long-term commitment to evolutionary change processes, is likely to be problematic both from the standpoint of funding support and faculty durability. In some communities, of course, relationships with university-based change programs have not been especially satisfying. The community mental health center is more likely to have an integrated relationship with the community, if it has survived this long since the origins of such centers; but few mental health centers have a sufficient research capability, and their commitment to involvement in community change processes is likely to be quite limited in many communities.

Although not made explicit in the examples presented here concerning intervention and research, the ecological model in the community requires participation by a number of individuals with varied competences representing a number of different fields, not just psychology or even those disciplines traditionally associated with the helping professions. One setting that is a promising possibility for employing the ecological model is the urban and regional planning facility. Indeed, planners seem to have shown more of an interest in aspects of psychological methods than psychologists have shown in concerns with problems of planning (Michelson, 1975). The planning setting comes as close as any currently available to meeting the criteria for such a setting. Catalano and Monahan (1975) have discussed how psychological research could be employed in developing behavioral impact studies of planned new developments, a function that could logically originate from a planning facility.

Rappoport and his associates (1975) have developed a community psychology action center that, while associated with a university program, is planned as a community setting. Although not explicitly based on an ecological model, the early work with the development of this setting is an attempt to find alternatives to what Rappoport calls person-blaming and environment-blaming philosophies, an approach that could be accommodated within the ecological conception of community processes.

A variety of potential settings for the ecological model, then, present a number of opportunities and limitations. The multiple methods for coping with a variety of problems may ultimately work as well through some sort of cooperative arrangement that involves persons from a variety of settings coming together to work with the community on enhancing its ability to cope with the challenges of evolutionary change processes.

Assessment of the Model

The ecological model conceptualizes community processes as subject to natural, evolutionary change. This assumption places a time perspective in a prominent place within the model and also has important implications for the planning of successive interventions. It is not necessary, then, to create forces for change according to this model, but rather to channel resources in the environment to anticipate and deal with naturally occurring change.

The model places explicit emphasis on values that arise within the setting, with interventions designed to meet local conditions. A high value is placed on participation in the model, with this role for citizens including the assessment process. These provisions for participation build accountability to the members of the setting into the structure and process of the model.

The survival value of the model appears to be high, provided that the criteria for its implementation are met. At the same time, meeting these criteria in the initial establishment of the model can be seen as its most serious problem. The model does address these problems directly, however, in its provisions for dealing with locally defined problems through member participation. Morevover, the ecological model takes specific account of the problem of survival through the principle of succession, in which an attempt is made to establish a continuing function for the anticipation of change within the setting. In this sense, the problem of survival is tied to the expectation of change and to the survival of the setting.

The ecological model is a point of view, an analytic framework, within which a number of approaches to understanding adaptive behavior and developing specific interventions can be incorporated. In its specific attention to the behavior setting and its concern for the interrelatedness of behavior and social systems, it provides a perspective with a high potential for integrating views of the individual and the community. In these respects it is unusual among psychological viewpoints. Its use of multiple criteria for different forms of adaptation is at variance with the single-criterion idealized standards that derive from a universalized intrapsychic view of behavior as exemplified by personality theory, in which the environment is assumed to be relatively uniform. Accordingly, the further development of the model will depend more on opportunities for and the willingness of psychologists to become involved in the ongoing problems of live behavior settings rather than a series of more quickly generated laboratory studies. Here the question is as much a question of the survival of the psychologist as of the model itself, since the model requires a new definition of criteria for the work of the psychologist in both university and community settings.

References

ALTROCCHI, J., SPIELBERGER, C. D., AND EISDORFER, C. Mental health consultation with groups. *Community Mental Health Journal*, 1965, *1*, 127–134.

BARKER, R. G. On the nature of the environment. *Journal of Social Issues*, 1963, *19*, no. 4, 17–38.

BARKER, R. G. *Ecological Psychology*. Stanford: Stanford University Press, 1968.

BARKER, R. G. AND GUMP, P. V. *Big School, Small School*. Stanford: Stanford University Press, 1964.

BLOOM, B. L. A census tract analysis of socially deviant behaviors. *Multivariate Behavioral Research*, 1966, *1*, 307–320.

CALHOUN, J. B. Population density and social pathology. In L. J. Duhl (Ed.), *The Urban Condition*. New York: Basic Books, 1963.

CARTWRIGHT, D. Introduction to K. Lewin, *Field Theory in Social Science*. New York: Harper & Row, 1951.

CATALANO, R., AND MONAHAN, J. The community psychologist as social planner: Designing optimal environments. *American Journal of Community Psychology*, 1975, *3*, 327–334.

DEEVEY, E. S., JR. General and urban ecology. In L. J. Duhl (Ed.), *The Urban Condition*. New York: Basic Books, 1963.

DESOR, J. A. Toward a psychological theory of crowding. *Journal of Personality and Social Psychology*, 1972, *21*, 79–83.

FRIED, M. Grieving for a lost home. In L. J. Duhl (Ed.), *The Urban Condition*. New York: Basic Books, 1963.

GANS, H. *The Urban Villagers*. New York: Free Press, 1962.

GEDDES, P. Cities in evolution. In D. R. Weimer (Ed.), *City and Country in America*. New York: Appleton-Century-Crofts, 1962. Originally published 1915.

KELLY, J. G. The mental health agent in the urban community. In L. J. Duhl (Ed.), *Urban America and the Planning of Mental Health Services*. New York: Group for the Advancement of Psychiatry, 1964.

KELLY, J. G. Ecological constraints on mental health services. *American Psychologist*, 1966, *21*, 535–539.

KELLY, J. G. Towards an ecological conception of preventive interventions. In J. W. Carter (Ed.), *Research Contributions from Psychology to Community Mental Health*. New York: Behavioral Publications, 1968.

KELLY, J. G. Naturalistic observations in contrasting social environments. In E. P. Willems and H. L. Raush (Eds.), *Naturalistic Viewpoints in Psychological Research*. New York: Holt, Rinehart & Winston, 1969.

KELLY, J. G. The quest for valid preventive interventions. In C. D. Spielberger (Ed.), *Current Topics in Clinical and Community Psychology*, vol. 2. New York: Academic Press, 1970.

KELLY, J. G. The socialization of competence as an ecological problem. In Symposium, "Social competence and mental health," American Psychological Association, 1971a.

KELLY, J. G. The coping process in varied high school environments. In M. J. Feldman (Ed.), *Studies in Psychotherapy and Behavior Change*, no. 2. Buffalo: State University of New York, May 1971b.

KELLY, J. G. Longitudinal study of person-environment interaction. *Community Psychology Monograph Series*, Laurence Erlbaum Associates, Hillsdale, N.J., in press.

LEVINS, R. The strategy of model building in population biology. *American Scientist*, 1966, *54*, 421–431.

LEWIN, K. *Field Theory in Social Science*. New York: Harper & Row, 1951.

LINDORFER, D. The relationship between demographic variables and deviance. Unpublished doctoral dissertation, University of Texas, Austin, 1972.

MANN, P. A. Residential mobility as an adaptive experience. *Journal of Consulting and Clinical Psychology*, 1972, *39*, 37–42.

MANN, P. A. *Psychological Consultation with a Police Department*. Springfield, Ill.: Charles C. Thomas, 1973.

MICHELSON, W. (Ed.). *Behavioral Research Methods in Environmental Design*. Stroudsburg, Pa.: Dowden, Hutchinson & Ross, 1975.

MOE, E. O. Consulting with a community system: A case study. *Journal of Social Issues*, 1959, *15*, no. 2, 28–35.

NEWMAN, P. R. Persons and settings: A comparative analysis of the quality and range of social interaction in two suburban high schools. Unpublished doctoral dissertation, University of Michigan, 1971.

PRICE, R. H., AND BLASHFIELD, R. K. Explorations in the taxonomy of behavior settings: Analysis of dimensions and classification of settings. *American Journal of Community Psychology*, 1975, *3*, 335–352.

PROSHANSKY, H. M., ITTELSON, W. H., AND RIVLIN, L. G. (Eds.). *Environmental Psychology: Man and his Physical Setting*. New York: Holt, Rinehart & Winston, 1970.

RAPPOPORT, J., DAVIDSON, W. S., WILSON, M. N., AND MITCHELL, A. Alternatives to blaming the victim or the environment. *American Psychologist*, 1975, *30*, 525–528.

RAUSH, H. L., DITTMAN, A. T., AND TAYLOR, T. J. Person, setting, and change in social interaction. *Human Relations*, 1959, *12*, 361–379.

RHODES, W. C., SEEMAN, J., SPIELBERGER, C. D., AND STEPBACH, R. F. The multiproblem neighborhood project. *Community Mental Health Journal*, 1968, *4*, 3–12.

TRICKETT, E. J., KELLY, J. G., AND TODD, D. M. The social environment of the high school: Guidelines for individual change and organizational redevelopment. In S. E. Golann and C. Eisdorfer (Eds.), *Handbook of Community Mental Health*. New York: Appleton-Century- Crofts, 1972.

WEIMER, D. R. (Ed.). *City and Country in America*. New York: Appleton-Century-Crofts, 1962.

Part III

Implications for a Psychology of the Community

8. The Study of Community Life

Before moving to a comparative summary of the models we have examined, it is instructive to review the historical context in which these models have developed. Community psychology began to develop its first self-definitions in the context of the community mental health program. The reader may wish to note that, prior to this program, the role of the clinical psychologist in the mental health field and in relation to the rest of psychology was not entirely clear. A number of conferences had been held to attempt to develop the appropriate training for a professional role, which evolved in a discipline that had previously been concerned largely with research (Hoch, Ross, and Winder; 1966; Raimy, 1950; Roe, Gustad, Moore, Ross, and Skodak, 1959; Strother, 1956). The development of new challenges for psychologists in the mental health field, entering an arena of discourse in which there was already considerable uncertainty, may have added to the confusion, as these new challenges did generally in the mental health field. The development of additional "community" programs undoubtedly increased this confusion. In this chapter and those that follow, an attempt will be made to clarify some of these points of uncertainty.

The review of the various models has underscored the variability in the concept of community that is employed in them. Yet these differences have more often been overlooked than understood. Recall from Chapters 4 and 6 that the community mental health programs and the community action programs had quite separate developmental histories, yet their aims often seemed to psychologists to be the same. While these programs are similar in their common concern with the community, the mental health and social action models are, as we have seen, distinct in their assumptions, interventions, and goals. How then could this confusion have arisen? Aside from the possibility that some of the personnel of these programs were not clear or explicit about their assumptions and goals, there appear to be two compelling and interrelated factors that have contributed to the lack of clarity. One of these is the paucity of relevant theory and research in the field of psychology that was applicable to the enormous challenges of mental health and poverty. The other was the deceivingly compelling sociological theory and history on which the community action programs were based.

As Marris and Rein (1967) have noted, the theoretical base on which the early Ford Foundation and government programs to combat delinquency were based was a circular conception of poverty as the basic cause of a multitude of psychological and social deficits that in turn led to more poverty. Thus, one could assume to be correcting virtually any of these social problems by fighting poverty. Not only did this circular theory make it unnecessary, and perhaps impossible, to set priorities; it also blurred the distinctions between different approaches to the problems assumed to be linked to poverty. When the community action program concept became translated into the more generalized war on poverty, these blurred distinctions were carried along with it.

In addition to this conceptual murkiness, there was also strategic confusion concerning national policy toward poverty. Rein (1969) has traced in detail how what started out to be a services approach to the problem of poverty was transformed gradually into an income transfer policy. Originally, the services approach was designed to correct what were seen as personal limitations of the poor to take advantage of the opportunities available to them. At the same time, as we saw in Chapter 5, an effort was to be made to make social institutions more reponsive to the needs of the poor. The linking strategy between these two different levels was the concept of participation. However, as we have discussed previously, the increase in benefits and in the numbers of eligible persons, coupled with a serious, perhaps fatal, failure to actually expand employment opportunities, resulted in increasing resources going to what was in fact an income supplement policy rather than one of psychological and social transformation of the poor.

Accordingly, both theoretical and strategic disjointedness contributed to another significant problem: a confusion of boundaries between the various enterprises involved in these programs. Kahn

(1969) has discussed this problem in a particularly illustrative way in regard to community psychiatry and community mental health, and his analysis is applicable to this discussion. The heart of Kahn's proposal is that the boundaries of activity should be defined by particular competencies and by expectations of relevant publics. Resolution of the boundary problem thus requires not only a recognition of domains of expertise within a field, but also the limits of those domains and of the competencies of others in related or different fields. This analysis is reminiscent of Knudson's suggestion (see Chapter 1) that psychologists should avoid concern with broad and vague topics such as mental health and should specify the types of problems in which they are interested; and it also underscores Reiff's exhortation (quoted in Chapter 1) that psychologists should make explicit the basis of their participation in social programs. Thus, there are two concerns for community psychologists as we review the features of the various models: one is the applicability of each model to different community problems; the other is the legitimation of the community psychologist's role in approaching these problems. Having reasserted the significance of these observations, we can now proceed to a comparison of the implications of the models for studies of community life.

Dimensions of Community Psychology Research

The four models of community psychology reviewed here have important similarities and differences both with respect to the types of research that they generate and the types of interventions that derive from each. The implications for interventions will be considered in the next chapter, but despite the separation of research from intervention for purposes of discussion, the reader should keep in mind that these models require both research and intervention as integral parts. Our purpose here is to identify the particular utility of each model for its contribution to studying the community.

DOMAINS OF INQUIRY

In discussing the mental health model, the uses and problems of epidemiological research were identified. It should be noted that while this methodology developed in the context of disease studies, it is applicable to studying the incidence and prevalence of any social problem that can be identified by the number of individuals affected. Thus, one could also speak of the incidence and prevalence of delinquency, divorce, unemployment, or other categories. Its use serves as a social problem identifier, and in the context of evaluating preventive mental health interventions it is critical for the assessment of changes in the distribution of mental disturbance. However, as we noted, its systematic use is no more well developed than are the data systems for the other kinds of social problems mentioned above.

The limited use that has been made of epidemiological studies is a critical shortcoming for the mental health model. These studies are a necessary counterpart of preventive mental health services. New regulations governing the funding of community mental health programs (P.L. 94-63) require that 2 percent of the budgets of mental health centers be devoted to program evaluation, and this regulation, if enforced, may provide some incentive to conduct further epidemiological studies. However, evaluation in the community mental health centers has consisted largely of management-oriented, cost-control, and evaluation-of-effort data collection so far, and a major shift in emphasis will be required to employ more meaningful epidemiological forms of evaluation. In addition, many more individuals trained in this methodology will need to be employed by or available to mental health centers than is presently the case.

As we noted in Chapter 4, the use of extended time-series designs could enhance the inferential power of epidemiological studies; so could such monitoring over time enhance the evaluative power of this method. In fact, the extension of time dimensions both historically and into the future is a major theme of the type of research that is badly needed in all of these models.

Epidemiology is a limited method, however, when it comes to attempting to assess changes in "positive mental health." Here the criterion problem becomes infinitely more complex than it does in defining cases for epidmiological study. One source of criterion ambiguity is the time-honored yet uncorrected cliche that mental health is more than the absence of disease. This is a phrase with which it is easy to agree, but its meaning is difficult to fathom. Probably nowhere is it more important than at this point to dispense with the notion of "mental health" and to develop specific criteria for defining outcomes of specific interventions. And, as Kahn (1969) suggested, it is here that one encounters the boundary between mental health and the other models under consideration.

There is a natural tendency to confuse the domains of health and disease. This confusion has implications for what is sometimes referred to as the medical model problem, but which is more properly referred to as the "disease model" (Cohen, 1971). The medical-practice laws of most states regulate the dispensing of prescription drugs and the performance of surgery, limiting such practice to those legally qualified to perform such services. Thus, the medical profession controls the treatment of disease, including the facilities and allied personnel involved in treating disease. However, if health is more than the absence of disease, then medical practice can lay either legal or expert claim to jurisdiction over only a part of the health field. Yet society's institutions, the health insurance industry, and increasing amounts of social resources are allocated to the disease treatment segment of the health field. This is true in regard to public health's relative slice of the general health field pie, as well as in regard to the preventive activities portion of mental health resources (Brown and Stockdill, 1972).

Aside from the legal and considerable political forces that tend to maintain this situation, it is nevertheless true that progress in the nondisease segments of both health and mental health activity will not be furthered unless specific criteria of behavioral and social goals are developed apart from a disease-oriented model. Increasing need for developing this aspect of the health field has been recognized in the middle 1970s (APA, 1975). This is an area where psychologists have the potential to provide legitimate contributions.

It seems more likely that this specification of problems and criteria for community psychologists will come from an understanding of the other models presented here than from the mental health model. As comparatively rich as psychology's association with mental health has been, the concept of disease applied to what are essentially psychosocial problems is a severely limiting factor, both conceptually and organizationally. Thus, as Kahn (1969) suggested, we should draw a boundary between research related to disease problems and the delivery of services for those problems, and other activities designed to promote and enhance the benefits of community life.

Of the models we have considered, the ecological model presents the broadest theoretical framework for the conduct of meaningful research. Moreover, the framework provides guidelines for the identification of research problems, assigning of priorities, developing a time perspective, and establishing boundaries for the scope of the work. In comparison, the social action model provides no such theoretical perspective, while the organizational model's perspective is more limited in its capability of reaching community processes. This is not to say that these other models do not have important contribuitons to make to the meaningful study of community problems, but rather that a perspective is needed that is more precise on the one hand and more comprehensively articulated with community processes on the other. This perspective is crucial to drawing the distinction referred to in Chapter 2 between "societal" and "community" problems and solutions. These distinctions are necessary not only for defining an appropriate and meaningful area for research, but also for selecting the appropriate level of intervention, a problem to be considered further in the next chapter.

LEVELS OF ANALYSIS

The anchoring of the ecological model in behavior settings affords the community psychologist with a starting point that is real in both time and space. Moreover, it is a reference point to which others, professionals and citizens alike, can readily be directed. Although seemingly a simple idea, in fact it is no insignificant consideration in implementing a study or planning process. The concept of linking behavior settings with each other and with human interaction lends itself to a systems approach in which the interpersonal, organizational and community levels can be defined explicitly. Finally, ecological theory, as described in Chapter 7, provides a set of principles that guide the definition of problems and point to appropriate areas of research. It is possible, then, within this framework to identify problems that lend themselves to organizational analysis within the community system, including analyses of interaction patterns (Newman, 1971), studies of interpersonal relations and effects on the development of self-concept (Barker and Gump, 1964; Kelly, 1971a), and studies of organizational output or effectiveness in different settings. The social action model underscores the importance of the role of the citizen in the research and planning process, and calls attention to the role of nonpsychological factors, such as political and economic structures, in shaping behavior. These concerns are also part of the ecological model.

In reviewing the organizational model, it was noted that the criteria for organizational effectiveness were difficult to establish outside of a profit-defined productivity framework. In the context of the ecological model, however, the emphasis on enhancing adaptive behavior in specific settings makes this definition somewhat more attainable. Care must be taken at this level, however, not to fall into the trap of using problem-alleviation, such as reduced conflict, absenteeism, or complaints, as the sole criteria of organizational effectiveness. The problem here is similar to the disease-reduction vs. enhancement-of-health problem in the mental health model. Desired outcomes, such as enhanced adaptation in other settings for school graduates, or improved effectiveness of social case workers or policemen, need to be defined and measured.

Principles of the social action model can alert the community psychologist to define the appropriate professional role for the psychologist, the psychological competencies that are relevant to that role, and the definition of the social and psychological issues involved. From this analysis, important distinctions can be made between problems that are amenable to solution within the local community and those that require modification of social policy. Rappoport and Kren (1975) have performed a useful service by bringing this question to the attention of psychologists. They suggest that a critical analysis of past work and principles is needed to develop a meaningful relationship between psychology and social problems. They point out that psychology is not relevant to every social problem, and not everything to which psychology is relevant necessarily leads to social solutions. They cite the example of the studies of the effects of television viewing on aggression as a short-sighted approach to the problems of crime and violence. Their recommendations are similar to those presented above, in that they call for the development of priorities for the evaluation of social problems and of "systematically organized ways of converting the knowledge we may have about social issues into publicly meaningful action" (1975, p. 841).

Thus, the psychologist may be appropriately engaged in social policy analysis, and in the design and testing of alternative social policies. This is, however, a different order of endeavor than that referred to above in the ecological model. While the ecological model seems quite well suited to studying the problems of the local community, the community psychologist leaves many of the assumptions and methods of that model when he approaches the broader questions of social policy. The reverse may also be true; that is, the social policy analyst leaves the boundaries of the social policy model and enters the ecological domain when dealing with problems of the local community, including the application of social policy there.

While there are numerous examples of psychologists' involvement in social policy issues, including Kenneth and Mamie Clark's (Clark and Clark, 1947) contributions to the 1954 Supreme Court decision on public school desegregation, an excellent recent example is provided by Goodwin and Tu (1975). These authors undertook a survey of a representative sample of citizens concerning their attitudes toward the support of the Social Security System. While methodologically sound from the usual conventional points of view, their study added some important dimensions that are especially commendable from the perspective being developed here. Prior to conducting the study, these authors examined the historical-psychological basis on which the program was assumed to be supportable by the public; i.e., the financing of the program out of income contributions by the participants. They also spent, by their account, nearly a year interviewing persons knowledgeable about the Social Security System as a basis for designing their survey format and defining an appropriate sample population. While the authors do not claim final definitiveness for their study, they are able to cite some possible psychological bases for policy change, as well as to point out some danger areas that might be anticipated with the program. Their approach seems to represent a more sound approach to defining possible bases for public support of social policy than is now utilized, and it represents a needed addition to the field of social policy analysis.

We have, then, identified three distinct fields of inquiry from our review of the four models, and the boundaries for these fields can be specified. One is the study of mental health problems and programs within the disease-oriented model of the mental health delivery system. Not all of the activities of those who presently identify themselves with community mental health are encompassed by these boundaries, nor are all of the problems included in this domain community-wide in their extent. Some problems of this nature are more properly studied at the interpersonal or group level. A second field is the major area of the study of person-environment interaction in community settings, following the framework of the ecological model. This work consists of some studies presently conducted within the framework of mental health, but not in a disease-oriented conception of the problem, and some organizational and social action problems. It is important in this domain to specify the behavioral and adaptational properties of the problems under consideration, and to separate those issues occurring at the level of adaptation in specific settings from issues at the level of larger social policy. The latter comprise a third field of inquiry in which the level of analysis and intervention is different, as are the historical and analytic methods. Thus, an important organizing principle for knowledge in community psychology is the specification of both the domain of inquiry and the level of analysis.

To illustrate these alternative approaches, let us consider an event that occurred some years ago in a moderate-sized midwestern community. In the spring of the year, a serious disturbance broke out in the high school in this community. Open conflict erupted between black and white students, and between black students and the school administration. The immediate focus of this incident was a protest over treatment of black students by white administrators, teachers, and students. Police were called to maintain order after fights broke out between black and white students, black student leaders presented demands and complaints to school administrators accusing teachers of racism and met with the administrators to press these demands. Tensions ran high, to say the least, and some students remained away from school because of their own or their parents' fears. The scene was not an unusual one for the times, as such disturbances occurred in many communities. How would a community psychologist approach such a situation?

The assumptions of the mental health model would define this situation as a crisis growing out of deficient knowledge, skills, confidence, or objectivity among the teachers for relating to minority-group students. In this instance, one would look for racist attitudes that interfere with the objectivity of teachers in their relationships with minority students. Within an organizational model, similar assumptions would be made concerning racial insensitivity, again defining the situation in terms of interpersonal relations. The social action model would identify racism as a significant social problem, related to social and economic structures, and manifesting itself in this conflict.

On the basis of these assumptions, the mental health model would prescribe consultative intervention of the consultee-centered type. Training sessions in human relations involving groups of teachers and students with mixed racial backgrounds would follow from the organizational model. The social action model would define interventions that involved organizing the minority community to press for greater involvement in educational policy, possibly pressing for more recruitment of minority teachers, or, in concert with the organizational model, demanding more training in racial sensitivity for school staff.

Within their own assumptions, and on the basis of the presenting situation, each of these approaches is valid. It is especially interesting that in this particular situation as it actually occurred, all three of the above approaches were actually implemented in direct response to the disturbance. Shortly after this disturbance the school superintendent, a sensitive, well-intentioned, and competent school official, resigned. Within two years the same school was rocked by an even more serious disruption that resulted in the closing of the school for several days.

The ecological model was not employed in this situation, but we can hypothesize how one would approach the situation from that model. One would begin with an analysis of the school setting. Approximately 10 percent of the community population was black, with a similar percentage represented in the school population. The community itself was largely upper middle class with relatively high average levels of income and education. The black residents of the community included many who were long-time residents, although the average level of education and income for blacks was significantly lower than that for whites. While there were some minority teachers on the staff, it is not known whether they were proportionately represented; probably they were not. Politically, the community would probably be described as moderate, alternately electing candidates from each party. In general, the stance toward local candidates tended to be more conservative than that toward national office holders. While a major university was located in the community, the community itself was significantly more conservative than the university population.

Within the school, one would want to assess the function of the school setting in establishing adaptive behavioral criteria, examine the interdependencies among persons in the setting and between persons and the environment of the school, assess the resources available within the setting, and consider the past and likely future problems of minority-group integration within the school system. While this assessment process might draw upon knowledge from other settings, the focus would be on this particular local community and its school.

While the author happens to be familiar with this particular situation to the extent already described, it is clear that more detailed information than is presented here would be required for further definition of the problem. However, it is known that a committee of teachers and students was established to study the problem and make recommendations for further action. Those solutions implemented as described above grew in part out of this committee. In addition, the committee called attention to the fact that the predominant orientation of the school was toward college preparation, and that those students who shared that orientation commanded a preponderance of the resources and rewards, status attainments, and satisfactions of the school. This finding implied that at least half of the students (the percentage of students not going on to college) did not share this orientation. This group included both white and black students, with white students being a numerically larger portion of this group. In this sense the issue was one of social class as well as race, or perhaps instead of it. Given this information, the ecological model would examine the availability of appropriate settings and resources that could be created within the school for the non-college-bound student, work with the faculty to create increased opportunities for success for such students, and plan for successive curriculum and extracurricular modifications to meet these needs.

Admittedly, this portrayal simplifies the first three models presented, yet it describes faithfully the kinds of approaches that would, and indeed did, follow from them. Furthermore, it is not the intent of this comparison to diminish the importance of the problems that might be identified or the solutions that might be proposed from the assumptions that these models make. Increasing human relations skills among students and staff and encouraging increased participation among minority members of the community in school affairs are important in themselves and could be part of an ecologically defined intervention. The point is that the other models are insufficient in themselves to deal with the multiple and complex problems contained in such a situation, especially at the level of community systems. It should also be noted that the first three models were very much in vogue among psychologists and other helping professionals, and issues of racism and inequality were highly salient in the public consciousness at that time. Still, it is well to remember that an adequate conceptual framework for the problems one faces is highly preferred to faddishness, and adequate humility in the absence of adequate theory is the best defense against foolishness.

TEMPORAL DIMENSION

Thus far we have presented considerations pertinent to domains of inquiry and to levels of analysis. Another important consideration is the dimension of time. We noted in Chapter 2 the observations of Boulding (1970) concerning the cyclical pattern of social change in response to revolutionary developments, and the continuous pattern associated with evolutionary development. Boulding suggests that information serves to enhance evolutionary processes. He states: "It is ignorance, rather than knowledge, which makes for dialectical processes. Once knowledge is achieved (disseminated and absorbed) the dialectical pattern disappears" (Boulding, 1961, p. 61). Duncan (1964) notes that the natural environment contains three types of resources: material, energy, and information. Of these, only information is not subject to conservation-of-energy laws; that is, information can be utilized without being used up. It is this characteristic of information that allows the evolution of human culture.*

Thus, many of the efforts to solve social problems during the 1960s, mounted more out of a sense of urgency than of adequate knowledge, may have enhanced the likelihood of initiating a cyclical pattern of social change. If such actions can be seen in the spirit of experimentation and knowledge generation, then it is clear that they have considerable potential for contributing to evolutionary processes, provided that the appropriate lessons are learned from them. This will not occur from a wholesale rejection of the ideas and concepts that were implemented during that period, nor from a precious and wistful clinging to those or older ideas. Rather, learning will come from a careful examination of their potential lessons.

These observations serve to underline the importance of social and community history to community studies. As Sanders has observed:

*Information is only relatively free of laws of conservation, since some energy and material is required for transmission and storage of information, as well as for converting it into usable form.

> The past definitely lives on in the present; without a knowledge of this past, contemporary events cannot be fully understood. The temporal factor should involve more than just tracing a sequence of events; it should also include some effort to reconstruct the interrelationships that existed at a given time in the past among important social units of the community and the relevance of such interrelationships to present behavior in the community. (Sanders, 1966, p. 28)

An example of such an analysis on a societal level is excellently represented in the Levines' (1970) examination of the relationship between social conditions around the late nineteenth and early twentieth century and the development of a variety of social services in the United States.

The temporal dimension of research has implications for the form and utility of the information beyond its mere factual usefulness. Biddle and Biddle (1965) distinguish between community research and community development research. The former is descriptive of present conditions and may leave the impression of inevitability, while the latter is descriptive of change and is more likely to support optimism about further change. They also emphasize that community development research should have practical utility to stimulate discussion and involvement with the community development process. Further underscoring the time dimension, the Biddles describe community development research as the study of ongoing social processes and their results, and include the research as part of those processes.

An additional and relatively undeveloped aspect of the time dimension is the construction and analysis of future events, including both natural evolution and planned intervention. In Chapter 7 a possible role for the community psychologist in assessing adaptational impacts of new community developments was suggested. On a larger scale, the widely publicized study by the Club of Rome (1974), population projections such as those of Ehrlich (1968), and efforts by biological ecologists to examine alternatives for environmental support of society (Odum, 1972) are examples of this kind of future modeling. However, in the area of human adaptation within local communities this function is largely undeveloped. The ecological model provides a framework for beginning this kind of analysis. To date, some tentative predictions can be made about the effects of the number and manning of behavior settings from Barker's work, and about the effects on adaptation of changing environments from Kelly's studies, but these represent only the bare beginnings of what is needed before community psychologists can generate empirically based models of future adaptation.

CITIZEN PARTICIPATION

A final dimension of importance to community studies involves the participants in and consumers of the research process. Biddle and Biddle (1965) describe the democratization of the research process as one in which the social scientist, citizen, and practitioner share responsibility. They describe this participation as a learning process for the citizen who can make increasing contributions to the process as a result of experience, but it is also a learning process for the social scientist and practitioner who can learn from the citizen and from each other. This dimension of cooperation and involvement has been stressed by Kelly (1971b). It is intimately linked to both effectiveness and accountability in community work.

The emphasis in the ecological model is on developing the natural resources of the community through the creation of competencies. Involvement of citizens in the research process is thus critical to defining problems that are salient to the local community, for gaining sanction for the work, and for providing an opportunity for citizens to develop their competencies. This sharing of both process and accountability is especially important for the community to develop a planning capacity of its own. If residents of the community are to become resources for each other, they must have the opportunity to learn about their community and to develop their own competencies.

Resistance to community studies is as real and nearly as frequent as is resistance to intervention programs. This fact has been recognized by anthropologists for some time. While a part of the community psychologist's task is to seek out and identify individuals who care about their community and who have made or can make a commitment to its development, uncritical acceptance of the process cannot be universally valued either. Kelly (1975a) has described how two schools in which a longitudinal research project of student development was conducted reacted to the implications of the research. One school, which had warmly welcomed the study and given the researchers every possible cooperation, was indifferent to feedback on the implications of the study for school modification; while another school, which had questioned critically nearly every step of the procedure and appeared to be quite resistant, was nevertheless quite interested in the implications of the findings for making changes in the school and proceeded to implement the changes that were suggested by the results. These two different responses indicate different expectations about the research process and, indirectly, about the commitments to the school setting.

Resistance opposed to change is one of the preconditions of revolutionary, cyclical patterns of social change processes. However, if Boulding's observations about the role of information in fostering evolutionary change are valid, then the important task for the community psychologist is not just to accumulate information, but to assist in its dissemination and absorption. As psychologists, we know that learning is enhanced by active involvement in the learning process. In this sense, the role of participation takes on important implications for the form of change that is likely to occur, as well as increasing the likelihood of change. It would be interesting to compare the durability of the changes implemented in the one school on the basis of Kelly's research with the durability of similar changes introduced into another school that were not based on a study of the setting. In the latter case, revoluionary process would be predicted that would lead to an eventual reaction against the change and a tendency to return to the former state.

The importance of developing shared expectations between professionals and community clients has been mentioned previously (see Chapter 2 and Glidewell, 1959) as a factor in overcoming resistance, or, equivalently, in establishing trust. As Kelly's example suggests, the development of shared expectations may take some time. Sharing of information through participation in the study process constitutes a ready vehicle for shared expectations to develop.

Sanford (1970) describes a process of "research-action," which involves the inhabitants of a setting in research and planning as part of an intervention strategy. This process is based on modifications of Lewin's concept of action research. Lewin (1947) describes action research as a process of both general research on social situations and research designed to diagnose a specific situation. The addition of the principle of participation in this process is an aid in providing a basis for work to overcome resistance to both the study and the possible alternative interventions, to insure that the problems defined will have meaning to the citizens involved, and to build utility of the results and accountability for the effects of both studies and interventions into the process. While Lewin's concept was to create change for the puposes of research, which could then lead to further changes, Sanford suggests creating research for the purposes of change.

The study of community life, then, must be defined with respect to four dimensions. This review has identified three *domains of inquiry*: the study of mental health problems within the disease-oriented system of mental health services; the study of person-environment interactions in community settings; and the study of problems of social structure and related social policies. These problems vary in their *levels of analysis*: mental health problems may be studied on an interpersonal or group level; questions of social adaptation, "positive mental health," and personal competency involve an examination of the community settings and systems in which these processes occur; and problems of social structure require analyses of societal processes and policies, frequently involving economic questions. The *time dimension* specifies the relevant historical, contemporary, and future analyses of ongoing processes, emphasizing that community psychology studies are studies of change, rather than of static conditions. The *participation and accountability dimension* is concerned with the sharing of information and developing expectations concerning the process and outcome of the study, with important implications for the type, degree, and durability of the change that results.

These dimensions have more than just the virtue of intellectual clarity to offer. They are essential to defining competencies and roles of community psychologists to themselves and their professional and community colleagues; they contribute to the meaningfulness and effectiveness of the community psychologist's work; and they define the measure of accountability for community studies.

Contributions to a Body of Knowledge for Community Psychology

At the end of Chapter 1, Table 1 presents an outline of the requirements for a body of knowledge for community psychology. The reader may wish to refer to that table for the following discussion. The first two columns of the table refer to categories of studies needed to develop this body of knowledge. We can now make some entries in those two columns with some of the studies that have been reviewed in order to exemplify the types of knowledge that fit those needs. The third column refers to interventions and will be discussed in the next chapter.

DEVELOPMENTAL CONTEXT: ANALYSIS OF SOCIAL PROCESSES

In Table 1, the focus of this column is on analysis of social processes and social policies across different time dimensions. In an evolutionary focus, social history accounts of the relationships between processes and policies are involved. Levine and Levine (1970) provide an outstanding example of a longitudinal analysis of this type, while Marris and Rein's (1967) more contemporary analysis of community action programs is another. Two papers by Katz represent especially comprehensive systems analyses of social movements (1967) and the social-psychological basis of social change (1974). Pettigrew's (1969) examination of the historical effects of racial separatism and integration in the light of contact theory in intergroup relations is a similar analysis. Pettigrew also goes on to illustrate the remaining two cells of this column in regard to that particular problem, by considering the then current state of affairs and developing a model from which predictions can be made about the effects of alternative future courses of action. Reiff's (1971) historical analysis of psychologists' participation in social policy also falls in this category.

In a contemporary time focus, evaluative analyses of current social programs comprise a major area. While these studies have a time dimension in a before-and-after sense, they are not of the sort ordinarily associated with the concept of longitudinal research. The time range is more restricted here, whereas the social-historical accounts compare at least two distinct periods or eras. One might say that these contemporary studies are too recent to have become nostalgic.

Examples of the contemporary type of research are the analyses of developments in the welfare program during the 1960s by Rein (1969), and of the war on poverty by Davidson (1969). Comparative program evaluation studies—such as those of Aiken (1969) comparing the adoption of community programs in cities with different types of power structures, and of Barbarik (1975) on the effectiveness of different strategies in community action programs—also belong here.

While none of these areas can claim an abundance of research, the future time focus is especially underdeveloped. The work here consists of model building and making predictions. The study of the Club of Rome (1974) and similar studies are quite ambitious examples. Pettigrew's projections in the area of race relations are especially instructive since he considers the effects of alternative courses of action. Perhaps his study can also teach us that adequate developments in future prediction are highly dependent on adequate understanding of the historical and contemporary processes.

INTERACTIONS IN SPECIFIC SOCIAL SETTINGS

While the previous discussion was on the level of societal processes, the considerations here deal with specific communities and settings within those communities. The evolutionary focus calls for the type of study described by Sanders, quoted earlier in this chapter. Examples of this type of research, which have been discussed here, are Seashore and Bowers' (1970) longitudinal study of the Weldon Corporation, and Kelly's (1976) longitudinal study of the high school environment.

In a contemporary time focus the studies are more numerous, since this is the temporal and spatial context of the majority of social-psychological research. A wide range of types are representative, such as Barker and Gump's (1964) comparative studies of high school size and interaction, Guttentag's (1972) evaluation of the community-controlled schools in Harlem, and numerous studies in the field of organizational development referred to in Chapter 5.

Future-focused studies are again in short supply. Research on the consultation process over time, to include behavioral effects on clients over time, is an approach to this type of study. Catalano and Monahan's (1975) suggestion for developing environmental impact studies from the standpoint of human adaptation represents another type in this category. Kelly (1970) has presented three different types of research designs that might be employed in evaluating processes in mental health consultation, organizational development, and community development. Drawing on concepts from

Campbell and Stanley (1966), these suggestions illustrate the use of extended time series designs in assessing the radiating effects of mental health consultation, nonequivalent control groups designs for studying the effects of organizational interventions, and a patched-up design for the assessment of community development processes.

It is worth repeating again that an effective community psychology depends on a continuous interplay among these different levels of analysis and different time perspectives, as well as with those dimensions relevant to intervention. Applying the ecological principles to this outline for the purposes of specific community psychology problems, one would think of the dimension represented by the rows in Table 1 as representing the interdependencies among the various processes, and the dimension representing the columns as bearing on the principle of succession in an evolutionary sense. The task remaining would be to identify the existing or potential resources pertinent to that problem, and the interaction between resources and human adaptation in the specific settings with which one is concerned.

The studies represented here include the work of social psychologists, community psychologists, sociologists, social workers, political scientists, and urban planners. The body of knowledge relevant to community psychology is interdisciplinary. It is nevertheless incumbent on the community psychologist to be clear about the nature of the contributions that he or she can make to this effort. Toward this end, we will now consider some suggestions for needed research in this context, and how it can be made meaningful.

Needed Research

Most historical novelists present as a matter of course the relevant social and local history in defining the locale of their stories. This is not typical of psychology. Besides a number of differences between novelists and scientists, perhaps one reason for this difference is that the methods of psychologists are subject to change and lack of standardization, so that longitudinal comparisons using psychological methods are difficult. This was notable in the Dohrenwends (1972) review of epidemiological studies (Chapter 4). Moreover, psychologists show a proclivity for preoccupation with methodological refinements that yield rather slow progress in accumulations of substantive knowledge. Of course, the adequacy of methods, designs, and criteria must precede standardization, and this is undoubtedly a factor in this state of affairs. However, psychologists could make more substantive contributions if they took more seriously Bordin's (1966) recommendation that they observe an obligation to return their focus to the real world from which they first derived their problems for laboratory study, and that they test out the adequacy of their results against the problem in its original context. According to Bordin's analysis of the problem, this would require that psychologists inhibit doubting to a degree, expand the range of their curiosity, and act more on compassionate motivation than is often the case.

The field of epidemiology in mental health represents an apt illustration of opportunities to apply this principle. The development of the twenty-two-item symptom questionnaire in the Midtown Manhattan study (Langner, 1962) has now received sufficient repeated use that it may be considered to be somewhat standardized in the field. Repeated sampling with this instrument over time under known changed social and economic conditions could make a significant contribution to epidemiological knowledge by relating rates of impairment to changing social processes rather than to static social conditions. Such knowledge could be expected to identify alternative areas for effective intervention much more clearly than can cross-sectional analysis, because it would provide clues to what change forces tend to influence rates.

A second kind of inventorying was suggested in discussing the ecological model. Most citizens are somewhat aware of the economic and employment resources of their community and may even have some conception of the rate of unemployment and average level of income of residents of their community. Few if any will have any conception of the number and range of behavior settings in their community or their influence, although some of them may be aware that their community seems to be an exciting or boring place to live, that it has few or many good places to go to eat or to be entertained, or that the community feels as if it is an involving or alienating environment. Yet from the standpoint of human adaptation such knowledge of the range and accessibility of behavior settings and their effects would seem to have considerable importance to both the community psychologist and the citizen in understanding the community. Kelly (1975b) refers to Barker's comparison of the behavior settings of Midwest and Yoredale, and notes that the fact that Midwest had many more behavior settings in which adolescents were active than did Yoredale has important implications for understanding the theory of socialization that is dominant in each community and the effects of living in those communities.

If we are to view people as resources for each other in conceptualizing community processes, then two additional important areas of inquiry emerge. One is the return of interest to the study of prosocial behavior (Wispé, 1972), and another related area is the study of the social-psychological basis of participation in community development. How persons interact with behavior settings of different characteristics to develop these orientations is an area of substantive concern for the field. Such questions as what needs and satisfactions are involved in community participation, what correlates of participation contribute to commitment and staying power while others are apathetic or discouraged early in the process can be analyzed according to the framework presented earlier in this chapter from both a historical and contemporary standpoint with implications for the creation of resources in the future.

The entire area of developing models for altenative futures based on various contingencies is, of course, a largely undeveloped and uncharted area. This work need be neither pie-in-the-sky nor crystal-ball gazing, but can consist of both computer-simulated models and actual social experimentation.

It can be concluded from this review that the major needs in the study of the community are for studies of social process, rather than social conditions. This may well be considered one of the defining properties of community psychology research, that it is process oriented. It is important to establish a baseline of principles and data, both historically and currently, in order to arrive at a starting point. However, the more information these and subsequent studies can tell us about change processes, the more useful they will be.

References

AIKEN, M. Community power and community mobilization. *Annals of the American Academy of Political and Social Science*, September 1969, *385*, 76–88.

AMERICAN PSYCHOLOGICAL ASSOCIATION, *Monitor*, November, 1975.

BABARICK, P. Field-force intervention strategies: Changing the educational status quo in a community. *American Journal of Community Psychology*, 1975, *3*, 47–58.

BARKER, R. G., AND GUMP, P. V. *Big School, Small School.* Stanford: Stanford University Press, 1964.

BIDDLE, W. W., AND BIDDLE, L. J. *The Community Development Process*. New York: Holt, Rinehart & Winston, 1965.

BORDIN, E. S. Curiosity, compassion, and doubt: The dilemma of the psychologist. *American Psychologist*, 1966, *21*, 116–121.

BOULDING, K. E. *A Primer on Social Dynamics.* New York: Free Press, 1970.

BROWN, B. M., AND STOCKDILL, J. W. The politics of mental health. In S. E. Golann and C. Eisdorfer (Eds.), *Handbook of Community Mental Health.* New York: Appleton-Century-Crofts, 1972.

CAMPBELL, D. T., AND STANLEY, J. C. *Experimental and Quasi-Experimental Designs for Research.* Chicago: Rand McNally, 1966.

CATALANO, R. AND MONAHAN, J. The community psychologist as social planner: Designing optimal environments. *American Journal of Community Psychology*, 1975, *3*, 327–334.

CLARK, K. B., AND CLARK, M. P. Racial identification and preference in Negro children. In T. M. Newcomb and E. L. Hartley (Eds.), *Readings in Social Psychology*, 1st ed. New York: Holt, 1947.

CLUB OF ROME. *The Limits of Growth*, 2nd ed. New York: Universe Books, October 1974.

COHEN, L. D. Health and disease: Observations on strategies for community psychology. In Division 27 of the American Psychological Association, *Issues in Community Psychology and Preventive Mental Health.* New York: Behavioral Publications, 1971.

DAVIDSON, R. H. The War on poverty: Experiment in federalism. *Annals of the American Academy of Political and Social Science*, September 1969, *385*, 1–13.

DOHRENWEND, B., AND DOHRENWEND, B. Psychiatric epidemiology: An analysis of "true prevalence" studies. In S. E. Golann and C. Eisdorfer (Eds.), *Handbook of Community Mental Health.* New York: Appleton-Century-Crofts, 1972.

DUNCAN, O. Social organization and the ecosystem. In R. E. Faris (Ed.), *Handbook of Modern Sociology.* Chicago: Rand McNally, 1964.

EHRLICH, P. R. *The Population Bomb.* New York: Ballantine, 1968.

GLIDEWELL, J. C. The entry problem in consultation. *Journal of Social Issues*, 1959, *15*, no. 2, 51–59.

GOODWIN, L., AND TU, J. The social psychological basis for public acceptance of the social security system: The role of social research in public policy formation. *American Psychologist*, 1975, *30*, 875–883.

GUTTENTAG, M. Children in Harlem's community controlled schools. *Journal of Social Issues*, 1972, *28*, 1–20.

HOCH, E. L., ROSS, A. O., AND WINDER, C. L. (Eds.). *Professional Preparation of Clinical Psychologists*. Washington, D.C.: American Psychological Association, 1966.

KAHN, A. J. *Studies in Social Policy and Planning*. New York: Russell Sage, 1969.

KATZ, D. Group process and social integration: A systems analysis of two movements of social protest. *Journal of Social Issues*, 1967, *23*, no. 1, 3–22.

KATZ, D. Factors affecting social change: A social psychological interpretation. *Journal of Social Issues*, 1974, *30*, no. 3, 159–180.

KELLY, J. G. The quest for valid preventive interventions. In C. D. Spielberger (Ed.), *Current Topics in Clinical and Community Psychology*, vol. 2. New York: Academic Press, 1970.

KELLY, J. G. The socialization of competence as an ecological problem. In symposium, "Social competence and mental health." American Psychological Association, 1971a.

KELLY, J. G. Qualities for the community psychologist. *American Psychologist*, 1971b, *26*, 897–903.

KELLY, J. G. The search for ideas and deeds that work. Keynote address, Vermont Conference on the Primary Prevention of Psychopathology, University of Vermont, Burlington, 1975a.

KELLY, J. G. The ecological analogy and community work. Paper presented at symposium, "Public Policy and Ecological Change," International Society for the Study of Behavioral Development Biennial Conference, University of Surrey, Guilford, England, July 1975b.

LANGNER, T. S. A twenty-two item screening score of psychiatric symptoms indicating impairment. *Journal of Health and Human Behavior*, 1962, *3*, 269–276.

LEVINE, M., AND LEVINE, A. *A Social History of Helping Services*. New York: Appleton-Century-Crofts, 1970.

LEWIN, K. *Resolving Social Conflicts*. New York: Harper & Row, 1947.

MARRIS, P., AND REIN, M. *Dilemmas of Social Reform*. Chicago: Atherton, 1967.

NEWMAN, P. R. Persons and settings: A comparative analysis of the quality and range of social interaction in two suburban high schools. Unpublished doctoral dissertation, University of Michigan, 1971.

ODUM, H. T. *Environment, Power and Society*. New York: Wiley, 1972.

PETTIGREW, T. F. Racially separate or together? *Journal of Social Issues*, 1969, *25*, 43–70.

RAIMY, V. C. (Ed.). *Training in Clinical Psychology*. Englewood Cliffs, N. J.: Prentice-Hall, 1950.

RAPPOPORT, L. AND KREN, G. What is a social issue? *American Psychologist*, 1975, *30*, 838–841.

REIFF, R. Community psychology and public policy. In Division 27 of the American Psychological Association, *Issues in Community Psychology and Preventive Mental Health.* New York: Behavioral Publications, 1971.

REIN, M. Choice and change in the American welfare system. *Annals of the American Academy of Political and Social Science*, September 1969, *385*, 89–109.

ROE, A., GUSTAD, J. W., MOORE, B. V., ROSS, S., AND SKODAK, M. (Eds.). *Graduate Education in Psychology*. Washington, D.C.: American Psychological Association, 1959.

SANDERS, I. T. *The Community*. New York: Ronald Press, 1966.

SANFORD, N. Whatever happened to action research? *Journal of Social Issues*, 1970, *26*, no. 4, 3–24.

SEASHORE, S., AND BOWERS, D. Durability of organizational change. *American Psychologist*, 1970, *25*, 227–233.

STROTHER, C. R. *Psychology and Mental Health.* Washington, D.C.: American Psychological Association, 1956.

WISPE, L. (Ed.). Positive Forms of Social Behavior, *Journal of Social Issues*, 1972, no. 3.

9. Intervention Strategies

Archimedes said, "Give me where to stand, and I will move the earth." No doubt many a well-intentioned change agent has felt some kinship with this remark in more frustrated or more expansive moments. There is a very real danger that the terms "consultant," "change agent," or "interventionist" may conjure up visions of moving the earth in the minds of some people. We have already reviewed how the excess of enthusiasm and urgency has outstripped theory, boundary definition, and establishment of clearly delineated goals in past community programs. While this state of affairs may not be entirely controllable, the serious student of community psychology must recognize the dangers in such expansive conceptions of interventions and interventionists. It is perhaps an all-too-ready assumption in society that because we have police there will be law and order, because we have physicians there will be health, or because we have schools there will be education. It is also easy to assume, then, that because we have change agents there will be change, and that such changes will produce the desired benefits. The truth is that we know all too little about change, in both its natural and deliberate forms. Much of science, including social science, has assumed a relatively static view of the world. If we are to apply what we do know about change and add meaningful increments to that knowledge, then clarity of theory, problem definition, and goal setting are needed to provide safeguards against the dangers of overexpansive thinking.

In this chapter we will explore some of the considerations that are relevant to the planning of interventions, based on the material reviewed in the preceding chapters. First, we will examine concerns that bear on the change agent's own role and setting, then consider factors influencing the recognition of the need for change and the definition of problems. Next, we will direct our attention to dimensions of intervention strategies derived from the previous chapters.

Role of the Change Agent

In discussing the models of community psychology, the typical settings for each have been mentioned. The setting is an important consideration not only as a potential base of operations for the would-be change agent, but also as a source of constraint on the range of alternative interventions that may be possible. The change agent's own base of operation will likely influence the points of entry into other systems that are available for beginning interventions, and the perceived role and purpose of the change agent's organization will determine at least partially the types of problems for which help is sought and the types of help that will be requested.

Even though consultation services have been an officially sanctioned part of community mental health center activities from the beginning, we noted in Chapter 4 the constraints that the largely direct-service, clinical-model setting has imposed on this activity. This lag has been recognized, and some added support is contained in the 1975 amendments to the community mental health centers act (P. L. 94-63). However, this support is aimed mainly at continuing present levels of effort, and it is not at all clear that preventive activities such as consultation have any significant sanction in the community mental health field to date (Snow and Newton, 1976). On the other hand, the community mental health center does have a degree of acceptance in many communities and, depending on local conditions, may provide a base for some innovative approaches, such as those outlined in Chapter 7. Sooner or later, however, the change agent can expect to be asked, "What does this have to do with mental health?" and the closer the community's definition of mental health is to treating cases of mental illness, the more constrained will be the alternative interventions available. Moreover, the new community mental health centers amendments expressly prohibit the use of consultation and education funds for community organization activities, such as those described in the social action model.

Internal support for the change agent's activities is also an important consideration. Glasscote *et al.* (1969) noted in their review of consultation activities at various community mental health centers that center directors had little faith in such activities and did not encourage staff who were interested to become involved in consultation work. Many mental health centers are staffed with persons trained mainly in clinical work, many of whom were hired before the more recently produced community-trained people and who are thus more likely to be in positions of influence. The community-oriented change agent in the mental health setting may therefore find little in the way of collegial support or persons interested in or capable of participating in community change efforts.

In university settings, as in community mental health centers, the types of innovation that are supported and rewarded will depend greatly on the availability of funds. However, sanctions for community activities will be influenced at least as strongly by the purposes and reward structures of the particular setting within the university from which the community psychologist operates. Demands for teaching and research, unless they are integrated with community activities that can provide learning opportunities for students, will often limit the community psychologist in the university setting to occasional forays as a consultant, with few opportunities for developing an identification with community settings, which is required for the longer-term demands of community work. On the other hand, where the academic setting supports this type of activity for psychologists and attracts students interested in preparing for community work, greater freedom to consider and explore alternative interventions may exist.

Another important dimension of the change agent's base of operation is whether he or she is located as an external or internal change agent in relation to the community system. An analogous problem has been examined by Lambert (1963) for school consultants. She noted that the internal consultant is more constrained to adopt operational patterns that are sanctioned within the setting and to undertake to work on problems defined by the system, while the external consultant may be more free to employ a wider range of methods and attempt to change the definition of problems. The internal change agent may enjoy greater familiarity with members of the community system and have more opportunities to develop close working relationships within the system than the external consultant, an advantage that may help especially in sustaining change once it has been achieved. Because the internal change agent occupies a legitimate role as part of the structure of the community setting, and the external consultant is by definition an outsider, those efforts that the internal change agent is able to make may generate less resistance than those of the external change agent. In examining the internal-external base of the consulting psychologist working with police agencies, Mann (1977) suggested that the outside consultant is likely to be called upon to fill a single role in regard to a change effort, while the internal consultant, employed by the police agency on a full-time basis, may be involved in a wider range of change-agent roles.

In either case, of course, the effectiveness of the change agent's work will depend on the quality of the relationships that can be established with members of the setting and the extent to which goals for change are shared among them.

Some additional concerns for the would-be change agent are suggested by Lippitt, having to do with the questions that the consultant should ask of him/herself before entering a consulting relationship:

> Question I: What seems to be the difficulty? Where does it come from? What's maintaining it?
>
> Question II: What are my motives as a consultant for becoming involved in this helping relationship? What are the bases of my desire to promote change?
>
> Question III: What seem to be the present, or potential, motivations of the client toward change and against change?
>
> Question IV: What are my resources, as a consultant, for giving the kind of help that seems to be needed now, or that may develop?
>
> Question V: What preliminary steps of action are needed to explore and establish a consulting relationship?
>
> Question VI: How do I as a consultant guide, and adapt to, the different phases of the process of changing?
>
> Question VII: How do I help promote a continuity of creative changeability? (1959, pp. 5–12)

Aside from the technical considerations in these questions, what is salient to the discussion here are questions 2, 3, and 4. In Chapter 1, reference was made to a set of postulates proposed by Levine (1970), one of which suggests that the values of the helping agent should be congruent with the values of the setting. Cherniss (1976) has discussed this cluster of concerns as critical "preentry" issues. His discussion is centered around three questions: whether or not to intervene, whose interests will be served, and what will be the focus of intervention. As Cherniss notes, these are critical, but all-too-often unexamined, issues.

Their critical nature concerns the ambiguity that often surrounds and impedes intervention efforts. Though Cherniss discusses these issues in the context of consultation, they apply equally to any strategy of intervention. Clarity about the purposes of the intervention and the role of the change agent cannot be expected on the part of the constituents of a program of change if these questions are not clear and present in the mind of the change agent. Moreover, they are of strategic significance to the planning of change. We have mentioned repeatedly the important role of congruency of expectations between change agents and constituents, with regard to roles, values, and goals, in the planning and conduct of intervention programs.

Thus, the consultant who cannot answer the questions concerning congruency of expectations affirmatively must consider not intervening, along with alternative forms of intervention. In addition to the question of expectations, the change agent must consider whether he or she has the technical expertise, and whether the setting and the change agent together have, or can produce, the resources required for change. Cherniss notes that the typical danger here is to underestimate the resources required or to overestimate the resources available. Among other things, these resources are closely related to the institutional or organizational freedoms and constraints operating on both the change agent and the client, the change agent's previous training and experience, and his or her personal style and aptitude for certain types of change efforts.

These considerations should be taken as calls for thoughtful reflection, rather than warnings intended to intimidate. The author has observed would-be change agents decline opportunities for intervention on the grounds of lack of resources, including personal training and experience, when such decisions appeared to be based more on personal values or lack of imagination, as often as he has seen change agents enter into a change program that they were not equipped to conduct. Often a more adequate knowledge base, both in formal training and personal experience, about the processes of natural and deliberate change can help to overcome such inhibitions. However, it is an important part of that knowledge to recognize that not every change agent should attempt to move every world, even if they do have a place to stand.

We move now to an effort to develop further that knowledge base by considering processes that influence the recognition and definition of the need for change.

Factors Bearing on the Definition of Problems

Archimedes did not indicate whether the fact that the world was moving already had any role in his plans, but community psychologists must first be cognizant of the fact that change does occur in community processes with or without consultants, change agents, or interventionists. Accordingly, it is important to recognize the difference between methods of intervention and processes of change. The former are deliberate, explicit, and optional; the latter are naturally occurring, implicit, and inevitable. Neither plans for intervention nor evaluations of outcomes can be made meaningfully without taking these distinctions into account.

In reviewing the four models of community psychology in the foregoing chapters, we have found that each makes certain assumptions about how opportunities arise for intervention. While phrased somewhat differently, each model assumes that some failure of adaptation occurs that is of sufficient magnitude to warrant consideration of a change effort. Each of the models portrays the failure of adaptation as occurring on different levels. In turn, these assumptions lead to different definitions of the problem to be resolved. The mental health model assumes that adaptational failure occurs in the form of a crisis arising for a person in a key care-giving role. This crisis contributes to adaptational problems for the caregiver's clients, and provides a strategic point for the mental health consultant's intervention. The organizational model assumes that the adaptational failure occurs in relation to the organization's performance of its function, and that improved interpersonal relationships within the organization, in the form of communication, interpersonal perception, and cooperative problem solving, requiring the intervention of a change agent skilled in promoting these processes, will help the organization to better fulfill its purposes. The social action model assumes that the failure of adaptation is in the social structure, which fails to distribute resources so as to meet basic human needs, and that those who are thus deprived need to be organized to press their legitimate claims for changes in the social structure. This definition of the problem requires the introduction of a community organizer. The ecological model assumes that the adaptational failure lies in the relationship between structures and functions in the community ecosystem, and that the inhabitants of that system must be engaged in the redevelopment of an adaptation-promoting relationship of elements of the system.

The mental health, organizational, and social action models assume that the failure of adaptation is due to a characteristic, recurrent, and predictable attribute of the locus of the problem, even though that locus varies from one model to another. The ecological model recognizes explicitly that the adaptational failure results from some naturally occurring change, either within the community ecosystem or in its relationship to the surrounding environment. Also, the ecological model is alone among this group of approaches in that it does not specify a method of change to be employed. The ecological model does not have within it a method of change that is unique to it, but may employ a variety of methods according to the problems encountered. There is always the danger, of course, that the existence of personnel trained in a particular method of change will exercise an influence so that problems tend to be defined to fit the method that is available, whether or not these definitions are most appropriate. By specifying the need for a range of alternative interventions, the ecological model comes closest to avoiding this difficulty of the models we have considered. What is needed is a point of view that can help in providing an understanding of how problems are defined independently of a particular method of change.

A little reflection suggests that the notion of "naturally occurring" change must implicitly play a part in the decision to initiate change programs in any of these models. Natural change processes may be as subtle as a personal acquaintance with a change agent, as superficial as a key member of a setting learning about change programs that have been implemented in other settings, or as dramatic and imposing as a serious disruption of the function of the setting, such as a real or threatened loss of resources, or riotous or rebellious behavior among the inhabitants of the setting. For the most part, these are proximal indicators of the need for change. Knowledge of more distal forces impinging on the structure and function of a community setting is taken into account only by the principles of interdependence and succession in the ecological model. Thus, changes in population such as age structure and migration may produce natural change processes in a community setting. So may changes in adjacent social systems, such as an upstream community changing water usage from a river, or a windward community implementing a cloud-seeding effort to produce rainfall, in the natural environment; or the opening of a new highway, or the opening of new shopping or employment facilities in adjacent communities, in the social environment. Examples of other such influences were discussed in Chapter 7.

One such example is worthy of further discussion here. The social policy decision to reduce state hospital populations and return former patients to the community affects both the many receiving communities and those whose economic base may be dependent on the large institutions. This decision was made in an effort to solve the problem of chronic patienthood that tends to occur in large mental institutions (Goffman, 1961; Mechanic, 1969). The failure to develop adequate programs of community support and social integration, however, produces an influx of persons into the community system who may then overload other support systems, such as local health care, law enforcement, and welfare systems. In this instance, solutions brought about by following one model, on one level of intervention, create problems on other levels. Seen from this perspective, these are ecosystem problems, rather than mental health, welfare, or law enforcement problems.

How are needs for change recognized in community settings? While a number of "real" indicators of change in adaptability may be present, the critical ingredient for the initiation of meaningful, deliberate change is on a psychological level. In Katz and Kahn's (1964) terms, this ingredient is some change in the feedback input that members of the setting receive. As Reiff (1968) has put it, changes in social forces may lead to changes in expectations, creating a perceived need for changes in conditions that, though no different, had been accepted previously. Thus, a critical first question for the development of an intervention strategy is not just, What needs to be changed? but rather, What changing conditions have led to a perceived need for change?

It does not follow, of course, that changing conditions will lead to a perceived need for change, or, if the need is perceived, that persons in the setting will agree on what needs to be changed. Feedback processes may vary greatly among members of a particular setting, according to the structure of information processing within the setting and the access and receptivity to feedback of individual members. Accordingly, an important corollary to the question above is, Who perceives the need for change, how widely shared is this perception, and how did these persons come to its realization? There are a few research findings that are relevant to this question. Sonnenfeld (1966) found that the non-native is more likely than the native to prefer change in the environment. Kelly (1968, 1969) suggested that fluid environments, because they are undergoing change, are more amenable to innovation. These findings suggest that persons with shorter tenure in a setting may be more receptive to feedback about the need for change, or may feel more free to act toward change. Mann (1972) reported that those lowest in social power within an organization are more accessible to a change agent than those higher in social power, and Aiken's (1969) research suggested that communities with diffuse power structures, associated with more diverse populations, adopted innovative programs sooner and to a greater degree than those with more centralized, pyramidal power structures. Thus, the centralization of power and the position of a given individual or group in relationship to the power structure may also influence either their access to feedback information, their interpretation of it, or their tendency to act on it. In general, these findings are consistent with research findings on the diffusion and adoption of innovations, which have been summarized by Rogers (1962) and by Rothman (1974). However, these findings do not help us to distinguish readily between the influences of feedback processes and freedom to innovate, on a social system level, or between these factors and personal histories of exposure to diversity.

Some hypotheses can be suggested from behavior setting theory and social systems theory. Barker (1968) found that students in small (undermanned) settings were engaged in more deviation-countering actions than those in larger settings. Social systems theorists assume that deviation-countering actions are triggered by negative feedback processes, those that provide information to the effect that a system is deviating from its state of equilibrium, while deviation-amplifying processes are stimulated by positive feedback processes, those that do not provide information about deviation from equilibrium (Buckley, 1968). Accordingly, the following hypotheses can be generated:

1. Those in undermanned settings have more access to, or are more attuned to, negative feedback processes than those in overmanned settings.
2. Those who have longer tenure in a setting, and/or those who

are closely related to centralized power structures, have more access to or are more attentive to, negative feedback processes.

3. In settings with centralized power structures, persons closely related to centers of power are affected by feedback processes in a manner analogous to those in undermanned settings; i.e., they receive more negative feedback and engage in more deviation-countering behaviors than those not so closely related to centers of power. The latter may engage in more deviation-amplifying processes and are more likely to receive negative feedback as relayed to them by those closer to centers of power. The latter form of communication represents deviation-countering behavior on the part of those closer to the center of power.

While these hypotheses do not allow exact derivations as to the way problems of adaptation may be defined in a setting, they do suggest generally that negative feedback processes in undermanned or centralized settings will probably generate problem definitions that call for deviation-countering interventions, while in overmanned, diffuse settings the need for change may be defined more often in ways that call for innovative, developmental changes. These directions are similar to the predictions that Kelly (1968) made for constant and fluid environments. Clearly, additional research would be needed to support these hypotheses. If supported, they could provide information that would be useful for diagnostic purposes in planning alternative interventions.

We cannot leave this discussion of who defines problems and how without mentioning another phenomenon of considerable importance to designing interventions. The values that members of a setting hold, and the degree to which members of the setting participate in its affairs, are germane to the assumptions about values and participation that each of the models of community psychology makes. We saw in our review of these models that the mental health model is based largely on values of prevention of disease, rational decision making, and economic efficiency, while participation of citizens is of limited concern. This is not to deny that community mental health policy encourages citizen participation, but rather to note that citizens' roles are usually seen as subsidiary to those of the professionals in this model, and that concern with citizen participation comes from models other than the mental health model. The other three models place more importance on participation, with the organizational model valuing humanistic self-actualization and the sharing of power, the social action model valuing human needs over economic and political ones and emphasizing freedom and self-determination, and the ecological model placing no explicit values within its framework but advocating attention to the values of the setting.

These considerations are more than just democratic or egalitarian concerns. History indicates that significant innovations in public programs have been the work of citizens who are not professionals in the fields involved. Dorothea Dix's championing of the cause of humane mental patient treatment, Clifford Beers's founding of the National Association for Mental Health, even President Kennedy's taking the political initiative to introduce the subject of federal involvement in community mental health centers, are well-known examples of this phenomenon. In other areas too, this has been the pattern. Citizen initiative in the civil rights movement, the activities of foundations and government in developing social action programs, and the actions of enlightened administrators in establishing human relations training programs in a number of public institutions have not been the result of professional intervention. Rather, professional intervention tends to follow citizen initiative.

At the same time, the Dixes, Beerses, and Kennedys are relatively rare phenomena. The Great Man theory of social change, when put into practice, is a little like a western movie where the citizens of a frontier town wait for the straight-shooting, heroic marshall to ride in from afar and save them from their intimidation at the hands of lawless rowdies. Cohen (1976) has suggested that the expectation that citizens will exercise significant influence in their participation in large-scale bureaucratic institutions is probably unreasonable, but that this possibility should not cause one to overlook the fact that many citizens do participate willingly and effectively in a number of smaller settings. Thus, expectations for the role of citizens in problem-definition and decision making should not be compared to highly visible but rare national figures, but should take into account the issue of the scale of participation in relation to the size of the setting. All of the foregoing is relevant to the topics to which we turn now—considerations of the dimensions of intervention strategies.

Selection of Levels of Intervention

In Chapter 3 we introduced the concept of community social systems being organized on several different levels, and the models we have discussed have approached problems on these different levels: interpersonal, group and organizational, community, and societal. From a social systems perspective, a problem occurring on any one level can be assumed to be operating also on at least one other level (Hoffman, 1971). Moreover, as Hoffman points out, actions that may be deviation countering on one level may be deviation amplifying on another. As an example of this phenomenon, Hoffman cites the diagnosis, labeling, and treatment of a mental patient on the individual level as an effort at deviation-countering action. If one assumes, however, that deviance serves a positive function for larger social systems by providing a marker for the limits of normality (cf. Erikson, 1964), then this action serves a deviation-amplifying purpose on this level, providing the deviant individual with positive feedback in the role of "deviant individual" at the social system level. Processes of social separatism may operate in a similar manner. If a subgroup of a larger population is considered deviant within that larger system, forces may arise that push toward the establishment of separate identities for the members of the subgroup and the remainder of the larger group. These elements may then withdraw their identifications with the larger group and establish separate social systems based on their separate group identities. Pursuit of the characteristics that are thought to distinguish the two groups by their members provides positive feedback within each group, while amplifying the differences between the groups. Any movement toward perception of similarities between the groups would produce negative feedback and deviation-countering actions within each subsystem. Overlooking differences and emphasizing similarities at the larger-system level would be needed to provide positive feedback at this level, which would be deviation amplifying at the level of the subgroups. Characteristics that provide these distinctions may be racial, sexual, ideological, economic, or nationalistic. This process may well provide the basis for Pettigrew's (1969) maxim, derived from social-psychological research findings, that separatism breeds more separatism.

While these considerations make the problem of levels extremely complicated, they do emphasize the importance of the consideration of levels in designing interventions, and they also provide a means whereby the would-be interventionist can consider possible unintended consequences of intervention. At the risk of whipping a dead horse, we have noted already how changes at the social policy level in the community mental health centers legislation introduced problems of deviance at the community level. We can also observe that this model, by failing to provide for the political and economic interdependencies at the local level, short-circuited the effectiveness of its assumption that local sources would be willing to pick up the tab for mental health services once the virtues of this approach were seen. By 1973, ten years after the passage of the initial legislation, the median level of support for 272 federally funded centers from local funds was 5.1 percent, and from state funds was 22.4 percent, of total funds for each center (NIMH, 1974). The total of these percentages is only slightly higher than the 20 percent of local funds required to match the federal share to begin receiving federal funds in the first year of a center's operation, with the amount of federal contribution declining in subsequent years.

On another level, let us consider an early-identification-and-treatment program aimed at secondary prevention of mental disorders among school children as an example. On the level of the individual, such a program assumes the effectiveness of early treatment techniques, but on a social system level the potential unintended consequence of this type of intervention may be to create a class of deviants among those who are not treated successfully. On a social action level, attempts at community organization may create polarization, and if polarization results in an increase in organization among the dominant community structure, those on whose behalf the organizational activity was undertaken may end up being more oppressed and deprived than they were originally. This result would seem to be more likely when confrontation strategies that are not seen as legitimate by the larger group are employed. Of course, from the vantage point of the oppressed, they may see their condition as putting them in a "nothing to lose" position, so that such considerations as unintended consequences would have little meaning.

In facing these realities, what frame of reference could be helpful to the would-be interventionist? The principle of interdependence in the ecological model would seem to be a logical starting point. An application of Barker's method for identifying behavior settings is relevant to the question of identifying levels of intervention. The first part of this procedure would be to identify the interdependent factors associated with a particular problem. A second part of the procedure would be to reduce this list to those factors that have a greater degree of interdependence with this particular problem than with other problems. This process need not be an exclusive one; that is, several factors may show greater interdependence at a societal level, while several others may be more interdependent at a community level. The degree of independence between these sets of interdependencies, then, would indicate whether one or the other or perhaps both levels of intervention would be required to solve the problem. The same procedure can be extended to the organizational and interpersonal levels.

In addition to defining the problem, a similar process needs to be carried out with regard to resources that are available, or can be created, for dealing with the problem. Resources, too, occur on different levels. They may include the availability of funds and the regulations and controls on the receipt and utilization of those funds, the talents and availability of persons needed to work on the problem, and the psychological climate of readiness to engage in change processes in relation to the problem.

The level-of-intervention question also turns in part on a concern raised earlier: the constituency of interest to be served and to whom the change program will be accountable. The knowledge and technology required to answer many of these questions as precisely as might be desired is not well developed. However, pursuing the questions within the framework suggested here can at least avoid some of the confusion that results from too-facile assumptions and provides the potential for generating further knowledge to serve the purpose of selecting levels of intervention.

This process of analysis can be illustrated by considering a situation that might be presented to a psychologist in a mental health role. A psychologist was asked by a school system to assist in establishing a special class for nonachieving children.* On its face, this request could be approached as a problem for program-centered administrative consultation in the mental health model. Let us assume for purposes of illustration that this community and school system were largely middle class. Observation of the setting from an ecological perspective might suggest a number of related, "naturally occurring" change processes that could contribute to the presentation of this request. Suppose that a new factory had been established in the community, which in turn generated an increase in working-class families moving into the school district. Or suppose that the school system had been ordered to accept an increased

*The author is indebted to James Kelly for bringing this example to his attention. The program and research data were produced by Kelly and his co-workers, but the suppositions suggested for purposes of illustration are supplied by the author. Kelly and his associates are not responsible for the treatment given the example here.

number of black students as part of the desegregation process. In either case, this change in the population structure of the setting could be viewed on several different levels.

The psychologist might hypothesize that this population change had produced a crisis for teachers by activating theme interferences that all working-class or black students are intellectually inferior. According to this hypothesis, intervention would consist of consultee-centered case consultation. This intervention would be at the interpersonal level and might be called the individual stereotype hypothesis.

However, the request coming from the school district as a whole suggests that the level involved with the problem is broader than the interpersonal level. One might hypothesize that the problem results from a discrepancy in expectations between the school and the parents and/or children. The problem might still be seen as stereotyped classism or racism, but at a collective or institutional level. Accordingly, human relations training for the school staff and community members might be undertaken. This intervention assumes that the problem results from institutionalized roles within the school as an organization.

This progression of levels could be followed to examine the prevailing attitudes in the community, based on the assumption that its suburban location was associated with isolationist or "white flight" tendencies. According to this hypothesis, the school system could be seen as an institutionalized expression of this community stance, with the special classes representing a form of internal segregation by social class or race. One could go further still to see the community's position as a reflection of a societal structure based on segregation and deprivation of the poor and minorities through structural inequities. Of course, all of these hypotheses are based on a presumption of interrelatedness between the supposed population change and the request for the special class. While this is a plausible assumption, given the suppositions put forth here, data on the population change and supporting observations within the school setting would be needed to support the assumption.

Each of the suggested interventions might be valid, given the hypotheses advanced at the different levels. The critical point, however, is whether the level of intervention selected has ecological validity for this setting. Moreover, the psychologist must still be responsive to the problem and solution defined by the setting in the original request.

In the actual situation that suggested this hypothetical discussion, one consideration behind the request was that the state government would reimburse schools for establishing special classes, and the school system had identified a number of children who were of normal intelligence but were underachieving significantly. The response of the mental health team was to suggest a demonstration program in which some of the children were assigned to a special classroom, and the rest were assigned to two other groups and remained in their regular classrooms. The latter two were "groups" only in the minds of the researchers, not being otherwise separated from their peers. In addition to assignment to special-class status, parents of the special-class children attended group guidance discussions with a psychologist, centered around positive parenting. A home-visiting program using a mental health nurse was conducted for special-class children's families and for the families of children in one of the regular classroom groups. Children in the third group received no services and served as a control condition. The teacher of the special class received regular mental health consultation from a psychologist, who also met with other school personnel to coordinate mental health services within the school setting.

It was discovered that there were many resource personnel in the school setting, some of them school-based and some of them community-based, whose skills were not being utilized as effectively as they could be, and whose efforts were not coordinated with each other. The group guidance sessions and home-visiting program were deliberately tailored to a format that would allow their continuation after the mental health team terminated the demonstration phase by using the skills of these persons in the school setting.

Evaluation of the program indicated that the achievement of both the special-class children and the first alternate group improved significantly during the program. It was also found that parents of the special-class children developed more negative attitudes toward their children and the children's abilities than the parents of the other children, and that the children not assigned to the special class had negative attitudes toward the special class. Following the demonstration period, all children were returned to regular classrooms and were adjusting satisfactorily (Kelly and Boone, 1964).

The significance of the program was that by selecting appropriate levels and forms of intervention it was shown that adequate services could be provided using the resources of the setting without requiring additional funds. Moreover, by using regular class placement supported by services, the negative attitudes associated with labeling and within-school segregation could be avoided. Accordingly, whether or not the suppositions about the school's difficulty in integrating population changes were correct in this situation, the intervention did accomplish a functional integration within the school setting that left it better able to accommodate to differences should they occur in the future. From an ecological perspective, the bringing together of functional units in the ecosystem with the ultimate goal of producing greater structural integration also contributed to the adaptation of individuals in the setting. Activities that increased parental involvement in the school setting, which were continued after the demonstration period, reached the level of the community social system. Bringing together the various internal and external helping persons to improve coordination among services increased the utilization of resources in the school setting, and the subsequent decision not to continue the special class freed resources that would have been devoted to it. Finally, the intervention reached the level of individuals by bringing about an increase in achievement among the students.

This example points up the importance of ecological criteria in establishing the validity of community interventions. While it would be interesting to have available more detailed information on the effect of the particular setting and the specific resources available in it on the selection of interventions, it does serve as a good illustration of the process of selecting levels of intervention. While methods of intervention have been mentioned throughout this discussion, they will now be given more specific attention.

Selection of Media, Channels, and Modalities of Intervention

The alternative methods of intervention will have been determined in part by preentry considerations and by the level of intervention selected. While data on the effectiveness of the methods discussed in this book are sparse and just beginning to be developed, one can at least ask conceptual questions about the effectiveness of alternative methods. These would include:

1. Does the method reach conceptually the interdependencies by which the problem is defined? Problems of intergroup relations

are not likely to be resolved by individual consultation; nor are social problems heavily intertwined with economic differentials likely to yield to improved human relations. At the same time, problems of recalcitrant attitudes of relatively isolated individuals or groups may not be improved by changes in social structure.

2. What types of resistances does the method tend to generate, and does the method make adequate provision for dealing with such resistances satisfactorily? The resistance-generating effects of coercive change are well known, but there may be other, more subtle, resistances that may tend to nullify or reverse changes that have been accomplished, by reasserting their influence at a later date. Sacon's (1971) data on the deterioration of attitude changes following intensive human relations training for policemen (cited in Chapter 5) are a case in point.

3. Related to question 2, what secondary and perhaps unanticipated consequences tend to be generated by the method of intervention? Here the ability to answer the question turns on how one can anticipate the secondary adaptations that may occur in the social system that is subject to the change effort.

We have seen how each of the models discussed employs different methods. Here the concern is with relating the media of intervention to particular problems in specific settings. A knowledge of the media of intervention that have been successful in solving problems in a setting is important information. One should seek to understand why such approaches have been successful in the context of the attributes of the setting. If past efforts have been unsuccessful, a similar effort to determine the reasons for failure is in order. For example, if outside funds are likely to be required to support the intervention, one will want to know what the attitude of the community is toward such funding. Many communities oppose federal or state funding because of a fear of loss of local control. One must ask whether this fear is grounded in actual experience, or whether the fear can be overcome through broad local representation in the planning process, and what local, state, and federal prerogatives may be attached to such funding.

It will also be important to know what the setting's history of self-help efforts has been, and what the likely response to outside or internal change agents will be. Of special importance here is the identification of inhabitants of the setting who can be counted on to support or participate in change programs. Are there other helping or change agents engaged in the setting, and, if so, what are their roles and purposes? Will there be confusion, conflict, or competition between their efforts and those that are planned? Can and should they be enlisted in cooperative actions with the change effort?

It is of more than passing interest that the selection of a method of intervention has not been a significant concern for individual psychologists in the past. Rather, the psychologist typically applied his or her method, with which he or she was closely identified, with relatively little assessment of the problem independent of the method. It is probably accurate to say that there has been more concern with broadening the application of preselected methods than with attending to problems in such a way that new, alternative methods might be suggested. This approach can easily lead the unwary into a variety of interpretations about the resistance of the problem, the patient, or the community on the grounds that the problem does not yield to the psychologist's method. While resistance of a systemic, and perhaps of a personal, nature is to be expected, the consultant or change agent must take care that his or her investment in a particular means of change does not create additional sources of resistance. This development can be minimized by striving to develop an appreciation of the inclinations of the inhabitants of a setting toward problem solving. Aside from the effectiveness of a particular method in a general sense, support for the method, and perhaps its effectiveness, can be increased by taking into account these questions about the compatibility of the method with the setting. This process would also seem to be enhanced where it is possible to identify those sources and processes of natural change that are contributing to the problem and select methods that have the potential to use those change processes as an aid in producing planned change.

Another important dimension of the media of intervention is the personnel to be employed. Issues concerning the training and availability of community psychologists will be considered in the next chapter, but it can be noted here that the availability of persons skilled in the planning and conduct of alternative interventions is one of the requisites of the type of activity being discussed. Also, the need for and availability of persons indigenous to the setting must be examined. Is there a role for trained nonprofessionals (see Chapter 6), what training will they require, and how will the training be conducted? What will be the role of citizens in the planned intervention? These questions lead to another part of this dimension of interventions, since the selection of personnel may be related strategically to the channels for intervention.

Channels for intervention are assessed in part according to the persons and groups involved in the social system, and their relationship to each other, the system, and the problem. The channels by which these persons and groups are accessible to intervention, with particular attention to differences in accessibility, will define in large part the channels through which the intervention will be planned. Differences in communication patterns, access to social interaction among various groups, differentials of status and power, and reference or interest group identifications are relevant to these considerations.

In discussing the theory of channels, Lewin observed:

> Social and economic channels may be distinguished in any type of formalized institution. Within these channels gate sections can be located. Social changes in large measure are produced by changing the constellation of forces within these particular segments of the channel. The analytic task is approached from the point of view of psychological ecology; nonpsychological data are first investigated to determine the boundary conditions for those who are in control of various segments of the channel. (1951, pp. 185–186)

Lewin considered these gate sections to be of critical importance to changing behavior in social settings. Access to channels is controlled either by impartial rules or by gatekeepers, either of whose function is to control access to the setting.

One of the first orders of business in planning an intervention in a setting with a formal social structure will be to obtain sanction for the work from those persons who are in authority positions, such as a school principal or superintendent, a mayor or police chief, or persons with record-keeping responsibility where documentary data may be employed in a research-based intervention. This sanction should include approval of a plan to accomplish the next step, which is to obtain access to those key persons in the setting who will be involved in the intervention process. Contacts made at this point in an intervention often prove critical to subsequent progress. Such persons may act as facilitators and traffic managers, key informants, and critical gatekeepers to the social system (Lewin, 1951).

It is a difficult but important task at this level for the would-be interventionist to have in mind, and to be constantly refining, a cognitive map of the social structure of the system. The chief danger here is the tendency to oversimplify one's conception of this structure. Grossman and Quinlan (1972) describe many of the pitfalls encountered in a consultation effort in a small hospital that result from this error, while Mills and Kelly (1972) describe the complexities involved in assessing the culturally based attributes of different Mexican Indian communities preparatory to designing alternative interventions. Key gatekeepers are often distributed according to the unofficial, and real, social structure rather than the official positions, and they are not always at the top or executive position.

On a more mundane level, arrangements must be made for assuring the availability of, and scheduling contacts with, those persons who are to be participants. A psychologist consulting to a school found that few teachers voluntarily sought consultation with him because several other helping resources were scheduled to be at the school at the same time. Consultation with police personnel may be difficult because of limited time when a significant number of them are available (Mann, 1973).

On an organizational level, commitments are required for scheduling groups of people for meetings, and such commitments may interfere with work schedules. Such issues as whether personnel are to be gathered together outside of working hours, and, if so, whether they will be paid for that time or rewarded in some other way, are important in determining accessibility. At the community level a similar issue occurs, although arrangements for paid participation will usually be inappropriate. Rather, the medium of exchange is likely to be through personal involvement with the problem, or through interpersonal influence. Kelly (1971) sees locating and bringing together persons who can become resources for the development of their own community as one of the central tasks of the community psychologist. The rewards are likely to be discovering new ways of functioning and of expressing their talents, as well as contributing to solving problems.

At a societal level the psychologist's contributions are likely to be conducted through the medium of research, defining support for and predicting consequences of alternative social policies, or demonstrating the linkage between policy and behavior (Back, 1974). The Society for the Psychological Study of Social Issues (SPSSI) represents one such collective effort by psychologists, in which examination of various social issues is disseminated through its publication, *The Journal of Social Issues.* Pertinent to the discussion here is the question of how such studies are consumed. For the most part, professional journals are read by other professionals, not by policymakers. Channels for distributing the results of research to relevant consumers are an important aspect of the use of research as intervention.

On the other hand, the account of the controversy aroused by the "Moynihan Report" (Rainwater and Yancey, 1967) illustrates the difficulties that can be encountered even when one has access to decision-making and action-producing capabilities. While Moynihan intended to draw attention to the destructive effects of poverty on the Negro family by compiling a host of data into a persuasive review of the problem, the solution, which was centered around efforts to support or "rebuild" the Negro family, was interpreted by many as an implicit blaming of the Negro family for its own plight. While the process that was involved and the reaction it generated were both complex, it appears from Rainwater and Yancey's review of the incident that the apparently unnoticed beginnings of the rise of black power and black separatist sentiment, along with a failure to discuss the implications of the research with black civil rights leaders ahead of time, contributed to the reaction that occurred. In terms of Lewin's theory, the black leaders functioned as unanticipated gatekeepers over an important channel, one controlling access to support from the black population for Moynihan's proposals.

Where one is dealing with social policy analysis, concern with the application of the considerations discussed here to the selection of channels for distribution of information, and with the choice of methods to be used for this purpose, are as important as the quality of the research itself. Such research must reach the appropriate consumers by the most effective means if it is to have an impact. These same considerations hold, of course, for research as intervention at any social system level.

Thus, Lewin's observations concerning the critical importance of understanding the social-psychological principles governing the gate section of channels to social settings appear to be valid still. One can imagine, as Lewin observed, that had Moynihan in the example cited above won the understanding and support of the gatekeepers, the same force that blocked access to the channel would have carried the idea along with equal intensity (1951, p. 187). Similar support at critical gate sections in channels in other social systems is important in any intervention, but the challenge for the community psychologist is first to identify those channels and gates.

The selection of media and channels for intervention will often define the modalities to be employed. The question of modalities is as much a concern within the change agent's own setting as it is in the social system for which intervention is planned. Much of what we have considered in this book refers to new modes of operation for professionals, and we have discussed repeatedly the need for sanctioning these new types of activity. Resistances to new modes of delivering services may arise as guild concerns or issues of control, as in the issues involving nonprofessionals discussed in Chapter 6, or as competition with existing patterns of practice and habits for professionals. We have mentioned already the need for the would-be change agent to scrutinize potential sources of support and resistance within the change agent's base of operations.

Considerations of modalities within the target setting must also take into account the compatibility of new forms with existing patterns of operation. One concern is the sanctioning of such activities, which makes this issue essentially a gatekeeper problem. Of more importance for the conduct of the intervention, however, is the appropriateness of the mode of operation for coping with the ongoing change processes in the setting and for bringing about the desired intervention outcome. Here the change agent faces a serious dilemma, for often those modalities that are compatible with existing patterns in both the change agent's and the community setting are insufficient to cope with the problem; they may, in some instances, contribute to maintaining the problem (Rhodes, 1972). Moreover, to the extent that an intervention may depend on perception of its unique character, by either change agents or inhabitants of the setting or both, similarities to existing patterns of operation may create confusion or reductionistic thinking about the change effort. Professionals are especially prone to assimilating new approaches to their existing patterns of operation—the old wine in new bottles phenomenon—and thus little change may result. Others may also view such efforts through the simplification implicit in such phrases as "So what else is new?" or "We tried that before and it didn't work."

Often this dilemma is resolved by the professional by conducting a demonstration project with the aim of making it a part of the setting, but the relatively low rate of survival and adoption of such projects suggests that additional considerations, such as those discussed concerning the utilization of research findings, are required. This is why we have made the survival value of a model one of the criteria for judging such efforts. This criterion, along with the principle of succession in the ecological model, emphasizes the importance of planning for sustaining a capacity for adaptation to change in the setting. The implication is clear: in addition to defining and selecting modalities for intervention, the community psychologist can anticipate the need to work to bring about change in existing modalities and to obtain legitimation for new ones.

Creating Resources and Organizing for Interventions

In Chapter 3 we discussed how maintenance forces in social systems create both a stability of ongoing processes and a resistance to change. In designing interventions, too, there is a tension between organizing forces and change forces. On a larger scale this tension is displayed in the conflict between planning efforts and reform movements. Traditionally, planning assumes some sort of orderly, predetermined, or controllable events. Master-planning connotes a set of contingencies imposed on a population by some superordinate group. To a greater or lesser extent, with more or less sophistication, democratization, or foresight, this is what different forms of government are all about. Implicit in this approach is the concept of social control that tends to inhibit change. Marris and Rein (1967) speak of the conflict between planning and reform at a societal level and note that while the reformer role is almost endemic in United States society, no one has legitimate authority in that society to assume a long-term master-planner role concerning the form of society. Rather, that role is dispersed among an array of voters, interest groups, and the like. Anyone who seeks change in the direction of reversing current trends, whether in a progressive or a regressive direction, may be considered a reformer from his own perspective. Governments are limited in the time periods for which they can commit funds by budget periods; changes in officeholders frequently signal changes in policies. Viewed in dialectical terms, planning efforts may be expected to generate forces toward reform in reaction to them, while reform forces may similarly generate reactions in the direction of planning.

On a community level as well, there is tension between organizing and change forces. The concept of organizing people in the community to bring about change has in it the potential for contradictory forces that both seek and oppose change. However, this view of conflicting forces tends to be cast in a revolutionary change perspective and assumes that other change forces are relatively constant. Yet not all changes are necessarily of a reform character. In reality, evolutionary change forces of a different nature underlie the conflicting revolutionary forces, but the pace of evolutionary change may at times be so slow as to be imperceptible, unless one also adopts the historical, contemporary, and future time perspectives that are advocated here.

One important potential resource in change processes is information. In Chapter 8 we noted the role of information in enhancing evolutionary change, and that information is a resource that is not subject to laws of conservation. However, the news media are full of information each day concerning the multitude of social problems that face communities, and few persons are stirred to action. Community organizers are quite familiar with the problem of motivation to deal with social problems among those most affected by those problems. But, periodically, information does lead to active efforts to bring about changes, and it is consistent with the framework presented here to assume that the more and better the information available, the more likely that the change that results will be of an evolutionary, rather than a revolutionary, character. On the other hand, change initiated on the basis of insufficient, inaccurate, or misleading information is likely to generate revolutionary change. Our concern here is how information may serve as a resource for change, and how it and change processes are related to the organization of communities.

Gamson's (1968) conception of the social influence and control processes between authorities and partisans is a useful starting point as an analogy to the processes that need to be considered. Gamson distinguishes among social groupings or quasigroups, the constituency or solidary group, and the interest or organized group in discussing the organization of potential partisans in influence structures. Social groupings are abstractions into which people may be categorized because of some common social characteristic they possess, such as social class, ethnicity, or religion. They are not groups in any functional sense, nor are they organized in any social-psychological way. Constituencies or solidary groups are composed of persons related to each other through psychological identification based on some common characteristics related to some political or social goal. Interest groups are formally organized groups that represent this solidary group in pursuing the latter's goals through specific actions. Interest groups are the agents of social action.

Gamson's framework specifies that the probability of a group's attempting to exert influence is a function of that group's trust that authorities will act in a way that favors, or does not diminish, their outcomes, and of the group's perception of the chances of exerting influence successfully. The implications of this framework for the role of information in promoting social change are several. Those individuals who perceive information about a particular social problem as relevant to themselves in a significant way may be expected to assess their trust that those in authority about such matters will act in the individual's interest.* This statement assumes that in order to perceive such information as relevant, these individuals will necessarily have to be aware of their interest in the problem. This factor may be an important part of the information. If such individuals do not possess a sufficient degree of trust that their interests will be served, they may consider the possibilities of exerting influence on the problem. Although some persons may be in a position to take individual action, ordinarily we conceive of this process as an assessment of their group memberships that are relevant to this problem, and an appraisal of the probability of any of those groups exerting successful influence on the problem.

Particularly in the field of human behavior and adaptation, these assessments are vulnerable to an overvaluing of the influence efforts of existing structures on the problem. Rhodes(1972) describes how a community's infrastructure of behavior-regulating institutions may serve as a defense mechanism that appears to control the problem but may fall short in the accomplishment. Thus, it may be assumed that the educational system provides for tasks of human development, when the school system does not see this as its function; or that an outbreak of physical illness will be controlled by the health system, when the medical society opposes any large-scale action.

It is in this context of social and psychological considerations that the problem of creating resources and organizing for change is addressed. A similar, although less detailed, conception has been presented by Sarason (1974, 1976) in his term "networks." However, the task for community psychology differs from the task of social influence and community organization in the political sense, and in the sense embodied in the social action model, in some subtle but significant ways. The community organizational work of the

*For many social problems there may be no particular authority who has the power to make binding decisions, or there may be several potential authorities who compete for that power.

community psychologist consists of creating networks, or solidary groups, across social groupings and constituencies. The task is based on a conception of common interests, or interdependencies, across these groups, and is not tied to single, organized interest groups. This notion requires a conception of community as a goal, which is probably best captured by the definition proposed by Biddle and Biddle: "Community is whatever sense of the local common good citizens can be helped to achieve" (1965, p. 77).

The task of creating resources through information is not an exclusive function of research. One may view the task of the mental health consultant, for example, as helping the consultee to discover new information about the client that reduces the consultee's "theme interference" and opens the consultee up to new sources of information. Certainly, the process of human relations training in the organizational model strives to increase interpersonal information through encouraging openness. The community organization work of the social action model increases information available to the community members, and also attempts to increase the flow of information from community members to those higher in the power structure. In the ecological model, explicit emphasis is placed on increasing information about the setting as a means of both solving problems and enhancing adaptation. In each of these models, individuals receive information from and about other persons. In an ecological sense, this process increases the resources available in the environment. The differences among the models with respect to information distribution are according to the level and extensity of the interdependencies about which they can create information.

But the models also differ in the goals this information serves. The mental health and organizational models both rely on direct, face-to-face work with individuals who are to be changed in such a way that the changes radiate to other interpersonal relationships. The social action and ecological models involve direct participation by the change agent with the members of a community. This is seen as a developmental process that does not involve radiation to another setting but seeks to change both the people and the place in reciprocal fashion; the former through personal development and enhanced adaptation, the latter through changes in behavior settings.

Accordingly, the task of organizing for change differs in its purposes, as well as in the interdependencies involved, in each model. The task of the mental health consultant and the organizational consultant is to establish a relationship with an existing organization. The task of the social action agent and the ecological psychologist also involves establishing relationships, but it requires further the work of creating and facilitating new organizational forms and new relationships among existing organizational forms.

The role of the community development specialist as an "encourager," described by the Biddles (1965), provides an excellent example of the professional involved in this organizational task. Besides functioning as a resource and facilitator to help community members define or redefine problems, and to assist them in exploring their own resources for dealing with these problems, the community developer may at times assume the role of researcher to generate additional information relevant to the problem. Community members also participate in this task, increasing their skills and increasing the resources in the community in the process. As distinct from much traditional community development work, this ecological perspective provides the potential for achieving an increase in the community's capacity for monitoring and adapting to change.

The Biddles describe the organizational process as beginning with a small core group, or nucleus, of concerned citizens who conduct the initial exploration of the problem and community resources. This process includes an exploration of the issues presented earlier in this chapter. It also includes a phenomenon familiar to any group or organizational worker: a period of stagnation and discouragement. Where the community group is willing to suffer through this period and continue the process of development, a new level of organization evolves, which the Biddles refer to as the larger nucleus. It is this group that becomes capable of internal organization, division of labor, and the cycle of action research: answering questions that have implications for action, taking the action, answering questions raised by the action, further planning and organization, and so on.

A question may be raised as to whether this process requires any professional who is very different from capable, well-informed citizens, who might conduct the process by themselves. Aside from the obvious answer that citizens seldom engage in this type of process to the degree described here, and that they may not have (although they may acquire) some of the expertise required, there are other important factors involved.

The community psychologist typically enters this process as a member of an outside setting, or as a representative of a setting or group that is not central to the influence processes of the community. This fact gives the community psychologist a different set of freedoms to act than is true of community members, although it should be observed that this does not necessarily mean more absolute freedom. In addition, as Sarason (1976) has observed, the community psychologist does in fact do many things that community members could or may do, but does them more consciously and more expertly.

On the other hand, it is not the goal of the community psychologist to maintain such distinctions between him or herself and members of the community. Rather, the acquisition of increased capacities on the part of the community's members is one of the goals of the community psychologist's work. Accomplishing this task requires a self-conscious attention to the problem of overvaluing expectations toward the psychologist by the community, at the same time as the psychologist encourages the community development process. The community psychologist must seek to become dispensable to the center of the community development process as the community acquires its desired level of competence.

Defining Accountabilities for Interventions

Although we are dealing with the question of accountability in a future time perspective, it is a concern that must be observed throughout the intervention process. In discussing accountability in the context of intervention strategies, we are also emphasizing that it is an integral part of any intervention, not just an afterthought. While these statements may seem merely obvious, they are often not observed in the actual conduct of many intervention programs.

The reader will find that many of the elements of the accountability process have been discussed already in this chapter. Biddle and Biddle (1965) mention that while it would seem to be something that would be done as a matter of course, few programs begin with an adequate assessment of baseline data concerning the problem or problems to be addressed. In the context of accountability, the collection of such data, as well as the kinds of specifications that have been alluded to earlier about the interdependencies of problems and settings, will provide an empirical definition of the problem without which the accountability process is limited greatly.

A concern with evaluation research is, of course, central to the question of accountability. We will not discuss here issues of specific research methodologies, but we will concern ourselves with concepts concerning the evaluation process and make reference to major sources that discuss methodology in more detail. It is essential to recognize that evaluation as discussed here goes beyond assessment of effort or the analysis and description of individual cases or projects, although these activities may play a part in the evaluation of outcomes that are the heart of the accountability process.

It is usual for most writers on the subject of evaluation research to make distinctions between what are variously called process evaluation and outcome evaluation, formative evaluation and summative evaluation, or evaluation of effort and evaluation of achievement (see for example, Schulberg, Sheldon, and Baker, 1969; Washington, n.d.). While evaluations of achievement, outcome evaluations, and summative evaluation are all roughly the same, process evaluation, formative evaluation, and evaluation of effort are not similar to each other. The former three, which we will refer to here with the general term *outcome evaluation*, are usually assessed in relation to the achievement of some prestated goal or set of goals that are set for the project. To the extent that these goals can be stated explicitly, they can be assessed empirically, and the outcome of the project can be stated in terms of accomplishment of these goals. However, if the goals are not attained, or are attained partially or with some ambiguity, outcome evaluation by itself provides no explanation of the results. We will use the term *process evaluation* to refer to monitoring of the conduct of the program during its existence. Process evaluation may serve as an evaluation of effort, to assess the resources allocated to the program, to determine if key elements of the change process actually took place, and to determine partial outcomes in achieving intermediate goals that are essential to the achievement of final goals. Only in this way can one hope to determine why final goals were or were not achieved.

However, process evaluation may be used in another way. Frequently one is unable to obtain a sifficiently clear or extensive definition of the problem, level of intervention, and the required methods and resources for addressing the problem at the beginning. Process evaluation may indicate the need to make modifications in the conceptualization of the problem, the fact that some key intermediate goal has not been attained, or that different methods and resources are required. Used in this sense, process evaluation serves program development, in what is sometimes called formative evaluation.

Schulberg, Sheldon, and Baker (1969) note that most evaluation is conducted according to a goal-attainment model in which process evaluation and program modification are seen as antithetical activities. Yet most program evaluation research is not experimental research in the true sense (Campbell and Stanley, 1966), and the tensions that often arise between evaluation and program development can be minimized through an adequate specification of intermediate goals and by provision for modifications in program elements in the research design. Such an approach also permits the use of time-series designs (Campbell and Stanley, 1966), which offer advantages in the evaluation of many programs over simple goal-attainment models. Using this approach, evaluation research and action research become part of the same package.

While the adequacy of a research design is an important question, community psychologists are more likely to be confronted with issues that are in reality based on resistances to evaluation and accountability, sometimes phrased in methodological terms. Resistance may arise from two different sources. Internal resistance within an agency or program stems from a fear that the results obtained will make the agency look bad. This type of resistance is likely to be increased, and realistically so, if the members of the agency staff feel that the researcher does not understand the philosophy and workings of the program, or that the research design does not appear to reflect the program accurately in its translation of program elements into measurable attributes. In some instances, also, agency staff may distrust the personal motives or values of the researcher, especially if the researcher is an outsider who is not also involved in the workings of the program.

External resistance may arise from the community because of objections to the program or because of fears of invasion of privacy, but again the objections may not be voiced in those terms. Sufficient resistance has arisen, for example, over the issue of psychological testing in the schools over the years to illustrate this phenomenon. While the manifest issue concerns the right to privacy—a legitimate issue—such objections may also represent objections to the role of the school in acting on the basis of psychological test results in the form of some program, an issue that should be open to debate.

This latter issue is of particular significance to community psychologists, since any research that attempts to estimate the incidence or prevalence of a social problem through the use of survey methods may generate such objections. Care should be taken not to equate such resistance with mere stubbornness or reactionism. At least some of the resistance may result from misunderstanding or lack of information about the purposes of the research. Other portions of the resistance may arise from a sense of imposition or exploitation by a project to which the resisters do not feel related. The long history of research conducted in communities, not just by psychologists but by others as well, with no feedback to the community and no provision for making the results useful to those who have participated, provides ample precedent for this feeling.

Whether one is dealing with internal or external resistance, the solution to these problems is the same for research as it is for program development. The researcher must be aware that, no matter what his or her beliefs and values are about scientific objectivity, research is a form of intervention. Acceptance of the evaluation process is enhanced if those involved in or affected by the evaluation have some say in the development of the research, and have some understanding of and agreement with the ways in which the results may provide some payoff to them. As with program development, participation of agency and community members in the evaluation process is often critical to its success in obtaining meaningful results. Such participants can often suggest questions, criteria, and procedural refinements that will yield better results, and distortions in responses to such instruments as surveys are likely to be reduced.

These considerations have implications beyond the conduct of the evaluation process that show accountability to be more than just evaluation. It is one thing to demonstrate the effectiveness of a particular intervention in bringing about desired change, and another, larger, task to interpret the impact of the change on enhancing the adaptive capacity of the community. As is the case with interventions, an important part of the accountability process is the congruency of expectations concerning evaluation between the interventionist-evaluator and the constituency or client group. Thus, the question of accountability is more than just bookkeeping and more than just the creation of change. The standards of the community for evaluation, in keeping with the community's standards for the change program, are important prior considerations. These include social and psychological satisfactions as well as financial expenditures and economic gains. It is in this sense that Washington (n.d.) suggests that cost-benefit analysis, which is phrased in economic considerations, is inappropriate and too limited a framework for the evaluation of human service programs. Washington proposes the concept of cost-effectiveness as a more comprehensive framework that can take psychological and social factors into account. That is the term that has been used here. Again, community participation is necessary if one is to gain a sense of what these psychological and social sources of satisfaction may be.

Accordingly, accountability consists of a process of evaluation of progress toward desired changes, guided by a congruency of expectations concerning the evaluation process among change agents, constituents, and researchers, which assesses both the costs and gains of the change program and the impact of that change program on the community system. Of the models we have considered in this book, only the ecological model provides explicit principles for the future perspective by which the accountability process can be guided.

The principle of succession in the ecological model calls attention not only to processes of naturally occurring change, but also addresses two concerns frequently encountered in change programs, which other change theories do not address. One of these is the question of unanticipated consequences of the intervention, or of the interaction between the change program and ongoing changes in the community ecosystem. The second is the question of the expected life cycle of the change program, and whether and to what degree changes should be maintained or institutionalized. In a sense these questions are interrelated, but in another sense they can be seen to relate to different ecological principles.

In addition to the principle of succession, unanticipated consequences are also tied to the principle of interdependence. Changes introduced into one part of the ecosystem will effect changes in other parts. The ecological model assumes that such effects introduced by deliberate change programs can be anticipated through an assessment of the interdependencies of the problem and the setting. While not all sources of change in the ecosystem can be anticipated, with increasing knowledge of the community ecology the ramifications of changes to other parts of the ecosystem can be anticipated once they occur in one part of the community, and adaptive measures can be implemented.

The capability of adapting to unanticipated changes is closely related to the question of the life cycle of interventions. Biddle and Biddle (1965), for example, describe the community development process as they conceive of it as different from other approaches in some important respects. They differentiate community development from social work in that community development is concerned with a growth in competence rather than the alleviation of misery; from community organization in that it does not deal only with problems of social structure; and from T-groups and organizational development in that these approaches deal with short-term issues and not with the common good outside the group, which is the focus of community development. In their view, community development is concerned with a long-term growth in the capability of people to create their own resources, and they see the process of organization merely to demand new services or to create a concrete agency or center as a hindrance to this process. They place more emphasis on developing the capacity of citizens to modify existing programs to fit changing needs than on the institutionalization of new programs.

Similarly, Marris and Rein (1967) noted that the Community Action Programs, which began with a goal of reform, shifted to a goal of increasing resources in the form of increased funding when resistance to reform was encountered from the existing political and agency structures. Both Marris and Rein and the Biddles see institutionalization as an impediment to change and development.

Yet the establishment of some visible form of accomplishment, often in the form of a building or a place, is a strongly compelling force with considerable historical precedent in society. People wish for a sense of stability and continuity as well as for development and change, the facts of psychology and biology notwithstanding. This is a recurrent tension in any society. The extent to which a society leans in one or the other direction undoubtedly has something to do with the quality of life in that society, especially in the form of the psychological and social satisfactions mentioned above.

Marris and Rein take a social-structural view in asserting that "progress depends on sustaining independently: (1) executive social planning, (2) marshalling protest against exploitation and neglect, (3) advocacy and advice, [and] (4) applied research on service and structure of social welfare" (1967, p. 231).

They feel that purposes, rather than procedures, should be institutionalized, and that this requires new forms of accommodation to the dilemmas of social life. In their view, it is the freedom to innovate, rather than the Marxian assumption of internal contradictions, that keeps change going.

In a similar theme, the Biddles believe that the capability of innovation, in the form of the personal development of individuals and their encouragement of local initiative, is essential to the maintenance of change that is meaningful to them. Neither of these views, however, is cast in a framework that takes into account the sort of ecological changes that affect both the need and the capacity to achieve desired changes. While this additional perspective may add understanding to the process of change, it is not a magical solution. The tough, fundamental question remains the extent to which and the form by which human beings can become more the masters of their fate. Human institutions have been designed on the premise that they make this task easier. Whether or not they can be modified and redesigned to enhance the adaptation of individuals, by adapting to changing requirements, is a persistent dilemma that forms the substance of the accountability process. The emphasis on participation in both the change and the evaluation process has been presented here as a measure that enhances alike the possibility of change, the direction of change toward desired goals, and fulfillment of the obligation for accountability. If community members are to learn to obtain satisfactions from change processes in forms other than concrete structures and places, this participation will also have the desired effect of providing the opportunity for community members to become more sophisticated consumers of evaluative data, through which they may develop the capacity for more effective participation in planning and taking action for their community.

The outline for the segment of a body of knowledge for community psychology discussed in this chapter can do little more than sketch a framework that suggests a direction along which knowledge needs to be developed for this field. This outline is more at the level of theory, maxim, and professional lore, and less at the level of substantive data, than the author would wish. Hopefully, however, it can improve on past definitions of what a community psychology would encompass. As numerous other writers have observed, the essential difficulty of the task is to be able to do and to think about what one is doing at the same time. An analytical framework such as the one presented here is of help in conducting that difficult task.

The discussion has, at several points, defined the need for the creation of new settings for community psychologists, and for the redefinition of criteria for community psychologists in existing settings. A beginning toward the development of these criteria is captured in Kelly's (1971) statement that the community psychologist works to solve a community problem but (and this is the distinguishing feature) does so in such a way that the solution also contributes to the development of the community. It may be that community psychology as it now exists and can be defined is a transitional form of activity. If so, pursuit of criteria for community psychology settings and efforts directed toward their creation may contribute to the information needed for the further evolution of the new form of psychological endeavor that is to emerge.

References

AIKEN, M. Community power and community mobilization. *Annals of the American Academy of Political and Social Sciences*, September 1969, *385*, 76–88.

BACK, K. Human nature, psychological technology, and the control of population growth. *Journal of Social Issues*, 1974, *30*, 279–295.

BARKER, R. G. *Ecological Psychology*. Stanford: Stanford University Press, 1968.

BIDDLE, W. W., AND BIDDLE, L. J. *The Community Development Process*. New York: Holt, Rinehart & Winston, 1965.

BUCKLEY, W. (Ed.). *Modern Systems Research for the Behavioral Scientist*. Chicago: Aldine, 1968.

CAMPBELL, D. T., AND STANLEY, J. C. *Experimental and Quasi-Experimental Designs for Research*. Chicago: Rand McNally, 1966.

CHERNISS, C. Preentry issues in consultation. *American Journal of Community Psychology*, 1976, *4*, 13–24.

COHEN, M. W. Citizen participation in the decision-making activities of formal social service agencies: An unreasonable goal? *Community Mental Health Journal*, 1976, *12*, 355–364.

ERIKSON, K. T. Notes on the sociology of deviance. In H. Becker (Ed.), *The Other Side*. New York: Free Press, 1964.

GAMSON, W. A. *Power and Discontent*. Homewood, Ill.: Dorsey, 1968.

GLASSCOTE, R. M., SUSSEX, J. N., CUMMING, E., AND SMITH, L. H. *The Community Mental Health Center: An Interim Appraisal*. Washington, D. C.: Joint Information Service, 1969.

GOFFMAN, E. *Asylums*. Garden City, N. Y.: Doubleday, Anchor Books, 1961.

GROSSMAN, F. K., AND QUINLAN, D. Mental health consultation to community settings: A case study of a failure to achieve goals. In S. E. Golann and C. Eisdorfer (Eds.), *Handbook of Community Mental Health*. New York: Appleton-Century-Crofts, 1972.

HOFFMAN, L. Deviation-amplifying processes in natural groups. In J. Haley (Ed.), *Changing Families*. New York: Grune & Stratton, 1971.

KATZ, D., AND KAHN, R. *The Social Psychology of Organizations*. New York: Wiley, 1966.

KELLY, J. G. Towards an ecological conception of preventive interventions. In J. W. Carter (Ed.), *Research Contributions from Psychology to Community Mental Health*. New York: Behavioral Publications, 1968.

KELLY, J. G. Naturalistic observations in contrasting social environments. In E. P. Willems and H. L. Raush (Eds.), *Naturalistic Viewpoints in Psychological Research*. New York: Holt, Rinehart & Winston, 1969.

KELLY, J. G. Qualities for the community psychologist. *American Psychologist*, 1971, *26*, 897–903.

KELLY, J. G., AND BOONE, D. *Mental Health Services for Non-Achieving Children*. East Adelphi, Md.: Mental Health Study Center Reports, National Institute of Mental Health, August 1964.

LAMBERT, N. Variants of consultation service to schools and implications for training. Washington, D.C.: American Psychological Association, 1963.

LEVINE, M. Some postulates for practice in community psychology and their implications for training. In I. Iscoe and C. D. Spielberger (Eds.), *Community Psychology: Perspectives in Training and Research*. New York: Appleton-Century-Crofts, 1970.

LEWIN, K. *Field Theory in Social Science*. New York: Harper & Row, 1951.

LIPPITT, R. Dimensions of the consultant's job. *Journal of Social Issues*, 1959, *15*, no. 2, 5–12.

MANN, P. A. Accessibility and organizational power in the entry phase of mental health consultation. *Journal of Consulting and Clinical Psychology*, 1972, *38*, 215–218.

MANN, P. A. *Psychological Consultation with a Police Department*. Springfield, Ill.: Charles C. Thomas, 1973.

MANN, P. A. Ethical issues for psychologists in the law enforcement system. Paper prepared for the Workshop on the Police, Task Force on the Role of Psychology in the Criminal Justice System, American Psychological Association, Berkeley, California, 1977.

MARRIS, P., AND REIN, M. *Dilemmas of Social Reform*. Chicago: Atherton, 1967.

MECHANIC, D. *Mental Health and Social Policy*. Englewood Cliffs, N. J.: Prentice-Hall, 1969.

MILLS, R. C., AND KELLY, J. G. Cultural adaptation and ecological analogies: Analysis of three Mexican villages. In S. E. Golann and C. Eisdorfer (Eds.), *Handbook of Community Mental Health*. New York: Appleton-Century-Crofts, 1972.

NATIONAL INSTITUTE OF MENTAL HEALTH. 1973 profile for federally funded community mental health centers. Rockville, Md. Survey and Reports Branch, Division of Biometry, National Institutes of Mental Health, 1974.

PETTIGREW, T. F. Racially separate or together? *Journal of Social Issues*, 1969, *25*, 43–70.

RAINWATER, L., AND YANCEY, W. L. *The Moynihan Report and the Politics of Controversy*. Cambridge, Mass.: MIT Press, 1967.

REIFF, R. Social intervention and the problem of psychological analysis. *American Psychologist*, 1968, *23*, 524–531.

RHODES, W. C. *Behavioral Threat and Community Response*. New York: Behavioral Publications, 1972.

ROGERS, E. *Diffusion of Innovations*. New York: Free Press, 1962.

ROTHMAN, J. *Planning and Organizing for Social Change*. New York: Columbia University Press, 1974.

SACON, S. An intensive training program for a police department. Washington, D.C.: American Psychological Association, September 1971.

SARASON, S. B. *The Psychological Sense of Community: Prospects for a Community Psychology*. San Francisco: Jossey-Bass, 1974.

SARASON, S. B. Community psychology, networks, and Mr. Everyman. *American Psychologist*, 1976, *31*, 317–328.

SCHULBERG, H. C., SHELDON, A., AND BAKER, F. (Eds.). *Program Evaluations in the Health Fields*. New York: Behavioral Publications, 1969.

SNOW, D. L., AND NEWTON, P. M. Task, social structure, and social process in the community mental health center movement. *American Psychologist*, 1976, *31*, 582–594.

SONNENFELD, J. Variable values in space landscape: An inquiry into the nature of environmental necessity. *Journal of Social Issues*, 1966, *22*, 71–82.

WASHINGTON, R. O. *Program Evaluation in the Human Services*. Milwaukee: Center for Advanced Studies in Human Services, School of Social Welfare, University of Wisconsin—Milwaukee, no date.

10. Implications for Manpower and Training

The development of conceptual models and strategies for modifying community systems and institutions requires a significant amount of attention to the training and availability of persons who are knowledgeable and skilled in community psychological work. Many of the training issues in community psychology were mentioned in Chapter 1. The reader may wish to review part of that chapter, which discusses the highlights of the series of conferences that were held to discuss issues in training. Here we will review the main points of a variety of training conferences with a view toward assessing the direction of progress that is occurring in training programs, compare those directions with the conceptual framework presented in the intervening chapters, and make some suggestions for further directions that could bring training activities more clearly in line with needs in the field.

Developments in Community Psychology Training

While the Swampscott conference (Bennett, *et al.*, 1966) first articulated the term "community psychology," which implied that psychologists go beyond work with individuals to work with community systems, it was at the first Austin conference that the status of the new field was examined in terms of progress and problems that had occurred in training programs. In their report of that conference,

Iscoe and Spielberger (1970) noted the necessity for change in training programs if psychologists were to be prepared for new roles.

As part of that report, Golann (1970) provided results of a survey of graduate training programs that indicated that community mental health course content increased from 20 percent in 1962 to 44 percent in 1967. During this same period, the number of psychology departments that offered a distinct curriculum in community mental health had increased from one to ten. But it was clear that a number of problems remained. Iscoe and Spielberger raised the question of whether altering current programs, which Golann's data addressed, could provide sufficient training for community psychologists, or whether new programs would be needed.

Embedded in this question were a number of issues, most of which Iscoe and Spielberger believed turned on the definition of community psychology. They identified five critical issues: (1) the definition of the field, (2) the relationship between clinical psychology and community psychology, (3) the definition of new role requirements, (4) the academic foundations for these roles, and (5) the appropriate field training experiences. They approached a definition of the field by stating: "Community psychology implies a strong commitment to the promotion of positive mental health, *and to the creation of an environment that will be more conducive to human growth and development and harmonious human relations*" (Iscoe and Spielberger, 1970, p. 229; emphasis added).

Although the participants at the first Austin conference would have agreed with Iscoe and Spielberger's general statement, it is not at all clear that all of them would have agreed at that time with the distinctions that have been drawn in this book. The easily endorsable but vague referents of the term "positive mental health" have been noted earlier, and there were few examples of how one goes about creating environments that accomplish the goals set out in Iscoe and Spielberger's statement. Approaches to these goals varied more widely among the participants than may have been apparent at the time.

Accordingly, a second Austin conference was held (Mann, 1971a) to deal specifically with these conceptual distinctions. That conference has been described in greater detail in Chapter 1, and many of the issues raised there were addressed to the issues raised by Iscoe and Spielberger after the first Austin conference. While the first Austin conference concerned itself with distinctions between clinical and community psychology, including community mental health, the second Austin conference was devoted to exploring distinctions between community mental health and other forms of community psychology. It was planned that the second Austin conference would be considered preparatory to another meeting to address the implications for training raised by the issues discussed at the 1971 conference.

In the meantime, another conference was held at Vail, Colorado, in 1973, to consider more generally the issue of professional training in psychology (Korman, 1976). Undertaking to examine a number of issues, including the long-standing tension between academic and professional training in psychology, the Vail conference affirmed the desirability of explicit professional training programs. This was a significant step, in principle at least, toward a resolution of an issue that had been considered recurrently since at least 1949, as discussed in Chapter 8.

In 1975 a third conference was held in Austin to pick up the unfinished business from 1971. The theme initiated in 1971 is presented in the statement of purpose of the conference made by Iscoe: "to critically assess the many problems facing community psychology and to examine community psychology's conceptual independence from both clinical psychology and community mental health" (1975, p. 1193). This conference explored much more explicitly than previous training discussions the broader questions of social intervention and change, values and ideologies, and the needed conceptual and technological capacities that emerge as community psychology moves beyond the mental health model; and it began to delineate the training program elements that the responses to these issues imply. Clearer definitions of the distinctions between community mental health and community psychology emerged (Sarason, 1976) even though definitions of the latter were not resolved entirely. The proceedings of this conference are presented in Iscoe, Bloom, and Spielberger (1977).

As an adjunct to this third Austin conference, another survey of current graduate programs was conducted (Barton, Andrulis, Grove, and Aponte, 1976). Questionnaires were sent to 341 masters and doctoral level training programs and 114 internship settings. Responses were received from 237 university programs (69 percent) and from 60 internships (53 percent). Of those responding, 59 percent of the programs (141) and 78 percent of the internships (47) provided some community psychology or community mental health content, representing further increases from the earlier surveys. Compared to the 50 programs offering some training in this area found in Bloom's (1969) survey, the 141 programs offering some community psychology or community mental health training in 1975 is a very significant expansion.

The mixing of masters and doctoral level training programs, together with the combination of community mental health and community psychology content, makes an interpretation of the qualitative significance of these changes difficult. An examination of the course content in these programs reveals offerings in thirty-six different areas, with the most frequently offered content concerned with community mental health, including mental health consultation, crisis intervention, and mental health program evaluation. While "prevention of mental disorders" ranked seventh in frequency in these offerings, courses in epidemiology ranked thirty-third. In nearly all areas where comparisons with Bloom's data were possible, increased offerings are found. Exceptions are represented by slight declines in such content areas as "group process," "social milieux and their relationships to emotional disorders," and "mental health manpower issues." Only 15 of the 141 university programs and 2 of the 47 internship settings reported distinguishable curricula or specialization in community psychology.

Among faculty in these programs, approximately 80 percent had a community mental health interest, while only 20 percent expressed a social or community perspective. Although a breakdown of program content by faculty interest is not available, the programs with distinguishable community emphasis are a smaller percentage of the programs (10 percent) than the proportion of faculty interest in a social or community perspective. Unless there are larger numbers of faculty in programs with a community perspective than in those with limited community offerings—an unlikely possibility—it would appear that program emphasis does not reflect proportionately the interests of faculty.*

A recent survey of graduate students in clinical and community psychology training programs at the doctoral level (Zolik, Sirbu, and Hopkinson, 1976) indicates that most graduate students in these programs do not consider their training and field experiences in the community area to have been adequate. These findings are consistent with a number of individual reports in symposia sponsored by the Division of Community Psychology at the annual meetings of the American Psychological Association in which recent graduates have reported that their graduate training often had little

*The discrepancy may exist because faculty with social and community interests are younger and have less influence on program emphasis.

relationship to the demands for professional activity that they encountered later. All told, there appear to be a large number of token offerings in the community direction, and a much smaller number of programs making a significant community effort.

These findings indicate that the realities of program offerings still differ significantly from the conceptualizations of community psychology, although considerable growth has been made. The mental health model is represented in a preponderance of the training resources in the community field. The distribution of course offerings suggests that there is some danger that the field may become overly and prematurely preoccupied with technological concerns, with insufficient attention to conceptual issues and empirical bases of knowledge. The directions of further growth will have substantial implications for whether or not this danger is avoided.

It is clear, then, that existing training programs fall far short of providing opportunities for the acquisition of the knowledge and skills needed for functioning according to the outline of community psychology that has been presented here. Before returning to the question of whether existing programs should be modified or new programs should be established, there are two other considerations bearing on the existing state of affairs, and the possibilities for change, that must be examined. Both considerations involve institutional constraints; one deals with the manpower needs of society, and the other with the university training setting.

Manpower Issues and Social Process

The anticipated need for psychologists to function in new community mental health centers that led to the Swampscott conference (Bennett *et al.*, 1966) and consequently to the development of the term "community psychologist" has not come to fruition so far in either numbers or functions at the level of community demand. It is worth noting that the question of numbers and functions was seen to be correlated at that time, in that it was clear that there could never be enough psychologists produced to staff the anticipated number of centers *if they were to function in the traditional direct-service roles that had existed up to that time.* New functions seemed to be required if foreseeable manpower resources were to even approach meeting community needs. As we have seen in our review, the number of anticipated centers has not even been closely approached by the number that have been established, and the functions of those persons employed in them have not deviated significantly from traditional patterns.

Snow and Newton's (1976) observations have already been noted, to the effect that the expectation that community mental health centers would become community platforms for the delivery of new forms of service and support systems for new kinds of professional activity is not borne out by an analysis of the history and purposes of the community mental health center movement. It should not be assumed, however, that these expectations were based entirely on erroneous perceptions or misunderstandings of the community mental health center movement. Rather, they can be seen as arising from the conscientious efforts of a few psychologists to outline a strategy for meeting community needs as they saw those needs. If there were any erroneous perceptions, they may have been in the tendency to confuse community needs with community demands, a distinction that requires continuous amplification. The definition of community mental health as a continuation of the clinical model also serves to perpetuate the definition of community needs according to a "blaming-the-victim" ideology (Ryan, 1971) in which the individual is held responsible for his or her problems. In turn, this definition supports a community demand perspective that assumes that more and more professionals must be employed in treating the victims. Accordingly, the view is perpetuated that if services are inadequate to meet community needs, it is because of a lack of money to support more direct service personnel, rather than because of a lack of consideration of alternative methods of intervention. While we have noted other considerations bearing on the limitations that have arisen in the number of community mental health centers serving communities across the country, this failure to redefine professional roles, whether or not it was provided for in the original thinking behind the community mental health centers, can be seen as one major constraint on meeting community needs.

The immediate issues confronting society have changed considerably from the 1960s to the 1970s, if one is to judge from those concerns that make up the conscious preoccupations of citizens and government officials. From a concern with redressing social injustice, society has turned to a preoccupation with scarcity. Present means of attempting to solve problems have become so expensive that means of effecting cost controls are sought out almost desperately. Under these circumstances, the prevailing assumptions of the clinical model and increasing cost-consciousness, the alternatives are limited to devising less expensive methods of doing the same thing, an alternative that may result in a reduction of quality and effectiveness of services. In this context, the prevailing approach to program evaluation emphasizes accounting methods and cost- effectiveness. However, one should not confuse accounting with accountability, and the really tough questions concern how well existing programs meet community needs compared to alternative programs, and to whom these programs are accountable. Accordingly, while developments in the community mental health field promise to define a need for more persons trained in program evaluation methods, this is a need that should be examined closely.

University programs, including community psychology training programs, have tended to follow government demand as expressed in the form of available training funds. In Chapter 2, we noted Green's observation that university responses to the needs of government policymakers contain the potential risk of contributing to a "present-ridden social theory," which does not provide adequately for the exploration of possible alternatives and tends to accept prevailing, but untested, ideological assumptions about existing theory and method. Renner (1974) has raised the important point that the ready acceptance by universities of the victim-oriented definitions of mental health programs—which acceptance is implicit in the use of training funds to prepare personnel along traditional lines—aligns university programs with approaches to human services that may be, at best, irrelevant and, at worst, oppressive to some of the intended recipients. For instance, responding to the demand to train program evaluators without also considering the need for defining alternative interventions and modes of accountability to intended beneficiaries of programs might contribute to this problem. Renner argues that this issue has serious implications for academic freedom and the role of the university in society, and that to raise such questions is not to introduce political factors, but merely to recognize the political processes that exist already.

The distinction between need and demand in manpower and training issues raises the question of whether universities do not have an obligation toward society to participate in developing alternative definitions of community needs, and, concomitantly, to define new professional roles and new criteria for professional activities. For example, considering manpower questions in terms of various combinations of numbers and functions, as did the early definers of the field of community psychology, could contribute to a situation in which the possibilities of generating alternative approaches that may be more effective in addressing community needs and more creative in solving manpower demands would be increased. Moreover, attention to both current demand and potential needs might contribute to training programs that could produce more flexible and adaptive graduates whose usefulness to society may continue even though social priorities and programs may change. This would be a contribution that could avoid creating a large number of inflexibly trained personnel, who may later resist needed changes because of their vested interest in the status quo, or who, because of narrow, present-defined, specialized training, may become casualties of changing social requirements, as has been the case with aerospace engineers in the space program, or teachers in the face of declining school enrollments.

The possibilities for universities participating in the task of defining social needs as well as meeting present demands will depend on their capacity for doing so, but it will also depend on their awareness of an obligation to do so.* The considerations discussed here suggest that this dual approach to manpower questions can contribute to the university's role as an institution for free inquiry in society, and would contribute, not incidentally, to the refinement of social policy and practices, to the improvement of their training programs, and to meeting the needs of students and of communities more effectively. However, a complete understanding of the possibilities for universities in this role must take account also of the constraints operating within the university as a social institution.

The University and Social Process

A long-held traditional position is that universities should be places for the development and exploration of ideas, unrestrained by the demands of current, practical affairs. Those who hold such views are likely to feel that universities should be devoted to basic research, and that involvement with practical problems leads to a misrepresentation of research to the public and the placing of un-

*Professional organizations, government, and community settings also contribute to this process and should not be overlooked. The university's role is highlighted here because of its close relationship to training programs.

wanted pressures on university faculty to slant their efforts in whatever direction society happens to want at the moment. The ultimate fear of those who hold this view is that public demands may lead to infringements on academic freedom.

However, a strict adherence to this view ignores much of the history of the university as a social institution, as well as present reality. Graduate programs originated in large measure to prepare teachers and researchers who met a social need in an expanding educational and knowledge-generating system. This process has created a knowledge base that has in turn generated a vastly increased number of professions, and the further development of professional schools and training programs within universities. While there continues to be a need to prepare some persons for faculties in universities and secondary schools, it has been many years since a majority of Ph.D. recipients entered careers in university teaching. Gould (1971) noted that the Ph.D. had become increasingly a professional degree in many fields, yet the faculty of graduate programs continued to act as if their major purpose was to produce more graduates in the teacher-researcher mold. Gould perceived a new role for graduate schools:

> Just as knowledge in the late nineteenth century had to be made more disinterested, scientific, and factual to free it from the fabric of beliefs, opinions, traditions, and superstitions of the time, so knowledge now has to become more interested in the human condition. There will always be a need for speculative inquiry without regard to current problems, of course; but the degree of pride in and emphasis upon remote, pure research that has been evident in graduate schools can no longer be socially justified. (Gould, 1971, p. 355)

A nonacadamecian, Charles F. Jones, advocated similar changes in suggesting that graduate education provide ladders for both the academically and professionally oriented student. He proposed:

> If ever there existed a laboratory worthy of study, it is the modern American city. Our nation has moved more or less haphazardly from an agrarian society to a densely populated urbanized one without the concurrent underpinning of knowledge which might have prevented many of today's urban crises. In the overall scheme of things, the problems of designing a livable metropolis—from all standpoints—

> has not received sufficient attention from our researchers. Only in the last few years have institutes for urban studies blossomed all over the nation, yet most of these organizations tend to limit themselves to the collection of data without giving compensating attention to the application of data to the problems.
>
> Let us have research, then, but let us make a stronger effort to identify those human needs which require the greatest attention. (1971, p. 364)

Jones's hope for the prevention of community problems recalls Green's criticism, quoted in Chapter 2, that present-oriented social theories had failed to predict any of the social crises that arose during the 1960s, and his call for attention to the problems of creating livable human environments and the definition of human needs underscores the approach advocated here for the role of the university.

The problems that arose during the 1960s do not command as much attention as they once did, but they have not gone away, and the potential for social disruption may not be as far away as the present-day actions of society might suggest. While other problems may be more immediately pressing for academics, it will not help to attempt to rewrite history, or to claim that academicians made a horrible mistake by becoming involved in social concerns during the 1960s, as some have attempted to do. Rather it is necessary to separate the excesses from the substance of these efforts, and to distinguish politicization from responsible and knowledgeable approaches to social problems.

Resolution of the dilemma of pure versus applied interests will not come about by a wholesale flight in one direction or the other, nor is such a prospect realistic. The reality is that the modern university is vastly important to modern society. The extent to which society operates today on a basis of knowledge and technology precludes the diminishing of the role of the university in societal affairs, regardless of anyone's wishes, except at great peril to that society and its inhabitants. It must also be recognized that the role of universities in practical affairs did not, in fact, arise during the post–World War II era, the 1960s, or even in times of national crisis. The university's role in society has an evolutionary history in which the relationship of the academic to the practical changes over time. The modern university cannot survive, any more than it ever could, by ignoring society's problems. Nor can society solve its problems by chasing universities away from them. In fact, the development of approaches to social problems requires a creative realignment of knowledge-generating and problem-solving resources, an eventuality that is not aided by retreat to traditional views of institutional roles. In many ways, the current problems of society and of universities stem from a retreat to narrowed definitions of social institutions that tend to separate them from creative, cooperative relationships with each other.

This analysis suggests that the university should be involved in present-day concerns, but that it should not do so unquestioningly. Moreover, the university's role should not merely be responsive to societal demands, but should participate in defining social needs and in demonstrating and exemplifying alternative approaches to social and community problems. However, in order for universities to fulfill these roles, policymakers must recognize that universities require resources that go beyond merely meeting present demands, and universities must recognize that the utility of new and creative approaches to social problems must be demonstrated before community needs can be transformed into demands. As Ray (1971) put it, to take a disinterested approach to these problems is not the same as taking no interest all.

What, then, can community psychology contribute to this process? As we have seen, there is a set of promising, innovative theories and methods, most of which are still in the process of development and in need of further testing. Much of what has been developed in the field has occurred in an atmosphere of crisis and urgency, a state that, in pushing toward premature solutions and over-valuing expectations also sows the seeds for disappointment. What is needed is a period of free inquiry detached from an air of crisis, although not detached from social and community problems, for the further development of the field. These developments also require programs for research and training new personnel, the details of which will now be explored.

Further Development of Community Training

The existence of fifteen distinct programs in community psychology is evidence that such programs can be created. However, fifteen programs is a small number compared to the 341 programs in psychology to which questionnaires were sent originally in the Barton *et al.* survey. How many more programs should be developed is an unanswerable question at the present time, as is the question of whether there should be 326 psychology programs that do not provide a community psychology option. In psychology, job opportunities relative to the supply of graduates have declined drastically in recent years, and more rapidly so for persons trained in the traditional experimental areas of psychology in academic settings than in the community field (Woods, 1976). It is clear that new roles will need to be created for psychologists simply to manage the problem of employability. Even though it is estimated that the need for psychological services in the population is significantly greater than present demand, in the form of job opportunities, it is not at all clear that meeting those needs calls for more traditional services or the preparation of more persons trained in traditional psychological methods. The expansion of psychology-as-usual to an increasing range of settings and problems may benefit psychologists more than it does society, and at best can be only marginally successful without also developing new perspectives, skills, and identities for psychologists.

The age and tenure of present psychology department faculty members make it unlikely that personnel conducting existing training programs will be replaced by others trained in new psychological approaches. Accordingly, the orientations of present psychology department faculty pose a limiting factor for the further development of community psychology programs other than those with a community mental health orientation. To return to the Iscoe-Spielberger question of whether new programs should be created or existing programs should be modified, it would seem that modification of existing programs would be a much slower process than the creation of new programs, and that the latter may serve to make clearer the distinctions from previous methods that need to be demonstrably visible. Moreover, if the development of community psychology requires the definition of new criteria for psychological work, it may prove extremely difficult to generate and apply these criteria in the context of existing programs where other criteria must be met also, and where the latter may take precedence.

Community psychologists may be able to apply some elements of their own theories and strategies to this question. One consideration that comes to mind immediately is that the course of further development of training programs should depend on the particular setting in many respects. Options may be the development of rather small programs within psychology departments, the establishment of professional schools that are separate from psychology departments but may be related to them, and interdisciplinary programs that are not distinctly psychological in character. The course of development may also parallel the community development process in some ways. The Biddles' conception, noted in Chapter 9, that the community development process moves from a small nucleus that explores issues and resources to a larger nucleus that organizes for further development, is applicable here. Community psychologists must judge when they are ready to move from the small-nucleus stage to the larger one, and decide how this can best be done. If this step requires the involvement of other psychologists, then the relationship of the program to a psychology department is important; if the step requires the involvement of other disciplines or community members, then the location of the program in relation to those resources becomes important. Beyond these particularistic considerations, there are some generalities that can be suggested concerning the design and content of community training programs, based on the models that have been reviewed.

PROGRAM CONTENT

Kelly (1975) has pointed out that the term community psychology involves a contradiction in itself. It may also seem a contradiction to suggest training in a field that does not have an established body of knowledge and set of techniques to be handed from faculty to students. However, these contradictions define a set of qualities for training in community psychology that are somewhat unique, although the uniqueness may be more apparent than real. Perhaps it is the case that the nature of community psychology forces one to face issues in training that are also important in other fields but are more easily overlooked. Be that as it may, training for community psychology must necessarily involve pursuit of knowledge in which ideas are valued, and it also must involve the development of action capabilities in which practical applications are valued. These two criteria are often hard to combine and are often viewed differently within universities and in community settings. Moreover, these pursuits require a more collegial relationship between faculty and students than is often the case because both are involved in learning about the phenomena under consideration. At the present stage of community psychology, the learning process needs to contribute to the body of knowledge as well as to pass knowledge along to students.

The qualities required for graduates of community psychology programs include both a clearly defined competence in solving problems in community settings and an intellectual and personal discipline that contributes to a capacity of the community psychologist for developing varied and changing approaches to enhancing the viability of community settings (Kelly, 1971). The development of these qualities may be approached in varied ways, but there are also some commonalities that mark the training as community psychology in character and differentiate it from training in other fields.

Programs that are based in psychology will normally include a coverage of the basic core areas of psychology and the development of specific skills in professional activity, research, and community work. Presented below is a listing of possible courses, divided according to those that have a unique association with particular models and those that should be common to preparation for working in community settings.

Unique

Model:
Mental Health: Consultation skills, crisis theory and techniques.
Organizational: Organization theory, consultation skills, human relations training.
Social Action: Theories of social structure, social policy analysis, community organization theory and skills.
Ecological: Behavior setting theory, ecological theory, consultation skills.

Common

Social systems theory.
Social history analysis.
Naturalistic observation and behavioral assessment.
Action research methods.
Techniques of multivariate analysis.
Survey research methods.
Community structure and development.
Human development in natural environments.

This is indeed an ambitious list, yet it may also be only minimally sufficient. Probably no program will embody all of these options, and many may specialize in one of the models combined with courses from the common area. It is for this reason that the common courses are presented in this way, since the review of the models has suggested that, with the possible exception of the ecological model, no one of the models by itself approaches what could be justifiably called a community psychology. At the same time, some of the course elements in the common area may be combined into single courses, and further experience may suggest that greater or lesser emphasis should be given to some of these areas.

FIELD TRAINING

Course content is only one element of a community psychology training program. Also required are opportunities for contact with community problems and for interactions with community residents. The author has suggested previously that appropriate training in community psychology requires a graded series of integrated academic and field experiences, in which there is an opportunity to examine the phenomena under study by observing manifestations of theory in the natural setting and reflecting on observations in the setting from a theoretical perspective (Mann, 1971b). Field training experiences present both rich opportunities and potential hazards. Rosenblum (1973) has reviewed the issues involved in field training experiences: defining the goals of training, selecting appropriate training locations, and providing adequate supervision. Ordinarily the trainee role will be a more circumscribed aspect of the professional role, but it is still important to provide a clear definition of that role, the learning experiences expected for the trainee, and the responsibilities and functions the trainee will assume. The expected role functions are also important to the selection of a training setting. The preentry issues surrounding intervention strategies apply here as well: such questions as congruency of values and expectations between the training program and the setting, the contributions the training program can make to the setting, and the costs and obligations incurred by the setting to accommodate trainees, are concerns that enter into the selection of and negotiation with potential training sites. Rosenblum observes that the potential for creating problems in the setting by trainee mistakes is probably greater and more damaging in community settings than in clinical training, and that the trainee is also probably more vulnerable in such settings. Moreover, complicated and serious ethical issues may arise that require all the tact and skill of highly experienced professionals, including issues that may lead to a decision to terminate the relationship with the setting. Accordingly, regular and timely supervision becomes critically important. Rosenblum recommends an apprentice relationship between a professional and a trainee who approach problems together, with the trainee observing the professional as role model and making contributions when appropriate. The trainee is introduced as a junior colleague, and the supervisory relationship reflects this conception of the respective roles.

For example, in introducing advanced community psychology graduate students as potential consultants to school settings as part of their field training, the author has made it a practice to point out that while the consultants were students, they had already had more psychological training and experience than many beginning school psychologists, and they could, if they chose, be working at that level for school systems. It is also important for the supervisor to clarify supervisory responsibilities to the setting, and to provide for the resolution of any misunderstandings that may arise. As the trainee becomes more familiar with the setting and more competent in the expected role functions, arrangements for increasingly independent activity need to be made. Rosenblum believes that this independence should occur more quickly in community training than in traditional training settings, and that, while continuous supervision and feedback should be provided, exposure to the risks of independent activity is an important contributor to growth as a community psychologist.

RELATIONSHIPS TO COMMUNITY SETTINGS

The criteria for community work outlined in the preceding chapters require that training programs develop relationships with community settings that have an ongoing life, rather than the occasional or opportunistic arrangement designed to fill momentary training needs. Long-term collaborative relationships offer many advantages. An economy of effort is achieved by reducing the need for repeated establishment of new training sites, gaining entry, and acquiring familiarity with the setting. While these processes must still be accomplished by new trainees entering the setting, long-term relationships provide a more controlled context for introducing the novice to this type of work.

In time, these long-term arrangements provide for acquiring a history of the setting and knowledge about effective behavior in different settings, and allow for assessing changes in criteria for adaptive behavior and alternative interventions over time. It is only under these conditions that students can be exposed to the requisite types of data referred to earlier in discussing community research and interventions. Equally important, long-term relationships are likely to increase the chances for assessing outcomes of interventions, assist in defining the process of accountability to the setting, and enhance the benefits that the setting will receive from the relationship. The long-term commitment reduces the likelihood of exploitative relationships, which are more probable in short-term training experiences.

These kinds of arrangements have been rare, but not entirely unknown, in training programs in community psychology and in other areas of psychology. A relatively frequent arrangement has been to combine research and demonstration projects with training opportunities for students, such as in the school consultation projects conducted by Cutler and McNeil (1966) and by Pierce-Jones, Iscoe, and Cunningham (1968), and in police consultation projects conducted by Bard (1970) and by Mann (1973). Similar relationships have been more common in research projects, of which Barker's (1968) Midwest Field Station is perhaps the best example discussed in the preceding chapters. However, each of these examples is more specialized in purpose and in the extent of community activity than would be required to provide a well-rounded set of training experiences.

Establishment of such relationships involves many of the difficulties involved in longitudinal research projects. Among these is providing for stability of staffing and funding, considerations that are not inconsequential. In part, the problem of staff turnover requires that a team of faculty and students be involved in the projected work, and that deliberate attention be given to the principle of succession as it applies to community psychologists. This concern also indicates that, where possible, the relationship should be built upon structural, and not just personal, commitments. This criterion requires interinstitutional arrangements between the training program and the community setting.

The selection of community settings for training purposes also requires some forethought. For several reasons, consideration should probably be given to establishing such relationships with a minimum of two contrasting settings. Not only will this arrangement provide a basis for nonequivalent control group designs for some types of research and evaluation, but it will provide other advantages as well. One problem in the selection of field settings is that the university's home community is often a readily available source in which relationships have been established already, and it is very likely to be chosen. However, university communities are not always representative examples of community systems. Moreover, the principles that have been reviewed in preceding chapters indicate the desirability of conducting studies and designing alternative interventions in different kinds of environments. A one-setting environment simply does not provide sufficient diversity for this purpose. Therefore, at least one community setting should be other than the university community.

The further development of community psychology training programs must grapple with a number of constraints, barriers, and problems. The structure of most existing training programs that do not provide a distinct community perspective make it seem unlikely that they will be able to meet the requirements for adequate training in community psychology. Therefore, new settings and new resources are needed, but at a time when resources seem to be diminishing. This is a problem that demands the best efforts of those qualities community psychologists like to think they possess. There are a number of possibilities for further development. In the next section, one possibility for integrating government programs, university research and training, and community development will be discussed, using the Agricultural Extension Service as an example.

The Agricultural Extension Service as an Example of University-Community Cooperation

The Smith-Lever Act of 1914 established the Agricultural Extension Service to promote and increase knowledge of agricultural and home economics practices among farm families. This act had been preceded by the Morrill Act of 1862, which established the colleges of agriculture, and the Hatch Act of 1887, which established agricultural experiment stations. The structure of the Agricultural Extension Service is a joint responsibility of the U.S. Department of Agriculture, on the federal government side, and the state agricultural colleges on the university side. A state Agricultural Extension Service, a division of the college of agriculture, is related to county extension agents and their staffs, who are supported by county governments. The county agent staff performs functions of community organization, home demonstrations, the 4-H club activities for youth, and extension work through subject-matter specialists (Loomis and Beegle, 1957).

The county agent, though perhaps trained in some specialty at the university level, is a generalist and change agent at the county level. He is a man of ideas at the local level. Historically, the county agent has carried the responsibility of introducing innovations into a local community, supported by a knowledge-generating base at the extension division of the state college of agriculture and at the agricultural experiment station. This example of university-community cooperation far precedes the academic debates begun in the 1960s over the "relevance" of university activity.

Importantly, the Agricultural Extension Service is an example of integrated cooperation among government at the federal, state, and local levels, and the universities and their community-based representatives. Such an integration overcomes many, although not all, of the difficulties that have been discussed in previous chapters concerning the relationships among these levels and perspectives. An important factor in making this integration possible was the provision in the Hatch Act that members of the Extension Service could not engage in political activities, as it was recognized that the nature of the county agent's work could provide for a powerful political base.

Although James Kelly (1964) introduced a parallel between the agricultural extension agent and what he called the urban mental health agent in the early days of the community mental health center planning, the analogy has not been developed further in community psychology, nor in the myriad community programs that followed. This oversight seems ironic, given the many parallels between the agricultural extension movement, particularly the discipline of rural sociology that it fostered, and the aims and concepts of community psychology. One can only speculate about the reasons for this development, but perhaps the linkage of the early community development programs to juvenile delinquency, and the traditions of the street-gang worker and settlement houses in the urban scene began the urban community programs with such a compelling focus as to preclude the historical example of agricultural community work. Also, at the time the urban programs were developing, they were responding to an increased rural-to-urban migration with an emphasis on socialization for urban, rather than rural, living. At the same time, these population shifts were placing considerable political pressure on efforts to obtain increased financial aid to cities when state legislatures were still dominated in many cases by representatives from rural areas. Finally, the sociological emphasis in these programs was heavily on the concepts of alienation and deprivation, which are popularly thought to characterize the urban scene but not the pastoral serenity of the countryside, the example of Appalachia notwithstanding. It seems plausible that the overlooking of the potential contributions of rural sociology may have been based in yet another conflict in American life—the ideological split between rural and urban interests.

This rift has a history as old as the nation itself. Thomas Jefferson said, in 1787, "We should allow just weight to the physical and moral preferences of the agricultural, over the manufacturing, man" (Plog, 1969, p. 288). Marris and Rein (1967) are critical of the current economic conceptions in the United States as more suited to a society of wealthy agricultural landowners than of current urbanized society. Yet these political and economic divisions are no excuse for an ignorance of an important and potentially useful part of intellectual and social history.

As for a concern with the disinterested development of ideas being mired in efforts to solve practical social problems, it should be recalled that most of the statistical methods employed in psychology and the social sciences were developed in the work at the agricultural experiment stations (cf. Snedecor, 1956). The research tradition in rural sociology has contributed some of the pioneering work in such areas as social organization and change, population distribution and environmental-planning and land-use policies, diffusion of innovations, and the effects of community organization and change on community cohesiveness (Loomis and Loomis, 1967).

There are, of course, limitations on transferring this model without modification to the problems of the modern, largely urban, community. But, as an analogy that has developed provisions for dealing with many of the obstacles and problems that have faced community psychology on both a conceptual and social level, as well as an important precedent, the example has considerable utility for the field.

Some Possible Future Directions

The integrated structure of the Agricultural Extension Service, while a bureaucracy, stands in marked contrast to the proliferated, sometimes overlapping, and unrelated collection of social programs for urban areas that characterize present-day community problem solving. These latter programs are also operated by bureaucracies. Moreover, the orientation of present social programs toward a competition based on political popularity, with little or no overriding policy, does nothing to encourage that psychological sense of community that could provide a basis for community development in a meaningful human sense. In fact, Public Law 94-63, which provides funding for community mental health centers, specifically forbids any community organization activity, while at the same time calling for explicit input of community members in assessing the mental health needs of the community. While not exactly self-canceling, these potentially contradictory provisions place a formidable obstacle in the path of community mental health centers' ability to reach a level of true community programming.

Under the impetus of funding for "community development" projects such as sewers, housing, and special revenue-sharing projects, many communities have developed special offices to receive and oversee the use of these funds. Most communities also have developed urban planning offices, or participate in regional planning activities. Few, if any, of these programs attempt to reach an ecological level of the community as described in previous chapters, either in planning and concepts or in actions. Such a level of conceptualization and action is not possible without some coordination among programs, but it is also not possible without an adequate knowledge base and appropriately trained personnel, and few communities can afford to support either or both. As we have seen, universities are unlikely to provide either the knowledge or the personnel under existing conditions.

This vicious circle of impossibility could be broken with the development of new resources. This development might well follow the example of the Agricultural Extension Service for community development. A model of such a new level of organization could employ many elements of existing structures, but would provide for new relationships among the several elements. With federal support, perhaps through the office of Housing and Urban Development, special community development divisions of universities could be developed with relationships to state-level offices of community development and to community development staffs at the local level. As one of its prime functions, this organization would have the goal of enhancing human development and adaptation in communities. Such an organization would not be populated by psychologists alone, of course, but would be a multidisciplinary organization at the university level and at the community level. Of considerable significance would be the potential for these integrated relationships to effect rearrangements among the departmental structures of universities and among scattered and uncoordinated efforts in the community. A distinct advantage that would accrue to this type of organization would be the explicit provision for an organized knowledge-generating component tied specifically to a set of community activities, unlike the haphazard, entrepreneurial grantsmanship that has attempted to provide a conceptual and empirical basis for previous community programs.

The linkage between university programs and community development staffs, the latter representing the local persons-with-ideas analogous to the county agent, could contribute to solving the inside-outside problem that many community psychologists experience, as well as creating settings and jobs in which community psychology could be applied in ways that present university and community mental health settings do not entirely allow. Moreover, the potential for increasing resources in local communities through both the addition of trained personnel via the availability of university linkages, and the enhanced development of capacities of citizens to become resources for each other, goes beyond the aim of previous efforts to contribute to the solutions of the problems of communities. This model provides a basis for providing additional support to university training programs to meet a clear social need, a step that not only has considerable precedent, but without which the ability of society to solve the problems of its citizens will be limited unnecessarily.

Tasks for Community Psychologists

The model sketched above is an idealized vision. While it could become a reality in some form, it would be a serious mistake to assume that further developments in community psychology cannot take place in its absence. It is unrealistic, as well as bad psychology, to assume that progress cannot be made without large-scale funding. The following are a few suggestions of tasks that can contribute to the further development of community psychology. Taken together, these tasks can be subsumed under the heading of creating resources, and may sensitize the reader to the fact that resources may take several forms.

A critical activity for the community psychologist is the development of local relationships. Seeking out and identifying citizens who are committed to the development of their communities is an essential activity for identifying the problems that citizens define as in need of solution. This activity requires that the community psychologist become conscious of the pressures toward the definition of their work in societal terms, which may not fit the local situation, through the medium of nationally circulated professional journals, and through membership in national professional organizations. In many cases this problem is greater for those in academic circles, whose welfare is tied more to the development of national recognition than it is to local affairs. At the same time, those community psychologists who are in academic settings have an obligation to participate in the definition of criteria for local responsibility for the university and for their profession (Kelly, 1971).

Such activities may occasionally lead to expanded opportunities for training and practice in the local community as an additional payoff. This development provides the basis for another important task for community psychologists, the creation and definition of roles for community psychologists. While the community mental health center provides a limited setting for many community psychology activities, increasing requirements for community needs assessment and program evaluation are real opportunities for the definition of the community psychologist's role as distinct from the clinical and mental health models. In these functions, community psychologists can make a substantive contribution in a major community institution. Similar opportunities are developing increasingly for program evaluation activities in many other community agencies and programs. Community psychologists can provide conceptual, methodological, and technical competence that can move such efforts beyond research designs and bookkeeping to the kind of accountability discussed in Chapter 9.

Additionally, where opportunities arise, community psychologists can contribute to community planning through the study of and development of guidelines for assessing the impact on human adaptation of changes in housing patterns and land use (Catalano and Monahan, 1975), the optimal location and design of human service facilities and programs, and the effects of community participation in health and social service programs. These activities, too, can contribute visible examples of the work of community psychologists that can further the definition of their roles and functions.

As Sarason (1976) has suggested, community psychologists need to put additional effort into the creation of networks among community psychologists to stimulate and support their work. This activity requires a specific commitment to the profession to foster the principle of interdependence that is a central concept in the field. One subgoal of this activity is the fostering and strengthening of relationships between community psychologists in university settings and in field settings. The practice of conducting planning for training programs without explicit participation by persons in field settings that may contribute an important element of that training is particularly shortsighted in view of the need to create and develop functional roles for community psychologists outside university programs. Additional subgoals of this activity would include a real effort to include both nonpsychologist professionals and citizens in such networks. Especially in training programs, these individuals may be able to make surprisingly helpful suggestions concerning the expectations they would hold for community psychologists (Kelly, 1975). To do otherwise is to perpetuate the parochialism in its own house, which community psychology attempts to overcome in the community. The development of these networks can serve as both a model and a form of continuing education and renewal for community psychologists. The development of linkages among university, field setting, and community representatives can approach on an informal basis the sort of integrated relationships suggested by the agricultural extension analogy, and could serve to enrich those in each role.

Finally, community psychologists must undertake to further the conceptual and empirical base of the field, drawing on inputs from each of the activities discussed above. Without such developments, the ability of the field to realize its goals to contribute to problems identified by the local community is severely limited. Expansion of community psychology's base of knowledge adds an important resource to the creation and definition of roles for community psychologists. This conceptual and empirical activity is likely to be fostered in turn from the networks that community psychologists create.

Together these activities comprise a set of interdependent activities that can contribute to an integrated field of community psychology that can create its own resources and opportunities. The activities of many individual community psychologists, and the integration of many of the principles of the models of community psychology into everyday activities in the human services indicate that these activities and principles are relatively well established and likely to survive. Whether community psychology as an organized field of professional psychological activity will survive to go beyond the stage of being a profession created by federal grants will depend on the individual decisions of those who identify with the field, in numerous settings, to make a commitment to the kind of integrated, mutually supporting, and personally satisfying modes of activity that they advocate for the residents of communities.

References

BARD, M. *Training Police as Specialists in Family Crisis Intervention.* Washington, D.C.: U.S. Department of Justice, 1970.

BARKER, R. G.*Ecological Psychology.* Palo Alto, Calif.: Stanford University Press, 1968.

BARTON, A. K., ANDRULIS, D. P., GROVE, W. P., AND APONTE, J. F. A look at community psychology training programs in the seventies. *American Journal of Community Psychology,* 1976, *4,* 1–11.

BENNETT, C. C., ANDERSON, L. S., COOPER, S., HASSOL, L., KLEIN, D.C., AND ROSENBLUM, G. (Eds.). *Community Psychology: A Report of the Boston Conference on the Education of Psychologists for Community Mental Health.* Boston: Boston University Press, 1966.

BLOOM, B. L. Training opportunities in community psychology and mental health: 1969–1970. Mimeographed. Washington, D.C.: Committee on Manpower and Training, Division of Community Psychology, American Psychological Association, 1969.

CATALANO, R., AND MONAHAN, J. The community psychologist as social planner: Designing optimal environments. *American Journal of Community Psychology,* 1975, *3,* 327–334.

CUTLER, R. L., AND MCNEIL, E. B. Mental health education in schools: A research analysis. Ann Arbor: Department of Psychology, University of Michigan, 1966.

GOLANN, S. Community psychology and mental health: An analysis of strategies and a survey of training. In I. Iscoe and C. D. Spielberger (Eds.), *Community Psychology: Perspectives in Training and Research.* New York: Appleton-Century-Crofts, 1970.

GOULD, S. B. A new social role. *The Graduate Journal,* 1971, *8,* 351–358.

ISCOE, I. National Training Conference in Community Psychology. *American Psychologist,* 1975, *30,* 1193–1194.

ISCOE, I., BLOOM, B. L., AND SPIELBERGER, C. D. (Eds.). *Community Psychology in Transition.* Washington, D.C.: Hemisphere, 1977.

ISCOE, I., AND SPIELBERGER, C. D. (Eds.). *Community Psychology: Perspectives in Training and Research.* New York: Appleton-Century-Crofts, 1970.

JONES, C. F. A new mission. *The Graduate Journal*, 1971, *8*, 361–368.

KELLY, J. G. The mental health agent in the urban community. In L. J. Duhl (Ed.), *Urban America and the Planning of Mental Health Services.* New York: Group for the Advancement of Psychiatry, 1964.

KELLY, J. G. Qualities for the community psychologist. *American Psychologist*, 1971, *26*, 897–903.

KELLY, J. G. Varied educational settings for community psychology. National Training Conference in Community Psychology, Austin, Texas, April 1975.

KORMAN, M. (Ed.). *Levels and Patterns of Professional Training in Psychology.* Washington, D. C.: American Psychological Association, 1976.

LOOMIS, C. P., AND BEEGLE, J. A. *Rural Sociology: The Strategy of Change.* Englewood Cliffs, N. J.: Prentice-Hall, 1957.

LOOMIS, C. P., AND LOOMIS, Z. K. Rural sociology. In P. F Lazarsfeld, W. H. Sewell, and H. L. Wilensky (Eds.), *The Uses of Sociology.* New York: Basic Books, 1967.

MANN, P. A. Mid-Winter Conference of the Division of Community Psychology, American Psychological Association, Division of Community Psychology, *Newsletter*, 1971a, 5, no. 3.

MANN, P. A. Integration of academic and field training. In symposium: *Advanced Training in Community Psychology*, American Psychological Association, Washington, D.C., 1971.

MANN, P. A. *Psychological Consultation with a Police Department.* Springfield, Ill.: Charles C. Thomas, 1973.

MARRIS, P., AND REIN, M. *Dilemmas of Social Reform.* Chicago: Atherton, 1967.

PIERCE-JONES, J., ISCOE, I., AND CUNNINGHAM, G. Child behavior consultation in elementary schools: A demonstration and research program. University of Texas, Austin, 1968.

PLOG, S. C. Urbanization, psychological disorders, and the heritage of social psychiatry. In S. C. Plog and R. B. Edgerton (Eds.), *Changing Perspectives in Mental Illness.* New York: Holt, Rinehart & Winston, 1969.

RAY, G. N. The idea of disinterestedness in the university. *The Graduate Journal*, 1971, *8*, 295–309.

RENNER, K. E. Some issues surrounding the academic sheltering of community psychology. *American Journal of Community Psychology*, 1974, *2*, 95–105.

ROSENBLUM, G. Advanced training in community psychology: The role of training in community systems. *Community Mental Health Journal*, 1973, *9*, 63–67.

RYAN, W. *Blaming the Victim*. New York: Pantheon, 1971.

SARASON, S. B. Community psychology, networks, and Mr. Everyman. *American Psychologist*, 1976, *31*, 317–328.

SNEDECOR, G. W. *Statistical Methods*. Ames, Iowa: Iowa State College Press, 1956.

SNOW, D. L., AND NEWTON, P. M. Task, social structure, and social process in the community mental health center movement. *American Psychologist*, 1976, *31*, 582–594.

WOODS, P. J. (Ed.). *Career Opportunities for Psychologists*. Washington, D.C.: American Psychological Association, 1976.

ZOLIK, E., SIRBU, W., AND HOPKINSON, D. Perspectives of clinical students on training in community mental health and community psychology. *American Journal of Community Psychology*, 1976, *4*, 339–349.

11. The Individual and the Community

In his customary manner of getting to the heart of things, Glidewell (1976) has said that what most people want from their community is a place to live, to work, to raise a family, and to have fun. Yet even a cursory examination of virtually any community shows both that individuals vary in their preferences in these matters and that members of a community find themselves in quite different circumstances in attaining their desires. Thus, the community must provide for diversity in taste, but it must also concern itself with inequality. It must reflect its unique character, but it must also insure to all its citizens rights guaranteed by the Constitution. The community must provide some sense of stability in the midst of processes of natural change, which means that it must to some degree be involved in planned processes of deliberate change that can maintain, and hopefully enhance, the quality of life of its members.

The desired qualities of a place to live, work, raise a family, and have fun address many issues of unfinished business in communities—housing, employment, education, human relations, recreation, and personal development—at a time when technological and social change continues to accelerate. The American Institute of Planners conducted a series of discussions on the future environment during the mid-1960s (Ewald, 1967, 1968a, 1968b) to consider the needs and prospects for community planning for the next fifty years. Ewald (1967) sounded one of the basic themes of these discussions by asking whether and how society would move beyond a concern with the minimally safe environment to consider the design of optimal environments.

These are challenges and problems of massive scale, made all the more difficult for the individual who seeks to control in some measure his or her life by the increasing crowdedness of the world and the increasing dependence of individuals on large organizations and immense concentrations of political power for the necessities of life, according to the view of Sir Geoffrey Vickers. As part of the AIP deliberations, he said:

> This crowded, urbanized world will call for qualities in its individual citizens different from those they needed in more individualist days; for more patience and tolerance; more intelligence, to understand far more complex situations; a wider sense of responsibility; more sensitivity to people; less of that aggressive maleness on which individualists so prided themselves and less of the qualities that go with it. (And why not, seeing that half the world are women?) It will curtail many opportunities that individualists valued and bring many new ones that individuals may value more. None of these changes are in themselves threats to "The Individual." On the contrary, they make room for individuals of far greater variety and require of them all higher intelligence, more capacity for human relations and greater self-control and offer them all wider opportunities for significant human life. (1968, p. 299)

Indeed, if the liberation of women succeeds only in making women equal to men, it will have failed society badly by missing the opportunity to bring human beings, men and women, closer to those human social qualities that Vickers addresses, qualities that have traditionally been attributed to women more than to men. But the important point of Vickers's remarks is to underscore the extent to which an emphasis on rugged individualism—and its associated characteristics of competition, opposition, and separatism—belies the fundamental interdependence of human life. Bringing human beings closer to the required human social qualities will not likely be accomplished through the exercise of economic and political processes alone, but will require the application of social-psychological knowledge, much of it as yet undeveloped, to our communities and social institutions, and to the socialization of individuals for human relationships. This is an area where psychologists may make legitimate and significant contributions to the planning process for society.

Should it develop, as seems likely, that working hours will be reduced in the future, the capacity of individuals to "have fun," and the development of appropriate behavior settings for such activities will assume increasing importance. The role of recreation in socialization experience, already an important one for young people in society, may assume as much significance for all members of society as work does at present. One danger in this prospect is that people may begin to take recreational activity too seriously, making it necessary to invent other forms of diversion. At the same time, increasing leisure time will very likely alter attitudes toward the centrality of work in our culture for some, while others who wish to enhance their economic standing may seek to work more, either through overtime or second jobs. Could it become necessary to limit the work a person is allowed to do?

There are competing tensions involved in the solution of any social problem. The ecological principle of interdependence indicates that every change has a set of associated costs and benefits. Economic considerations are only part of the costs and benefits, but allocating costs and benefits in human, nonmonetary terms is not typically provided for in the planning process. Thus, most human social programs are assessed against monetary cost savings effected in some other program or sector of society, rather than in terms of benefits to human life. The absurdity of this situation is illustrated by the government accounting process that assigns monetary values to services received through government programs and then counts these benefits as part of a person's income. According to this procedure, a person in abject poverty could rise to middle-class status by having a catastrophic illness (Harrington, 1977).

Besides helping to assess the costs and benefits of social plans in human terms, psychologists may also be able to contribute to the conduct of the planning process itself. As Myrdal noted in the AIP discussions:

> The first condition for planning in a democracy like the United States is to reach the people and enlighten them in regard to both the social and economic facts and to the policy conclusions to be drawn from the ideals and the facts. Without success on this popular level, all planning becomes nothing more than an intellectual exercise among a small sect of devoted planners, who will, moreover, remain under the constant temptation to compromise their planning in order to have something accomplished, however inadequate and perverted from the point of view of their professional program and the real needs of the nation. (1968, p. 262)

Among the facts of which Myrdal speaks, it would seem that two are of central importance. First, as population density increases and as facilities for rapid, widespread communication and travel improve, individuals and communities become increasingly interdependent. Second, the United States is a pluralistic society, and its political processes reflect that pluralism from the makeup of the central government to the regional and community differences it reflects. These facts have psychological, as well as social and political, implications. The planner or the program that ignores either runs serious risks of failure. Together, these facts represent a significant source of conflict in social planning and in social living.

Broad-scale social programs tend to assume a universalistic appropriateness and support of their goals. Certainly no one can argue reasonably that assuring rights guaranteed by the Constitution to all citizens is not an appropriate universal goal that deserves, if it does not always receive, universal support. But interdependence should not be confused with universalism. Interdependence may be the basis for opting for universalistic program goals, but it may also be the basis for choosing differentiated regional and community goals, each of which is interdependent with the other, and which, in turn, may result in some desired overall outcome.

Broad-scale economic planning, such as the control of the economy by the regulation of the supply of money and resources, or allocating funds for construction projects, serves more to control and restrict individual choices and community change than to promote human adaptation in any direct, positive way. The increasing dependence of individuals' welfare on these policies tends to link individual and social expectations to monetary considerations, creating optimism or pessimism about the future on the basis of perceived universals of affordability. While American society has not begun to approach what it can afford for human development, the problem lies more in the assignment of priorities and values, and in the better use of both natural resources and human talents, than in affordability. Psychologists are one of the few groups who can speak for the value of human development in the planning process, and for articulating the link between social systems and individuals—a psychological link with behavioral consequences.

Conflict between universalism and pluralism is one of the contributing factors to the revolutionary cycles of reform and reaction of which we have spoken. In discussing the Boston school desegregation issue, Featherstone notes:

> The fact that the residents of Charlestown and South Boston are resisting elite social planners, that they are defending community and

> neighborhood and even, in their prayer marches and American flags, the symbols of patriotic and religious nationalism, gives them a more respectable hearing now than they might have had five or 10 years ago. The contrast between the country's universal ideals and the actual diversity of its peoples, races and cultures has made for a history that swings between periods of universalism and periods of tribalism. The universal ideals of the republic often serve as a mask for nativist and racist definitions of America; this is why, periodically, they fall into disrepute. Periods of tribalism are often healthy responses to the failure of the American consensus to acknowledge the genuine pluralism of the culture. (Featherstone, 1976, p. 14)

It is often this tension between universalism and pluralism that underlies the disputes over local versus federal control discussed in Chapter 2. When the people Glidewell spoke of look at their community as a place to live, to work, to raise a family, and to have fun, it is to be expected that they will give at least equal weight to their individual and tribal preferences compared to the preferences of a universal and societal program. The more conflict that exists between these preferences, the more the individual will resist the changes embodied in the move toward universal goals. The point is not to champion localism or tribalism, but rather to promote the democratic process and the recognition that universal ends may be sought through different means.

From a psychological standpoint, optimism or pessimism reflects an individual's faith in the possibilities of change. On a social level, the participation of individuals in collective efforts at change depend not only on faith, but on the additional factor of some perceived stake in the outcome of change, and on a sense of trust that their interests will be treated more fairly by their participation (Gamson, 1968). Viewed in this context, the heavy dependence of many of the social programs of the 1960s on federal funding as their prime moving force, without an underlying support in the form of an organized psychological commitment at the community level, left these programs vulnerable to the changes in psychological outlook that occurred when economic policies changed and it appeared that the goals of the programs were not universally supported.

Thus, the pessimism toward social programs of the 1970s may be justified, but for the wrong reasons. It is not so much a question of the affordability of change as it is a matter of recognizing the need for psychological, social, and political preparedness for change among the populace. The popular outlook on the possibilities of change is badly out of line with the demands that evolutionary change processes are placing on our adaptive capacities. The fascination with elaborate theoretical systems, backed up by a complicated computerized technology, which marks so much of our social-planning efforts, creates an orientation toward problem solving with which few ordinary citizens can identify. If we persist in these directions without at the same time providing for the development of the individual in those characteristics that Vickers describes, the sense of alienation and pessimism is likely to be prolonged.

Change and the Community

In discussing the concept of optimal environments, it is well to bear in mind the importance of the pluralistic nature of society. Even the definition of the term "optimum environment" lacks any consensus (Ewald, 1967) among scientists, planners, or citizens. Moreover, the term can hardly be used before someone will come up with the question, "Optimum for what?" Such questions remind us that the environment is itself a complex system that serves many purposes. Whatever those purposes may be, however, it is also essential to recognize that both the environment and its purposes change over time whether or not any planning is involved. Preoccupation with the problems of change should not divert us from the real needs of the present, but the reverse is also true. A major problem implicit in planning is to better understand the causes and processes of change, and to make allowances for unanticipated changes. Thus, pluralism extends not only to diversity in the present, but to the temporary state of contemporary needs and purposes as well.

A major limitation on the adaptation of individuals to such conceptions of change results from socialization processes that tend to stress adaptation to given conditions as if they were permanent. In most instances, the task of parenting is carried out with reference to parental value systems and beliefs grounded in the parent's own earlier experience rather than in the future for which the child is being prepared. While this orientation provides a certain measure of stability to both family and social life, the price of adaptation must be paid by someone at some point. Similarly, while evolutionary changes tend to be gradual, they are also relentless, whereas changes in political and social processes tend to react grudgingly and reluctantly because of their orientation toward the past traditions of society. Despite the visions of political ideologists, the tumult of revolutionary change, and the impatience of the dissatisfied, political change and social change are likely to remain gradual processes (Katz, 1974).

Perhaps the advocacy of large-scale social change during the 1960s can be viewed usefully as a large-scale effort at socialization by paternalistic government. This is the image conveyed by Kearns's (1976) discussion of President Lyndon Johnson's views of the programs. While President Richard Nixon was dismantling many of these programs in the name of individualism, it is clear that his views were no less paternalistic (Horner, 1972). This paternalistic outlook, although imbued with different value systems under different administrations, is an analogue of McGregor's (1960) Theory X applied to society. Perhaps this is exactly what people object to in complaining about that perpetual social bogeyman, the federal bureaucracy.

If society is to meet the challenges of the future and avoid the limitations on individual and community development of paternalism, it is clear that changes in socialization experiences will be needed, not only for children, but for members of society at every age level. To accomplish this goal, changes will be required in the institutions of socialization: families, schools, churches, and governments. These changes will require not only an extension of conscious socialization practices to the entire age-range of society, but a reorientation of the concept of socialization to include the institutions themselves in mutual and cooperative learning. This is the analogue of Theory Y applied to society.

However, it would be ignorant of all that is known about socialization to assume that this process can occur to all persons in all places at the same time or to the same degree. To respect the diversity and pluralism of society is to appreciate the conditions of life in particular communities, and the differences among communities and individuals in their readiness for development. Accordingly, an evolutionary conception of community development would recognize that a process of development will have different effects on different needs, and that not everyone will arrive at the same place at the same time. This principle recognizes psychological, as well as cultural, pluralism.

These changes will not occur without conflict or without planning. They will require as a beginning some changes in professional conceptions of the planning role, and it is unreasonable to expect that citizens will find the functions of planning either acceptable or attractive until those changes in the role of the planner are accomplished. What is needed is a change in professional self-definition, from an elitism that professionals often recognize only dimly, to a participative, democratic, human development perspective (Kelly, 1970).

These considerations mean that rather than planning for a community that is perceived by the professional not to recognize, understand, or be capable of dealing with its problems, the professional must plan with the community so that it is able to do these things. In the process, the professional may come to recognize, understand, and be capable of dealing with those problems, too. These considerations also mean that the professional and the citizen alike will have to become involved in more than token ways in the life of the community as it moves toward the future.

To be so involved means unavoidably to be active in political processes, for both the professional and the citizen. It does not mean that political considerations are the basis for the professional's participation. Restraint from the appearance or the fact of partisan political activity will be strengthened in direct proportion to the theoretical and empirical contributions that the professional can offer, as well as the thoroughness with which the professional seeks the participation of all segments of the community. For the citizen, involvement is the key to whatever sense of self-determination individuals may achieve in a complex, pluralistic society.

Involvement also means exposure to diversity for both professional and citizen. For both, such involvement may provide the basis for the development of those characteristics Vickers described as necessary for adaptation to future conditions. Exposure to diversity provides a limiting factor on the development of narrow and preconceived assumptions and beliefs. Such experience may contribute not only to our ability to plan for the future, but to adapt to the changes it brings, as well. These challenges will be neither easy nor comfortable to meet, but they are inherent costs in a democratic society. As Bazelon (1968) observed, passivity is a greater enemy of democracy than is force.

The Psychologist and Community Change

In this excursion into the possibilities of a community psychology, we have explored the prevailing models in the field, attempting to clarify the confusions that sometimes arise among them and to identify the potential contributions that each model can make. The purpose of this exploration is to stimulate among students and psychologists a curiosity, and perhaps a commitment, to the further development of these possibilities. We have seen that each of these models approaches the community in different ways and to different degrees, yet they can all be evaluated against common criteria in their approaches to community life.

We have also outlined the possibilities for the participation of psychologists in the planning process as a legitimate professional role. Before that possibility can come to fruition there is much work remaining to be done. Further conceptual and empirical development of each of the models, and of the general strategies for community research and intervention, are required. It can hardly be doubted that the uncertainties of the future define a need for such work.

A colleague once remarked that psychologists are not society's heroes. In fact, little in psychology's history would suggest that psychologists are serious candidates for such a role. The development of a competence within psychology to contribute to community systems for human development will no doubt require heroic efforts, but self-definition of psychologists in heroic terms is contraindicated by the considerations that have been reviewed here. Progress in the ability of psychologists to contribute solutions to community problems that also enhance the development of the community will more likely depend on a difficult combination of zeal and humility, in which the psychologist is prepared to "give away the by-line" and not become indispensably heroic (Kelly, 1971).

But progress in community psychology will also depend on the mutual commitment of community psychologists to their collective enterprise. This developmental task requires a change in both the dominant preoccupations and orientations of many psychologists toward the subject of human behavior, and in their inclinations toward and criteria for professional activities. The task requires attention to the environmental setting and the ecological validity of the psychologist's work, rather than just the pursuit of universal laws of intrapsychic processes. It also requires mutual communication, critical examination, and support among community psychologists in both university and community settings.

In both its own practices and its own development, community psychology is a field in which the psychologist must both do and think about the doing, must both react and reflect. In going about the much-needed business of creating settings for community psychology, psychologists can learn much that may be helpful in contributing to the creation of settings for community residents (cf. Sarason, 1972). This should not be a narcissistic preoccupation, of course, but a self-conscious determination to learn by doing. At the same time, community psychologists must learn to appreciate the uniqueness of different settings in order to avoid inappropriate generalizations from one setting to another. If it can put together the task of building a sense of community with an appreciation for the diversity of human behavior and community settings, community psychology can assume a viable role in society.

Defining community by place, in terms of geographical boundaries, or by institutions that are located in communities, is insufficient for designing programs that contribute to community. The fact that services are provided or that professional activity takes place in a community does not define those functions as community programs or community activities. A true community program and, correspondingly, a true community psychology—on whatever level or in whatever form—is defined by its relationship to the community as a social system, and by its articulation with the social, psychological, and environmental characteristics and processes that link individual behavior with community systems and with the ongoing life of the community.

References

BAZELON, D. The new factor in American society. In W. R. Ewald, Jr. (Ed.), *Environment and Change*. Bloomington: Indiana University Press, 1968.

EWALD, W. R., JR. (Ed.). *Environment for Man*. Bloomington: Indiana University Press, 1967.

EWALD, W. R., JR. (Ed.). *Environment and Policy*. Bloomington: Indiana University Press, 1968a.

EWALD, W. R., JR. (Ed.). *Environment and Change*. Bloomington: Indiana University Press, 1968b.

FEATHERSTONE, J. Busing the powerless. *The New Republic*, January 24, 1976, 11–17.

GAMSON, W. A. *Power and Discontent*. Homewood, Ill.: Dorsey, 1968.

GLIDEWELL, J. Discussion of symposium, Community mental health activities in the midwest. Chicago, Ill.: Midwest Psychological Association, May 1976.

HARRINGTON, M. Hiding the other America. *The New Republic*, February 26, 1977, 15–17.

HORNER, G. D. Four more years: President Nixon pledges rigorous remedy for U.S. "crisis of spirit." *Washington Star News*, November 9, 1972.

KATZ, D. Factors affecting social change: A social-psychological interpretation. *Journal of Social Issues*, 1974, *30*, no. 3, 159–180.

KEARNS, D. Who *was* Lyndon Baines Johnson? Part 2. *The Atlantic Monthly*, June 1976, 65–90.

KELLY, J. G. Antidotes for arrogance: Training for community psychology. *American Psychologist*, 1970, *25*, 524–531.

KELLY, J. G. Qualities for the community psychologist. *American Psychologist*, 1971, *26*, 897–903.

MCGREGOR, D. M. *The Human Side of Enterprise*. New York: McGraw-Hill, 1960.

MYRDAL, G. The necessity and difficulty of planning the future society. In W. R. Ewald, Jr. (Ed.), *Environment and Change*. Bloomington: Indiana University Press, 1968.

SARASON, S. B. *The Creation of Settings and the Future Societies*. San Francisco: Jossey-Bass, 1972.

VICKERS, G. Individuals in a collective society. In W. R. Ewald, Jr. (Ed.), *Environment and Change*. Bloomington: Indiana University Press, 1968.

Index

A

B

C

N

O

P

R

S

T

W